PSYCHOLOGICAL, SOCIAL, AND EDUCATIONAL DIMENSIONS OF DEAFNESS

BARBARA R. SCHIRMER

Kent State University

ALLYN AND BACON

Boston ■ London ■ Toronto ■ Sydney ■ Tokyo ■ Singapore

Executive Editor and Publisher: *Stephen D. Dragin*
Editorial Assistant: *Barbara Strickland*
Senior Marketing Manager: *Brad Parkins*
Production Editor: *Christopher H. Rawlings*
Editorial-Production Service: *Omegatype Typography, Inc.*
Composition and Prepress Buyer: *Linda Cox*
Manufacturing Buyer: *Chris Marson*
Cover Administrator: *Brian Gogolin*
Electronic Composition: *Omegatype Typography, Inc.*

Library of Congress Cataloging-in-Publication Data

Schirmer, Barbara R.
    Psychological, social, and educational dimensions of deafness / Barbara R. Schirmer.
        p.   cm.
    Includes bibliographical references and index.
    ISBN 0-205-17513-9 (casebound)
    1. Deaf—United States—Psychology.   2. Deaf—United States—Means of communication.   3. Deaf—Education—United States.   4. Parents of deaf children—United States.   I. Title.

HV2551 .S35 2001
305.9'08162'0973—dc21

                                                                00-040132

Printed in the United States of America

10 9 8 7 6 5 4 3 2   05 04 03 02

To the two Jacks in my life, my husband and my dad.
I was certainly dealt the best possible hand.

CONTENTS

CHAPTER THREE

Language, Communication, and Culture   61

CHAPTER FOUR

Cognitive Abilities   97

CHAPTER FIVE

Personal and Social Development   119

CHAPTER EIGHT

Economic and Occupational Opportunities   223

CHAPTER NINE

Assessment   249

PREFACE

This book is a comprehensive and up-to-date treatment of the major psychological, social, and educational issues affecting the lives of children, adolescents, and adults who are deaf and hard of hearing and their families. It presents an inclusive description of current research and practice, complemented by the voices of individuals through personal essays that highlight and illustrate significant concepts and trends.

Professionals and preprofessionals preparing for roles in education, psychology, counseling, rehabilitation, interpreting, and speech and hearing science will, I hope, find this book timely, readable, and thorough. Each of the chapters focuses on a topic relevant to the broad scope of issues related to the lifelong development of individuals who are deaf and hard of hearing, including those who are born deaf or hard of hearing and those who acquire a hearing loss later in life. Each chapter provides in-depth explanations and offers a core body of current information to which instructors and students can apply both personal and professional experience.

The study of deafness and deaf individuals has been fraught with contention and dissension for virtually hundreds of years. I have made every effort to present a balance of perspectives on controversial issues, which I hope will enable readers to critically examine these issues and to draw their own conclusions. It is somewhat difficult to address issues that are so passionately debated. The terminology an author uses can be viewed as a predilection for one stance or another. I have chosen to use the term *deaf* throughout the book to refer to individuals with hearing losses ranging from mild to profound, in large part because it is so cumbersome to write *deaf and hard of hearing* each time the terms are used, and I feel that the initialized *d/hh* objectifies and depersonalizes individuals. Therefore, when I do use the term *hard of hearing,* I am referring exclusively to individuals with mild and moderate hearing losses. The same principle applies to my use of the term *Deaf* to refer to culturally Deaf individuals. When I capitalize *D,* I am referring exclusively to cultural identity.

When I was first asked to write this book, I was teaching at Lewis & Clark College, devoting most of my energies to preparing teachers of deaf children. Several editors later, I now devote most of my energies to chairing a large department in the College and Graduate School of Education at Kent State University. I want to thank my editor, Stephen Dragin, for the gentle reminder that "you owe us a book." I also want to thank his editorial assistant, Barbara Strickland, for carrying out the details that enabled the big ideas to come to life, and Amy Vessels of Omegatype Typography for managing the production of my book.

Between first and final drafts, the invaluable feedback from reviewers is both eagerly sought and fretfully dreaded. Lynn Woolsey (Ohio State University) offered a careful critique of each chapter, a perfect balance of constructive criticism and praise, and a coherent analysis of the book as a whole, even though I gave her the chapters out of order. I must have trained Lynn well when she was my student, given that she can think so clearly and logically in the face of chaos. Lynn's metamorphosis from teacher to teacher–scholar during her doctoral study has been wonderful to watch, and I am honored to be included in her life. I also want to thank the other reviewers for their thorough and thoughtful comments. They are as follows: Jack Foreman, University of Tulsa; Freeman King, Utah State University; Thomas N. Kluwin, Gallaudet University; Randolph L. Mowry, New York University; and Paula Sargent, Miami-Dade Community College, North.

During the writing process, several graduate students at Kent State assisted me with research and organization. I want to thank Christine Civiletto, Elizabeth Bender, Jennifer Beebe, and Lansing Cameron. I keep a cartoon on my desk that shows a man with a pink face, holding his hand on his mouth, with a book at his feet. The caption reads, "Everybody's got at least one book in him." Chrissy, Beth, Jen, and Lans know firsthand that books don't simply erupt from their authors in completed form, but rather involve months of stomachaches.

I also greatly appreciate the willingness of the individuals who shared their personal stories as essays. They are Lynn Woolsey; Jada Buczek; Tami, Ashli-Marie, and Keven Grant; Elihu Hirsch; Sheila, Sam, Dan, and Beth Owolabi; the students of Dynnelle Fields at the Learning Center for Deaf Children (Alexandra Ling, Jonathan Langone, Kristin Feldman, Erin McManus, Joey Cummings, and Randy Dewitt); Joe Henderson; David Brandel; Ruth Maddox; Cara Frank; Karen Clark; Gary Rollins; Tina Harrison; and Wendy Woods.

Most professionals in fields related to deafness have a personal story that connected them to a deaf person long before becoming a professional. We like to share these stories with each other, and we often ask new acquaintances what brought them into the field. I always tell about my grandmother. But the truth is, I became a teacher of deaf children because of my dad and not because my grandmother was deaf. I was a junior in college, studying elementary education and planning to teach young hearing children. Then, one day, while my dad was driving me to LaGuardia Airport, he said, "I guess you're kind of serious with that guy, Jack. I'll go along with this marriage if you get your master's degree first." First, I was stunned that he had broached an emotional topic. Our discussions were always intellectual and stimulating; they never touched on feelings. Second, I thought, it seems like a fair deal to me. So, of course, I agreed. Pursuing deaf education was natural for me because I was so comfortable with the one deaf person in my life, my grandmother. As an interesting aside, let me say that when I earned my master's degree, my dad said, "When are you going to get a Ph.D.?" And years later, when I earned my doctorate, he said, "When are you going to be a Dean?" He was a remarkable man, and I miss him very much.

While my dad held amazingly high expectations for me, my husband, Jack, helped me realize them. He has encouraged, supported, motivated, and galvanized me throughout our life together, and during the months of writing this book, he willingly put up with my relentless writing schedule. He is the reviewer I like the best because he thinks everything I write is wonderful. I'm glad that my dad "went along with this marriage to that guy, Jack."

CHAPTER ONE

DEAFNESS

FOCUS QUESTIONS

- Why is hearing loss difficult to define, and what distinguishes medical, educational, and cultural definitions?
- How has technology changed the ways that hearing loss is assessed and accommodated?
- What makes speech sounds so difficult to hear and understand for individuals who are deaf or hard of hearing?
- Why do the Deaf community and the medical community feel differently about cochlear implants?
- Do you think it would be more challenging to be born with a hearing loss or to acquire a hearing loss as an adult?

The difficulty with discussing deafness is finding terminology that does not imply disability. *Hearing loss, hearing impairment, hearing disorder,* and other such terms seem to presume that being a hearing person is positive and being a person without hearing is negative. In this chapter, and throughout the book, I will use the term *deafness* to refer broadly to all levels of hearing, from hard of hearing to profoundly deaf. I will also use the term *deaf person* to refer broadly to the range of individuals who are mildly hard of hearing to those who are profoundly deaf. On occasion, when it is important to distinguish between hard of hearing and deaf individuals, I will do so.

This chapter presents basic information about deafness that will enable you to understand information in later chapters about the psychological, social, and educational issues that are unique to individuals who are deaf.

CHARACTERISTICS

In order to understand deafness, we must understand hearing. This section will discuss the process and mechanism of hearing, the nature of sound, and how hearing loss is defined.

Process and Mechanism of Hearing

Hearing, which is sometimes referred to as audition, involves the gathering and interpreting of sounds. Each part of the ear serves a purpose in translating sound waves from the environment into meaningful information to the brain (Stach, 1998). As shown in Figure 1.1, the outer ear is the first point of contact between the individual and the sound. The outer ear, or auricle, gathers the sound and sends it down the auditory canal, or external auditory meatus. At this point, the sound enters the middle ear and sets the eardrum, or tympanic membrane, into motion. What started as acoustical energy in the outer ear is turned into mechanical energy in the middle ear. Between the eardrum and the oval window, which is the window to the inner ear, are the three smallest bones in the human body. The bones are called ossicles, and each bone has a name—hammer (malleus), anvil (incus), and stirrup (stapes). When the eardrum vibrates, the ossicles are set into motion, and the sound is carried through the oval window into the inner ear. The inner ear contains the cochlea and the semicircular canals. The cochlea is considered the main sensory

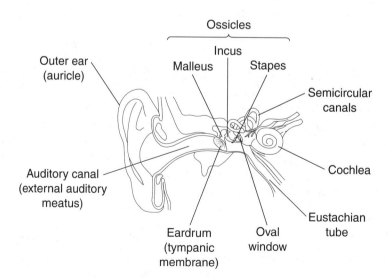

FIGURE 1.1   Anatomy of the Ear

organ for hearing. The fluid in the ducts of the snail-shaped cochlea moves in response to the mechanical energy sent by the ossicles. Tiny hair cells within the cochlea convert the mechanical energy into electrical impulses that are transmitted by neurons along the auditory nerve to the brain.

The eustachian tube, which runs between the middle ear and the back of the throat, controls air pressure in the middle ear. The semicircular canals in the inner ear control the sense of balance.

Nature of Sound

Sound waves are vibrations in the air. Sound is measured in units that describe the intensity and frequency of these vibrations. Intensity refers to the pressure of a sound. An increase in sound wave pressure is perceived as an increase in loudness. The intensity of a sound is measured in decibels (dB), named in honor of Alexander Graham Bell. Larger dB numbers represent increasingly louder sounds. The dB scale is also based on ratios. Each 10 dB increment represents a tenfold increase in intensity. Therefore, a 20 dB sound is one hundred times more intense than a 10 dB sound, a 30 dB sound is one thousand times more intense than a sound at 10 dB, and so on. Figure 1.2 shows the dB levels of common sounds. Leaves fluttering in the wind register zero dB, which is the lowest sound a person with normal hearing can perceive. Speech sounds range from about 20 to 55 dB.

Frequency refers to the number of vibrations that occur in one second. An increase in the number of vibrations is perceived as a higher sound or a higher pitch. The frequency of a sound is measured in a unit called *Hertz (Hz)*. If a vibration makes 100 up–down movements in one second, its frequency is 100 cycles per second, or 100 Hz. As shown in Figure 1.2, several speech sounds, a power saw, and a rock band have the same pitch, though very different levels of loudness.

Pure tones consist of one frequency only. Speech and environmental sounds are complex tones, and as you can see in Figure 1.2, they encompass a range of frequencies. The frequency range most important for hearing spoken language is generally considered to be between 500 to 2,000 Hz, though some sounds are at frequencies lower than 500 and higher than 2,000.

Definition of Hearing Loss

Hearing loss can be defined medically, educationally, and culturally. When defined medically, hearing loss is categorized at levels from slight to profound. When defined educationally, hearing loss is described in relation to the child's ability to learn language via audition and to perform academically. For example, the Individuals with Disabilities Education Act (IDEA)

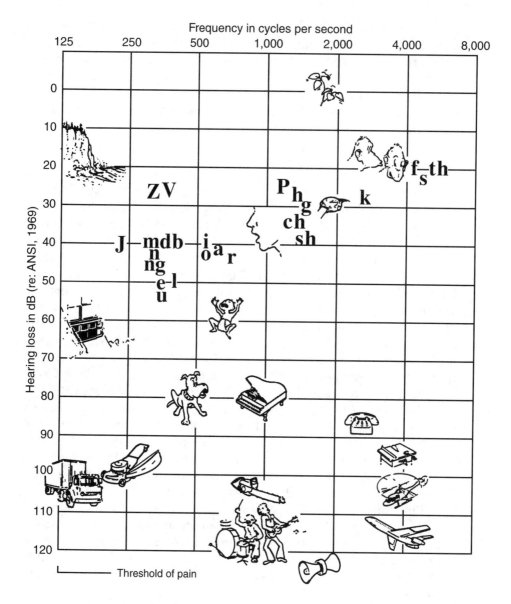

FIGURE 1.2   Frequency Range of Familiar Sounds

From J. L. Northern & M. P. Downs, *Hearing in children* (4th ed.), 1991. Reprinted by permission of J. L. Northern and Lippincott Williams & Wilkins.

uses *hearing impairment* as the category label and defines it as a loss that is severe enough to adversely affect a child's educational performance. When defined culturally, hearing loss is described in terms of a shared cultural identity among individuals who are deaf or hard of hearing.

The language that distinguishes between medical, educational, and cultural definitions can be confusing. When medical and educational definitions are used, it is common to refer to individuals who are deaf with a lowercase *d*. When cultural definitions are used, the term *Deaf* is used with an uppercase *D*, just as an uppercase letter would be used when discussing individuals who are Swedish, African American, or Muslim. In this book, I have capitalized the word *Deaf* whenever the term is used to refer exclusively to cultural identity.

The term *hearing impaired* is considered unacceptable because impaired implies a deficiency or pathology and carries a strong negative connotation. Although *people-first language* became the appropriate way to refer to individuals with disabilities subsequent to the passage of IDEA, people-first language is not considered particularly necessary when referring to Deaf individuals because, from a cultural standpoint, they do not consider themselves disabled.

TYPES AND CAUSES OF HEARING LOSS

The impact of hearing loss on an individual's life depends on the type and cause of the loss, which is discussed in this section, and the degree of hearing loss, which is presented later in the chapter.

Types of Hearing Loss

Hearing loss occurs when some part of the outer, middle, or inner ear is not functioning as described earlier. The two main types of hearing loss are conductive and sensorineural. Any problem of the outer or middle ear is called a *conductive loss*. Conductive hearing losses are often caused by disease that leaves fluid or debris in the middle ear, that causes wax buildup in the middle ear, and that leads to improper movement by the eardrum or ossicles. The most common type of conductive loss occurs when fluid collects behind the eardrum in the middle ear and becomes infected, perhaps because the person has a cold; the result is an ear infection and a conductive hearing loss. This is common among young children because of their susceptibility to upper respiratory infections and poor eustachian tube functioning. Often, the infection is treated successfully, but the fluid remains, causing a temporary hearing loss of 20 to 35 dB (Roark & Berman, 1996). Generally, conductive losses result in less-severe hearing loss than sensorineural losses, are often improved through surgery, and are likely to be improved by amplification.

Sensorineural hearing loss is caused by problems in the inner ear or along the nerve pathway from the inner ear to the brain stem. The outer and middle ear may be working properly, but the inner ear is not receiving the sound, or all aspects of the sound. Either sound is not delivered to the brain, the sound is delivered in a distorted manner, or only a little of the sound is delivered. Sensorineural losses can be aided through amplification, but the distortion of sound caused by the damage within the inner ear cannot be improved. Distorted sound without amplification is equally distorted with amplification, which is why some individuals have difficulty understanding speech even when it appears they should benefit greatly from their hearing aids.

The combination of both conductive and sensorineural losses is called a *mixed hearing loss*. Hearing loss can also be unilateral or bilateral. A unilateral loss is present in one ear only. A bilateral loss is present in both ears, but the degree of loss may be quite different in each ear. Children with a unilateral loss may have difficulty localizing sounds and listening in noisy or distracting settings, but they generally do not have any difficulty hearing and learning spoken language. Children with a fluctuating loss, such as children with periodic ear infections, may experience difficulty in learning language because of their limited ability to hear spoken language during periods of time.

Central auditory processing disorder does not cause hearing loss per se, but affects the comprehension of auditory information. It is caused by damage to the auditory nerve, brain stem, or auditory cortex. Individuals with auditory processing disorder generally demonstrate one or more of the following characteristics:

- Poor auditory attention
- Difficulty listening in the presence of background noise
- Impaired short-term memory
- Poor auditory integration
- Poor auditory sequencing skills
- Difficulty understanding rapid speech and other forms of auditory stimuli that have reduced redundancy
- Difficulty associating auditory with visual symbols (Hood & Berlin, 1996, pp. 235–236)

Causes of Hearing Loss

Hearing loss can occur before or after birth. Medically, hearing loss that is present at birth is referred to as *congenital;* hearing loss that is acquired later in life is referred to as *adventitious*. Educationally, whether the hearing loss is congenital or adventitious is considered much less important than whether it is prelingual or postlingual.

Causes of Hearing Loss in Children

Prelingual Causes.   A hearing loss that is present at birth or occurs before the child has learned language is called a *prelingual hearing loss (pre* for before and *lingual* for language). The majority of schoolchildren who are deaf or hard of hearing, approximately 95 percent, are prelingual (Commission on Education of the Deaf, 1988). Educators usually consider a loss to be prelingual if it occurred earlier than two years of age.

Although several hundred causes have been identified, the most common prelingual causes are premature birth or birth complications, heredity, maternal rubella, and congenital cytomegalovirus. Other causes include complications of pregnancy and RH incompatibility. Unknown causes account for about 33 percent of children with prelingual hearing loss (Center for Assessment and Demographic Studies, 1998).

Premature Birth or Birth Complications. Hearing loss is exhibited by some infants who are born prematurely with a low birth weight and some infants who experience hemorrhage in the brain or reduced oxygen to the inner ear.

Heredity. Between 150 and 175 types of hereditary or genetic deafness have been identified (Bess & Humes, 1995). Even though 90 percent of children who are deaf have hearing parents, approximately 30 percent have a deaf or hard of hearing relative (Moores, 1996). Because most hereditary deafness is the result of a recessive genetic trait rather than a dominant genetic trait, "the marriage of two deaf persons gives only a slightly increased risk of deafness in their children because there is small chance that two such persons would be affected by the same exact genetic deafness" (Northern & Downs, 1991, p. 90). It is important to note that although genetic counseling is available to parents, many Deaf parents would prefer to have Deaf children (Arnos, Israel, & Cunningham, 1991).

Maternal Rubella. Although rubella (often referred to as *German measles*) in children and adults is generally benign, it is dangerous in pregnant women, particularly during the first trimester, because the virus attacks the developing fetus, often causing hearing loss, visual impairment, heart disorders, and a variety of other serious disabilities. As a result of a 1964–1965 rubella epidemic in the United States and Canada, the incidence of hearing loss in children increased significantly and accounted for more than 50 percent of the students with hearing loss in special education programs in the 1970s and 1980s. It is important to remember that many of these students had concomitant disabilities, so the school-age population of deaf children changed dramatically during these years. The rubella vaccine was introduced in 1969, and since that time, the incidence has declined, although it continues to be a cause of hearing loss.

Cytomegalovirus (CMV). The cytomegalovirus (CMV) is a common virus that can remain in an inactive state in the body, possibly for the remainder of the person's lifetime. It can be contracted by the fetus within the uterus, through passage down the birth canal, or through breast milk. The most serious effects occur when the fetus contracts CMV before birth and when the mother has contracted the virus for the first time during pregnancy, rather than when the mother has experienced a reactivation of the virus (Strauss, 1999). It has been estimated that almost 50 percent of children who are deaf or hard of hearing may be as a result of CMV (Schildroth, Rawlings, & Allen, 1989). At present, there is no known prevention or treatment for CMV, though it may be detected through amniocentesis (Moaven, Gilbert, Cunningham, & Rawlinson, 1995).

Postlingual Causes.   A hearing loss that occurs after the child has developed spoken language is called *postlingual* (*post* for after and *lingual* for language). The distinction between prelingual and postlingual is important educationally because the child with a postlingual loss has an English language base for learning and communicating.

The most common causes of postlingual hearing losses are meningitis and otitis media. Other causes include side effects from medications, high fever, mumps, measles, infection, and trauma after birth. Unknown causes account for about 60 percent of children with postlingual hearing loss (Center for Assessment and Demographic Studies, 1998).

Meningitis.   Meningitis is a bacterial or viral infection of the central nervous system that may extend to other organs, including the brain and the ear. Children whose deafness is caused by meningitis generally have profound hearing losses, and many exhibit difficulties in balance as well as other disabilities.

Otitis Media.   Otitis media is an inflammation of the middle ear. It is the most common reason for visits to the doctor for children under age 6. Between 76 and 95 percent of children experience otitis media at least once by the time they are six years old, and approximately one-third of children experience three or more episodes (Bess & Humes, 1995). Medical treatment, including both antibiotics and surgical placement of tubes in the ear, is a common treatment. If left untreated, otitis media can result in a buildup of fluid and a ruptured eardrum, as well as other conditions, which can cause permanent conductive hearing loss. Vaccinations against several of the most common types of pneumococcal bacterias causing otitis media have recently been developed. Degrees of hearing loss are discussed in the section on assessment.

Causes of Hearing Loss in Adults

The most common causes of hearing loss in adults are noise, presbycusis, ototoxic drugs, Ménière's disease, and tinnitus. Other causes include impacted cerumen (ear wax) in the ear canal, eardrum perforation, trauma, tumors, otosclerosis (bone disease affecting the bone of the inner ear), and autoimmune inner ear disease.

Noise.   Repeated exposure to loud sounds, such as industrial noise, aircraft, guns, and amplified music, can cause significant hearing loss. Exposure to noise is considered to be a major cause of hearing loss among Americans (ASHA, 1999). Noise-induced hearing loss can be temporary or permanent. Almost everyone has experienced temporary hearing loss due to an evening of listening to loud music, exposure to the firing of a gun, or watching (and listening to) fireworks. Repeated exposure to these types of sounds can lead to permanent hearing loss.

Presbycusis.   Presbycusis is the deterioration of hearing as a result of the aging process. It is the leading cause of hearing loss in adults. It is difficult to separate the effects of aging from the effects of other causes, such as noise and ototoxic drugs.

Ototoxic Drugs.   Drugs are called ototoxic when they have an adverse effect on hearing. Many drugs that are administered to treat diseases, such as cancer and secondary infections resulting from HIV, are ototoxic.

Ménière's Disease.   Ménière's disease is a disorder of the cochlea. It was first identified by Prosper Ménière in 1861. It is characterized by sudden, unpredictable spells of severe vertigo, fluctuations in hearing, tinnitus, and pressure in the ear. Although not life threatening, it is incurable and can be quite incapacitating during attacks of vertigo. It typically occurs between ages 40 and 60, though it has been diagnosed in children younger than 10 and in adults older than 90 (Schessel, 1999). After repeated attacks, the hearing loss typically progresses.

In Essay 1.1, Lynn Woolsey describes her life from the moment she developed Ménière's disease.

■ ■ ■ ■ ■ ▬▬▬▬▬▬▬▬▬▬▬▬▬▬▬▬▬▬▬▬▬▬▬▬▬▬▬▬▬▬▬▬▬▬▬▬

ESSAY 1.1

Lynn Woolsey

I woke up early on the morning of November 23, 1984, with evidence of the worst hangover anyone could imagine. But I hadn't been drinking the night before. Lying flat on my back with my eyes on the ceiling, my head exploded with the racket of a jackhammer. I heard the incessant ringing of a distant phone and an eerie screeching, which I tried to muffle by pulling my pillow tight around

(continued)

ESSAY 1.1   CONTINUED

my ears. I felt a painful and rhythmic throbbing in my temples as I rolled over and faced the wall. Just the movement of rolling over brought on a tidal wave of nausea and an intense muscle spasm that emptied the meager contents of my stomach onto the hardwood floor next to my bed.

That was the day my life changed. That was the end of my normal hearing. That was the end of feeling "normal" at all. It was the beginning of a sojourn into the life of the "late-deafened."

It sounds dramatic, and it was. I couldn't stand alone. I couldn't hear anything in my left ear. Sounds reaching my right ear were distant and muffled, as though I was wearing ear protection. For three hours, all I could do was throw up and watch the room spin. I had no idea what was happening. I was frightened and felt helpless.

My mother happened to be visiting from the Midwest. It was her creative persistence that secured me a consultation with a neuro-otologist that very afternoon. Perhaps he was interested in the rapid onset of my symptoms and thought I might prove to be an interesting case. Maybe he just owed my physician a favor. Whatever the reason, he was like a savior for me that day. As I clutched a bucket close to my chest, he examined my ears, eyes, and body. He tried to get me to stand up, balance, and close my eyes; but I couldn't do any of these. The exam took a very long time because nearly every task brought on an uncontrollable wave of nausea.

I left the appointment armed with medication to reduce the nausea, and some reading material on conditions called Hydrops and Ménière's disease. Both involve a fluid imbalance in the inner ear, vertigo (dizziness), tinnitus (the sounds I was hearing, such as ringing), and sometimes, hearing loss. The medical emergency was over and with the medication, my symptoms were significantly reduced, but I could not drive or work. More tests were scheduled, and I simply had to wait for a definitive diagnosis.

The two weeks I waited for further testing were excruciating, but nothing like the test day itself. I endured a full day of probing, spinning, hearing tests, eye tests, and water tests. I left the appointment feeling as though I had experienced a sophisticated form of torture. If I had been privy to any government secrets, I would have begged to disclose everything to end the torture. I returned the next day for the results. I fully expected the neuro-otologist to write a prescription and tell me to rest for a few weeks. I expected to return to my normal life and chalk up this experience to a sensational medical emergency from which I fully recovered.

Instead, the tall Mediterranean-looking specialist in neurologically based hearing disorders and diseases leaned against the examination room counter and said, "Mrs. Woolsey, I have some good news and some bad news for you." I asked for the good news first. "Well, the good news is that you already know sign language. The bad news is that you'll need to use it. You have a progressive hearing loss that is complicated by balance problems. It is called Ménière's disease and there is no cure." Heartless. Simply heartless.

I was trained as a teacher of the deaf. Maybe he thought he didn't have to sugarcoat anything for me. It is true that I studied the ear and what happens when the hearing mechanism doesn't work as it should. I had a degree in deaf education, but nothing prepared me for this news. Nothing. The room spun again, and the nausea swept over me. This wave of nausea wasn't generated by any movement on my part. I was consumed by fear, dread, foreboding, panic, anxiety, grief, and a powerful dose of denial. I felt like throwing up all over his Gucci shoes. I screamed, "No" and started to plead. Was he sure? Did he really do all the tests? What was the chance that he was wrong? I couldn't be losing my hearing because much of it had returned in the two weeks of waiting. I was better, I told him. I was better. I wasn't feeling the dizziness as much. I was ready to return to work. I couldn't have Ménière's disease because those folks were older and I was young. And the one woman I knew who had Ménière's also had an operation to extract her auditory nerve, and she was left deaf in one ear. He simply had to be wrong.

But he wasn't. No, he wasn't wrong. I had Ménière's disease, and I was going to have to figure out a way to live with it.

There's a country song that describes a woman in denial about the loss of her man. She is called the "Queen of Denial," and so was I. While I could do nothing but survive the attacks of vertigo, I went into complete denial about the effects of the progressive hearing loss. I continued my life as it was. I participated in PTA meetings, I continued to teach childbirth classes, I worked part-time teaching American Sign Language, and I volunteered in the classrooms of my children. I coped by making excuses for my absence in large group meetings and by controlling conversations when I couldn't evade them. I avoided the phone but when I had to use it, I took advantage of our 20-foot cord and brought it into the front hall closet, where I could block out all other sounds. I began to isolate myself. I no longer accompanied my husband to business-related parties. Instead, I focused on the children. Lipreading them was an interesting challenge, but somehow we managed. I managed. I was doing just fine until one day, Ménière's disease forced me to abandon my fantasy for reality.

My son was five years old at the time. He was swinging on a tire swing hung from an enormous branch of the hundred-year-old maple tree that dominated our side yard. He was happily swinging. I watched him through the kitchen window as I unloaded the dishwasher. I was also tending to the laundry, which was in an open room just off the kitchen. It was noisy, I will admit, but if he needed me, I was certain that I would hear him. I went to take care of something on the stove and within five minutes, my cranky neighbor stood at my door with my screaming son, covered with dirt. "He fell off the damn swing and I had to come all the way over here to check on him. Where were you?"

I had missed it. I had missed my son's screams for help.

The next day, I made an appointment for a hearing test. Two weeks later, I was fitted with my first hearing aid. I inserted it in my ear, and I couldn't believe what I had been missing! I heard little things that I had lost somewhere along the way. The voices of my children were clearer. I loved it! I loved that hearing aid. It served me faithfully for several years, but true to the nature of the disease, I slowly lost more and more hearing. True to my own nature, I continued to function in denial. I became an even more skilled conversation manipulator and covered up my mistakes with the savvy of someone adept at concealing secrets.

Then I started graduate school. I was thrilled to be finally continuing my education. I took two courses that first semester. The instructor in one course

(continued)

ESSAY 1.1   CONTINUED

was a pleasantly boisterous former school teacher. He had a great, loud voice. The second instructor was a petite professor with a sweet and high voice. I could hear her voice if I strained. Then she turned on the overhead projector. Her sweet little voice disappeared. The mute professor emphasized concepts and clarified points with appropriate facial expressions, but not a sound from her voice reached my ears. No one else in the room showed any concern. It was me. I couldn't hear her. It so happened that there were some "real" deaf students in the class and a sign language interpreter was working in the front of the room. I snuck a glance toward him. I knew ASL and could understand his signs, but I wasn't deaf and I felt as if I shouldn't watch him.

Fifteen years have passed since my diagnosis with Ménière's disease. I have gone through three hearing aids and still wear them all my waking hours. I completed my Master's degree in Early Intervention–Deafness. I subsequently took more classes and received certification as a school principal. During the past fifteen years I have worked as a teacher of deaf children at public and residential schools, and as a principal at a state school for the deaf. I am still taking classes. I rely on interpreters, and I have learned how to make interpreting work for me, but I hate it. My grades as a student are inextricably linked to the skills of the interpreters who work in my classes.

My three children are nearly grown. They never learned sign language because I spent most of my time lipreading them. Enabler, extraordinaire. My first husband is long gone. He never got used to the idea that the woman he married was now deafened. He never wanted to learn sign language, and we lost our ability to communicate. I later married an interpreter. Our communication is spontaneous, smooth, and without barrier, as it should be.

When I was asked to write this essay, I reflected on the message that I wanted to convey. I realize that since my hearing loss was diagnosed, I have rearranged my life to ensure that communication is more accessible and clear. I worked in a residential school. I worked toward lipreading my children. I avoided noisy settings and social gatherings that inhibited my participation. I basically designed my life to reduce my communicative stress. I wonder if that is denial or coping, or a little of both.

I sometimes wonder what the future holds for me. In the early 1990s, I missed the sound of the dove but I heard the caw of the crow as music to my ears. I can't hear the crow's screaming call these days. I used to be able to hear the purr of a cat nestled in my lap. Now I can only feel its purr. I wonder, will I still be able to hear the voices of my children as they say "I do" to the partner of their dreams? Will I ever hear the sweet voices of my grandchildren as they call me "Granny" or "Nana"? I can't imagine trying to lipread the Cupid bow mouths of my children's children. I will get used to that, I know. I will figure out how to deal with it. That's what I do these days, and it isn't as painful as it once was.

There are a few things, though, that I think I will forever grieve. I miss music. It doesn't sound the same filtered through hearing aids and my sensorineural loss. I miss the sound of rain as it pelts on the window. I see it. I smell it and I feel it, but I can't hear the soothing pattern of sounds. Finally, I'll tell you what I miss the most. I will forever miss that time of the night when my husband turns out the light, turns to me, and whispers something sweet and tender.

Even with my hearing aid, I can't hear him. That's what I miss most, those loving and intimate whispers in the dark.

Reprinted by permission of the author.

Tinnitus.   Tinnitus is the sensation of noise with no outside stimulus. It can sound to the individual like ringing, hissing, chirping, roaring, and many other sounds or combinations of sounds. Tinnitus can be constant or appear intermittently. It tends to be more noticeable to the individual in a quiet environment and may be worsened by noise, certain medication, and stress (Epstein, 1999). Subjective tinnitus can be heard only by the individual. Objective tinnitus, which is quite rare, is typically caused by the sound of an abnormal blood vessel, joint clicking in the head or neck, or a muscle spasm in the palate, face, or neck.

Most incidences of tinnitus are associated with a hearing loss, and most individuals with a hearing loss experience tinnitus (House, 1999). When tinnitus is associated with an underlying condition that can be treated, such as otosclerosis, the tinnitus can be improved or eliminated. Sometimes amplification that improves hearing perception also reduces tinnitus. Often individuals are encouraged to use background music as a masking device for the tinnitus. Tinnitus retraining therapy teaches individuals to cope with tinnitus by eliminating it from their conscious awareness (Epstein, 1999).

ASSESSMENT OF HEARING

In adults, the earlier a hearing loss is identified, the more quickly the individual can receive appropriate medical treatment, habilitative services, and amplification. In children, the earlier a hearing loss is identified, the more quickly the child and family can receive early intervention services. Although the technology is available for identifying hearing loss virtually at birth, many hearing losses go undetected during infancy. Meadow-Orlans and her colleagues (1997) conducted a survey of parents of preschool deaf and hard of hearing children and found that parents suspected their children had a hearing loss at an average age of 17 months. The diagnosis was not confirmed until five months later, on average, although almost one-third of the parents received a confirmed diagnosis within one month. The more severe the hearing loss, the earlier the diagnosis was made. Children who are deaf had a confirmed diagnosis at a mean age of 14.5 months, whereas children who are hard of hearing had a confirmed diagnosis at a mean age of 28.6 months. More discouraging than the age at which the diagnosis was confirmed is the lag time between diagnosis and intervention. Children waited an average of 8 months to receive a hearing aid, 10 months to begin speech and auditory development, and 11 months to begin sign language instruction.

Assessment of Infants

Infants can be assessed in two ways. One approach is a diagnostic auditory brain stem response test. Sensors are placed on the baby's head and in the ear, computer clicks are sounded, and the baby's responses are measured. Another approach is otoacoustic immittance. A microphone is placed in the baby's ear canal, and it measures the sounds that the hair cells in the cochlea make when they vibrate in response to external sound. Both are screening procedures and do not provide specific diagnostic information about the infant's hearing status (Diefendorf, 1999). As of 1999, twenty-seven states had legislatively mandated newborn hearing screening programs.

Pure-Tone Audiometry

If an infant hearing screening is not conducted, the child's hearing loss may go undetected until the child's behaviors indicate that he or she is not hearing properly. Figure 1.3 shows the behaviors that should be expected at certain ages (Gleason, 1999; Northern & Downs, 1991).

When the parents, teachers, family members, or friends notice that the child is not responding to sounds, babbling, talking, understanding others, engaging in vocal play, or singing, it becomes apparent that the child needs a hearing assessment. An audiologist is a professional trained to evaluate hearing and recommend and fit hearing aids as well as assistive listening devices.

Children are certainly not the only age group that experiences hearing loss. This chapter discusses the diseases and conditions that cause adult-onset hearing loss. Adults may not always be aware of a hearing loss that develops slowly until it becomes severe enough to impair functioning. Once this happens, adults are assessed in quite similar ways to children.

Pure-tone audiometric tests are called *behavioral measures* because the individual's overt behavioral response to sound is measured. The audiologist uses an audiometer, which is an electronic device designed to generate pure tones at different levels of intensity and frequency. Pure-tone assessment can involve both air conduction and bone conduction. In air conduction testing, headphones are placed over the individual's ears. In bone conduction testing, a vibrator is placed on the bone behind the outer ear or on the forehead. In bone conduction testing, the sound bypasses the outer and middle ear.

FIGURE 1.3   Expected Auditory Behaviors in Infancy

ONE MONTH

Responds to sounds, such as a bell

Responds to voice

Begins vocalizing

THREE MONTHS

Turns to voices and may quiet to familiar voices

Stirs or awakens to a nearby, loud sound

Coos and babbles

SIX MONTHS

Responds by turning head to sound or voice

Engages in vocal play

Imitates sounds

Vocalizes for social contact

NINE MONTHS

Responds differentially to friendly and angry voices

Imitates speech sounds

Vocalizes recognition

Babbling acquires inflection

TWELVE MONTHS

Listens to familiar words

Turns head to locate sound

Responds to own name

Ceases activity in response to parent's voice

Stirs or awakens to nearby sound

Understands a few familiar words and phrases

Responds to music and singing

Says one word, such as *dada* or *mama*

Vocalizes emotions

Imitates sounds and words

Increases type and amount of babbling, and points while babbling

EIGHTEEN MONTHS

Comes when called

Responds to *no*

Follows simple commands

Uses 4 to 10 words other than *mama* and *dada*

TWENTY-FOUR MONTHS

Comprehends simple questions

Follows directions

Responds to rhythm of music

Shows understanding of many phrases

Plays with objects that make sounds

Has a vocabulary of 50 words or more

Combines words

Uses voice for expressing needs

Gives first name

Points to a named body part

Names a picture or object

Uses vocal inflection

The individual raises a finger each time a sound is heard and lowers it when the sound is no longer heard. The audiologist presents sounds at varying levels of intensity, from 0 to no higher than 120 dB, and at frequencies from 125 to 8,000 Hz in order to determine the individual's hearing threshold. A threshold is the level of sound so soft that it can only be detected 50 percent of the time. The audiologist plots the individual's threshold on an audiogram.

As shown in Figure 1.4, frequency is on the horizontal axis, and intensity is on the vertical axis. When you look at these audiograms, you can see that X represents the left ear and O represents the right ear. An X at 500 Hz and 80 dB means that the child was not able to detect this sound until it was 80 dB loud. In contrast, a child with normal hearing would detect this same sound at a level between 0 and 10 dB. The individual's hearing is tested in a soundproof booth, an ideal audiologic environment. Sounds that the individual can hear within the booth may be difficult to recognize and understand outside of the booth.

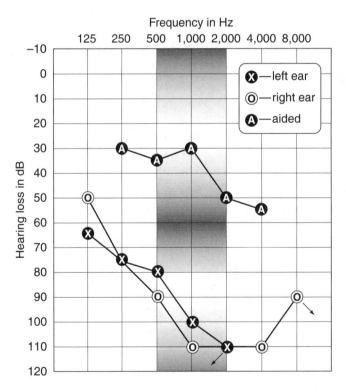

FIGURE 1.4 **Audiogram of a Child with a Profound Hearing Loss**

Young children and some individuals with severe disabilities are not able to follow the directions of conventional audiometric testing. Alternative assessments include behavior observation audiometry, visual response audiometry, and play audiometry (Madell, 1998). In behavior observation audiometry, which is typically used between birth and 6 months of age, the child is observed as sounds are presented. When the sound is loud enough to cause the child to suck more vigorously, blink, turn his or her head, or stop playing, the audiologist records the sound level. Visual reinforcement audiometry is typically used from 6 to 36 months of age. The audiologist trains the child to turn his or her head to a sound stimulus by pairing the sound with a lighted toy. In play audiometry, which is generally used after the age of 2 and a half, the child is taught to perform a simple, distinct activity each time he or she hears a sound during testing. For example, the child might put a peg in a board, put a block into a cup, or pick up a toy.

Two objective measures assess hearing without relying on behavioral responses. Transient evoked otoacoustic emissions assessment involves the use of electrodes for sensing slight electric signals generated by the auditory nerve in response to sound stimulation. In impedance audiometry, a small probe is inserted into the middle ear to detect sound reflected by the eardrum in order to identify middle ear problems.

Speech Audiometry

Speech audiometry tests the individual's ability to detect and understand speech. Speech reception threshold (SRT) identifies the intensity at which the individual can hear and identify one- and two-syllable words. Speech discrimination tests determine how well the individual can repeat monosyllabic words presented at comfortable listening levels. These tests use simple words presented in ideal conditions and do not represent the individual's ability to recognize and understand connected speech in normal conversational or classroom settings (Katz & White, 1992).

Degrees of Hearing Loss

Hearing loss is generally described in terms of the impact on spoken communication. With some variations, Figure 1.5 shows the categories that are typically used (Keith, 1996). Although hearing is categorized as slight, mild, moderate, moderate–severe, severe, and profound, in reality no two individuals have the same pattern of hearing even within these categories. And their ability to functionally use their hearing differs from individual to individual. It is also important to recognize that these categories are based on pure-tone audiometric testing without amplification.

FIGURE 1.5   Degrees of Hearing Loss and Impact on Communication

HEARING LEVEL	DESCRIPTOR	IMPACT ON COMMUNICATION
–10 to 15 dB	Normal	No impact on communication
16 to 25 dB	Slight	In quiet environments, the individual has no difficulty recognizing speech, but in noisy environments, faint speech is difficult to understand.
26 to 40 dB	Mild	In quiet conversational environments in which the topic is known and vocabulary is limited, the individual has no difficulty in communicating. Faint or distant speech is difficult to hear even if the environment is quiet. Classroom discussions are challenging to follow.
41 to 55 dB	Moderate	The individual can hear conversational speech only at a close distance. Group activities, such as classroom discussions, present a communicative challenge.
56 to 70 dB	Moderate–Severe	The individual can hear only loud, clear conversational speech and has much difficulty in group situations. Often, the individual's speech is noticeably impaired though intelligible.
71 to 90 dB	Severe	The individual cannot hear conversational speech unless it is loud and even then, cannot recognize many of the words. Environmental sounds can be detected, though not always identified. The individual's speech is not altogether intelligible.
91 dB +	Profound	The individual may hear loud sounds but cannot hear conversational speech at all. Vision is the primary modality for communication. The individual's own speech, if developed at all, is not easy to understand.

Individuals who use hearing aids may function quite differently than individuals who do not use amplification.

Figure 1.4 shows the audiogram of a child with a profound hearing loss. Eleni, like most profoundly deaf children, does not have an even hearing loss across all frequencies. At 125 Hz, she has a moderate loss in her right ear and moderately severe hearing loss in her left ear. At 500 Hz, the beginning of sounds most significant for understanding speech, her loss could be described as severe in both ears. At 1,000 and 2,000 Hz, she exhibits a profound hearing loss. Eleni's audiologist described her loss as a profound bilateral sensorineural hearing loss. At the time of testing, Eleni was five years old and too young for speech audiometry tests. She was fitted with binaural hearing aids, and when tested with her aids, the audiologist found that Eleni could hear within the range of normal conversational speech. At five years of age, it was not yet clear how well Eleni would benefit from amplification, but we can assume that she experienced some distortion in sounds. We also might assume that although she could hear within the range of normal conversational speech with her aids, at 30 to 35 dB she was going to miss much classroom discussion and hear conversational speech only at a close distance. We simply do not yet know whether she will be able to understand speech.

The categorization of hearing loss by degrees is one consideration. A second consideration is the shape of the audiometric configuration. The possible configurations are typically described as the following (Stach, 1998):

- Flat—thresholds are within 20 dB of each other across the frequency range.
- Rising—thresholds for low frequencies are at least 20 dB poorer than for high frequencies.
- Sloping—thresholds for high frequencies are at least 20 dB poorer than for low frequencies.
- Low frequency—hearing loss is restricted to the low-frequency region of the audiogram.
- High frequency—hearing loss is restricted to the high-frequency region of the audiogram.
- Precipitous—indicates steeply sloping high-frequency hearing loss of at least 20 dB per octave. (p. 107)

The effect on the individual's functioning is quite different for these configurations. For example, an individual with a high-frequency loss may miss the /s/ and /th/ phonemes, as in the word *thistle,* whereas an individual with a low-frequency loss may miss the /b/ and /d/ phonemes, as in *bad.* Typically, individuals with high-frequency losses have more difficulty understanding women's speech, and individuals with low-frequency losses have more difficulty understanding men's speech.

PREVALENCE

According to the National Center for Health Statistics (1999), approximately 22 million persons in the United States, or 8.6 percent of the population, have a hearing loss. The breakdown by age group is provided in Figure 1.6. The highest prevalence is among individuals 65 years and older, and the lowest prevalence is among children.

Estimates of severe and profound deafness range from .18 percent to .49 percent (National Center for Health Statistics, 1999). When the .49 percent prevalence figure is used, it is estimated that .10 percent of children

FIGURE 1.6   Prevalence of Hearing Loss by Age
Group in the United States

AGE GROUP	PERCENTAGE OF POPULATION
3–17	1.8
18–34	3.4
35–44	6.3
45–54	10.3
55–64	15.4
65+	29.1

are severely and profoundly deaf. This prevalence figure is the reason that deafness among children is considered a low-incidence disability.

Approximately 1.3 percent of all school-age students, ages 6 to 21, who received special education services during the 1996–1997 school year were served under the disability category of hearing impairment (National Center for Education Statistics, 1999). The other disability categories that are used by the U.S. Department of Education include specific learning disabilities, speech or language impairments, mental retardation, serious emotional disturbance, orthopedic impairments, other health impairments, visual impairments, multiple disabilities, deaf–blindness, autism and other, and preschool disabled. The prevalence of hearing loss reported above is undoubtedly higher given that some deaf children are counted under one of these disability categories because it is considered their primary disability. About 25 percent of students who are deaf and hard of hearing have one additional disability, and 9 percent have two or more other disabilities (Schildroth & Hotto, 1994).

AMPLIFICATION AND APPROACHES TO PROVIDING SOUND

Most individuals with a hearing loss are able to benefit from some form of amplification for two reasons. First, even profoundly deaf individuals can have some residual hearing at certain frequencies. Second, continued improvements in the technology of amplification have provided a range of ways to accommodate almost all types of hearing loss.

Hearing Aids

A hearing aid makes sounds louder. It is powered by a battery and operates by picking up sound, magnifying its energy, and delivering this amplified sound to the individual's ear. It has a microphone that converts acoustic energy into an electrical signal, an amplifier that increases the magnitude of the electrical signal, and a receiver that converts the amplified signal back into acoustic energy. It also has a control switch to adjust volume and tone. Some aids have a digital programming feature, which allows the person to adjust the aid for different listening situations by simply pushing a button or using a remote control device that activates one of the memories programmed into the hearing aid.

A hearing aid does not correct a hearing loss in the way that eyeglasses or contact lenses correct a visual impairment. Even with technological improvements, there is always some distortion of sound. And as you can see in Figure 1.4, the amplification provided by the hearing aid does not always bring the individual's hearing into the normal range.

Many types of hearing aids are available, including hearing aids on the body, behind the ear, in the ear, in the ear canal, and built into eyeglasses. A person can have a monaural aid in one ear or binaural aids in both ears. Most individuals with a binaural hearing loss wear binaural aids to maximize their ability to localize sounds and discriminate speech.

Cochlear Implants

A *cochlear implant* is an electronic device that compensates for the damaged or absent hair cells in the cochlea by stimulating the auditory nerve fibers. Unlike a hearing aid, a cochlear implant does not make sounds louder. Rather, it provides sound information to the individual by directly stimulating the functional auditory nerve fibers in the cochlea, thus enabling the individual to perceive sound.

The first cochlear implant devices had a single electrode, referred to as a channel. Subsequently, devices have been developed with multiple channels that are able to transmit increasingly greater amounts of sound information. As shown in the following photos, the cochlear implant has internal and external parts. The internal part is surgically implanted under the skin with electrodes inserted into the cochlea. The external part is worn in a way similar to a hearing aid.

Sound is picked up by a microphone in the external part, and a thin cord carries the sound from the microphone to the speech processor, which filters, analyzes, and changes the sound into coded signals. The coded signals are sent from the speech processor to the transmitting coil and then to the internal part of the cochlear implant. In the internal part, the signals are delivered to the electrodes that were inserted in the cochlea and stimulate the functional auditory nerve fibers, and the resulting sound information is sent to the brain.

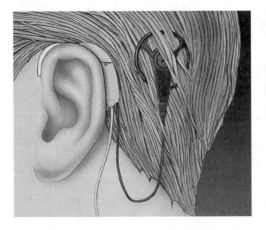 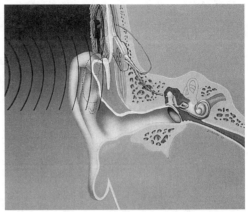

(a) The microphone in the headset of the ear picks up sound and carries it to the speech processor, which changes it into coded signals that are sent to the transmitting coil and then on to the cochlear implant under the skin.

(b) The cochlear implant delivers the signals to the electrodes inserted into the cochlea. The electrodes stimulate the functional nerve fibers in the cochlea, and the sound information is sent along the auditory nerve to the brain.

Photos courtesy of the Cochlear Corporation.

Much controversy has been generated about the cochlear implant because it is viewed by some individuals as an invasive procedure designed to change a deaf person into a hearing person. Given that many deaf adults view their deafness as a cultural difference and not a disability, the cochlear implant has been seen by the Deaf community as akin to a medical procedure designed to change a person of color into a Caucasian.

The medical community has viewed the procedure quite differently, of course. According to the Cochlear Corporation (1999), not all deaf individuals can benefit from a cochlear implant. Whether children or adults, they must have no medical contraindications. In addition, the following are the criteria for children, postlingual adults, and prelingual adults.

CHILDREN
- Profound sensorineural hearing loss in both ears
- Eighteen months of age or older
- Receiving little or no useful benefit from hearing aids
- High motivation and appropriate expectations
- Parents have high motivation and appropriate expectations.

POSTLINGUAL ADULTS
- Severe to profound sensorineural hearing loss in both ears
- Receiving limited benefit from hearing aids
- Desire to be part of the hearing world

PRELINGUAL ADULTS
- Profound sensorineural hearing loss in both ears
- Receiving no benefit from hearing aids
- Desire to be part of the hearing world

Assistive Listening Devices

Hearing aids provide maximum benefit when the environment is relatively quiet, the acoustics are good, and the individual is close to the speaker. In noisy environments such as schools, meeting rooms, and many workplaces, hearing aids do not work very well. Assistive listening devices can solve problems created by noise and distance. An assistive listening device picks up the sound at its source, amplifies it, and sends it to the individual who receives the sound through a receiver. Often, the receiver is the individual's personal hearing aid set to a specific frequency.

Assistive listening devices that use FM radio frequencies are often referred to as FM systems in educational programs. The teacher wears a wireless microphone, which enables the teacher and child to move around freely. In an FM system, the individual hearing aid will only pick up sound from the microphone, so activities such as group discussions can be cumbersome to carry out because the microphone must be passed from person to person. In Essay 1.2, Jada Buczek describes her amusing experiences with FM systems in school.

■ ■ ■ ■ ■ ▬▬▬▬▬▬▬▬▬▬▬▬▬▬▬▬▬▬▬▬▬▬

ESSAY 1.2

Jada Buczek

My name is Jada Buczek. I was born with a 65 decibel hearing loss. I'm interested in volleyball, ballet, music, reading, and writing stories. I have good grades in school, and I'm a hard worker.

In my family, it's not a problem to be hearing impaired. My Dad's entire immediate family is hearing impaired. For me it's easy to know that my impairment is hereditary. So, I know where to go for support in school and life.

I've worn the FM system ever since kindergarten. In fifth grade, I got a system called "the loop." It was a new experience because I was used to a cord going to my hearing aids. Now I'm in the seventh grade, and I have an "extend ear." I like it because it's kind of like a hearing aid and it's not as noticeable as the other two FM systems I've used.

I had a lot of fun with the FM. In the second grade, we had a student teacher who taught us about world travel. On the last day, she said good-bye and left. My teacher had assigned us a worksheet when I noticed that I heard strange noises like keys jingling and shoes clicking. I looked around and none of these things were happening. I raised my hand to tell the teacher that the microphone was still

(continued)

ESSAY 1.2 CONTINUED

on the student teacher. Mrs. Thompson ran after her and got the microphone back.

One time in the fourth grade, I had a male substitute. He left during work time to go to the bathroom. While I was working, I heard a whistling noise and a dribbling sound. When he got back, I laughed and told him that he didn't take off the microphone. He turned bright red! He was so embarrassed.

Reprinted by permission of the author.

Chapter 3 describes other types of devices that are assistive to living, such as ones that enable deaf individuals to enjoy television through closed-captioning, to use the telephone, and to realize when someone has rung the doorbell.

SUMMARY AND CONCLUDING THOUGHTS

This chapter discussed the nature of hearing and hearing loss, causes of hearing loss, hearing assessment, prevalence in the population, and approaches available for bringing sound to individuals who are deaf. Discussing deafness from audiological and medical perspectives is not easy because this type of discussion seems at odds with viewing deafness as a cultural entity. Is it possible to describe the characteristics of hearing and hearing loss without being accused of characterizing deafness as a disability? Ultimately, each deaf person, and each hearing person who interacts with deaf individuals, must figure out how to integrate medical models and sociocultural models in order to approach one another with respect and understanding. It seems critical to keep in mind that deaf individuals come in all ages, genders, ethnicities, races, and socioeconomic statuses. Some deaf individuals are born with a hearing loss and some acquire it later in life. Some are severely and profoundly deaf and some are hard of hearing with a mild or moderate hearing loss. Knowledge of the fundamentals of deafness is as important as knowledge of the other aspects that are discussed in the subsequent chapters of this book.

CHAPTER TWO

PARENTS AND FAMILIES

FOCUS QUESTIONS

- What are the most important qualities of communication between parents and their deaf children?
- Why do parents and professionals sometimes have conflicting views of what is best for the deaf child?
- What can teachers and other professionals do to support parents of deaf children?
- How are the experiences of hearing children of deaf parents and hearing siblings in a family with a deaf child similar?
- Can parents ensure the academic success of their deaf children by doing certain things?

When David Luterman wrote his seminal book, *Deafness in the Family,* in 1987, he began by noting that healthy families are characterized by the following:

1. Communication among all members is clear and direct.
2. Roles and responsibilities are clearly delineated, and the family allows for flexibility in role allocation.
3. The family members accept limits for the resolution of conflict.
4. Intimacy is prevalent and is a function of frequent, equal-powered transactions.
5. There is a healthy balance between change and the maintenance of stability. (p. 8)

When we apply these characteristics to families with a deaf member, several of the words take on special meaning—communication, flexibility, conflict, intimacy, change, and stability. From the moment of diagnosis and through all of the transitions that children and families experience, these characteristics are central to the healthy functioning of families with a deaf child. Securing and maintaining these qualities of family life can be a particular challenge for parents who have no prior experience with deafness.

This chapter discusses the issues involved in families with young deaf children, families with deaf adolescents, and families with hearing children and a deaf parent.

RESPONSE TO DIAGNOSIS

For hearing parents, a diagnosis of a hearing loss in their child is a medical determination. They are not likely to know about the debate in the field regarding deafness as a medical condition or a cultural identity. At the point of diagnosis, they are not inclined to appreciate the subtleties of the debate or the implications of the points made for pathologizing or depathologizing deafness. Although deaf parents may rejoice at the prospect of a deaf child, this response is typically beyond the understanding of hearing parents.

When parents are expecting a child, they have little information to assist them in understanding the real-life implications of having a child with a hearing loss. In order to find out how parents would initially learn about parenting a child with a hearing loss, Gregory (1991) examined a number of widely read baby books and found that they provided virtually no guidance about raising a child with a disability or hearing loss. The message for parents of exceptional children is that they are in a different category than other parents. Given this lack of information within the genre of general baby care books and the popular image of parenting children with disabilities as a noble and sacrificing endeavor, Gregory noted that parents are left with a contradictory image. "A disabled child is undesirable, but a mother of a disabled child is portrayed as loving and accepting her own child unconditionally" (p. 126).

The adjustment process is often described in terms akin to the stages of grief associated with death and dying that Kübler-Ross first identified in 1969. Although some parents may experience denial, anger, bargaining, depression, and acceptance, many do not respond according to this pattern. One reason is that the road to diagnosis can be a relatively lengthy one, and by the time it is made, the parents have had time to consider the possibility of a hearing loss and to learn about the implications. Sometimes, it is the parents who are reluctant to accept the concerns of others, but often it is the parents who are the ones pushing for confirmation of a suspected hearing loss; they can be relieved by the diagnosis, because they can now plan for the future and, sometimes, because they are grateful that something more serious is not wrong with their child (Boison, 1987; Gregory, 1991).

A second reason that parents vary so widely in their response to diagnosis is that they have such varying degrees of knowledge about deafness and experience with deaf individuals. A third reason involves the many variables that influence parents' understanding of their child's deafness. Kampfe (1989) found that parents' responses differ because their perceptions are so different. "Social status indicators such as parental age, gender and ethnic background might all have impact on the degree to which the event appears undesirable, disruptive, important, controllable or stressful" (p. 257). In addition, personality, coping strategies, general attitude toward life, personal career aspirations, sensitivity to others' opinion, education, finances, support from family and others, marital satisfaction, and the view of the parents' culture toward disability will result in different perceptions and differing abilities to adjust. Kampfe also found that perceptions can vary depending on the type, degree, and cause of the hearing loss.

A fourth reason involves the resources that parents have for responding to the diagnosis and the support they receive from professionals, family members, friends, the community, and other families with a deaf child.

Regardless of the differing responses among parents, most find the diagnosis initially to be a devastating end to their image of the perfect child. At first, they are almost always shocked. Grief, guilt, blame, fear, anger, and depression are common (Vernon & Wallrabenstein, 1984). Indeed, adoptive parents of deaf children have been found to respond similarly (Crittenden, Waterbury, & Ricker, 1985). (These responses can also surface later in the child's life, particularly during transition periods when the child may not be making the progress the parents had anticipated or hoped for.)

In Essay 2.1, one parent describes her experience in learning that her daughter is deaf. A major challenge for parents, and the first issue they confront, is communication with their deaf child.

■ ■ ■ ■ ■ ▬▬▬▬▬▬▬▬▬▬▬▬▬▬▬▬▬▬▬▬▬▬▬▬▬▬▬▬▬▬▬▬▬▬▬▬▬▬▬

ESSAY 2.1

Tami Grant

Ashli-Marie was our first child, and I didn't know what was normal and not normal. But when she wasn't talking by the time she was two, we had some concerns. When we voiced them, everyone said we were being paranoid and overprotective; kids talk at different times. One time we tried snapping our fingers to see if she would hear, and when she responded, we thought great, not thinking that she was responding because she could see us snap our fingers. Later, my mother-in-law admitted that she had suspected something was wrong but was afraid to say anything because we would think she was meddling. She

(continued)

ESSAY 2.1 CONTINUED

had a lot of guilt about that later, and we told her, there's no reason to have guilt. Her knowing wasn't going to change anything because Ashli was already deaf.

When she was two, we went to the pediatrician. And I'm really lucky because I didn't have one of those pediatricians who fought me. The pediatrician said, "Well tell me this, is she making syllable sounds?" When I said no, the pediatrician suggested we have her tested, and if nothing else, it will make us all feel better. Before this, Ashli had problems with chronic ear infections. We did have an idiot doctor at that point who told me if you can't cure it with antibiotics, it can't be cured. They gave Ashli so much antibiotics that she has staining on her teeth. I found another doctor that I liked, who put tubes in Ashli's ears. It took longer than it was supposed to, and when they came out, they told us that the liquid inside her ear had solidified. It was like someone had mixed maple syrup and toothpaste and put it in her ears. They had to scrape it all out. We thought that would help some of the issues, but it didn't. That was about a year before we had her hearing tested.

I had the test taken. I knew she was deaf because she was sitting on my lap throughout, and it was obvious. The day before, I found out my husband had diabetes. And the day after, I found out I was pregnant with my second child. It was a week! When they told me, I didn't say anything. They kept saying, "Mrs. Grant, do you understand what we're saying? Your daughter can't hear." And I kept responding, "Uh huh, uh huh, yes, I understand." I had seen the poster for the cochlear implant on the wall. I asked what it was. The audiologist was really honest. She said that her suspicion was that it was never going to be useful to Ashli because it doesn't seem as if she ever had any kind of speech or ever heard enough to recognize sound. And she immediately put us into contact with the University of Washington. They had a program that sends out parent trainers who work with parents and children on teaching sign, use of residual hearing, and things like how to test the hearing aids.

I cried all the way back to work. Once I got into the car, it kind of hit. My boss was also a good friend, and she said to me:

> You know what, Tami, I know you don't want to hear this, but let's put it into perspective. If you have to deal with some kind of disability with your child, and I don't know a lot about deafness, but it seems like deafness is not so bad because you can still drive a car, you can still function as an adult, you can still have friends, you can still run and play and jump and laugh and have a good time. Don't think about it right now, but later, I want you to think about it.

And then she sent me home. It took about two weeks of, I'm not going to have anything to do with this deafness thing. My brother-in-law is deaf and actually graduated from Washington School for the Deaf. He married my sister the year before we found out that Ashli is deaf. My sister said, "How about coming down here to the deaf school?" We were living in Edmonds, which is north of Seattle. That was in that two-week period, and I said, "Nope! She has to be part of the hearing world. We don't have a need for a special school."

My husband and I are strong in our faith, and we had someone come over to the house to give a blessing to my husband. And he turned to my husband and said, "Now you need to give a blessing to your daughter." And Keven said,

"No, I'm not going to do it. I don't think that I can let my personal wishes interfere with what God would want." And they went back and forth. When he gave her the blessing, he never said, "You're going to get better, you're going to get well." He said, "I'll bless you with patience with your parents while they learn how to communicate with you, know that I will remove stumbling blocks to your education, all things like that." And when it was done and the people left, my husband said, "That's it. From this day on, Ashli-Marie is deaf, and we learn to live with it and that's all there is to it. It's who she is, just like she has brown eyes. There's nothing we can do about it. But there's a whole lot we can do about her education." And from then on we concentrated on getting her the education that she needs and learning as much about sign language as we could.

Keven's mom gave us space the first two weeks, and when Keven called her and said, "This is it," she organized everybody in the family. His whole family got into taking sign classes. Everyone except the youngest cousins have taken at least one sign class. They just decided that Ashli is part of the family, and they need to be able to communicate with her. We feel really blessed that Keven has a family that way. They said they never want her to come and not be able to talk with them. A couple of years ago, Ashli didn't want to visit one of the cousins because she was afraid no one would be able to communicate with her. They had a family meeting and cried for a while and said, "OK, we've let our sign skills get rusty. We need to get back on track." They took refresher sign classes. We told them that you can't allow yourself to feel guilty because you're not around Ashli all of the time, and your sign skills will get rusty. Ashli is going through a period right now where she's not sure of new situations, and she'll work through it, too. I feel really blessed, and we're really fortunate. They've been very supportive.

When we had the opportunity to move to Vancouver, where the deaf school is located, we took it. We quit our jobs and gave up our house. I was down within two weeks, and Keven came down the next month.

I have one suggestion for parents. The minute you find out that your child is deaf, get a notebook and start keeping everything you get. Keep all of the information, including envelopes from the school so that you have original postmarks. Include the information on parent rights, the current IEP, the last IEP, audiograms, correspondence with the school, everything. When I go into IEP meetings, I have everything I need right there.

Reprinted by permission of the author.

COMMUNICATION BETWEEN PARENTS AND THEIR DEAF CHILD

Much of what we know about parent–child interaction when the child is deaf involves communication. It is interesting that researchers have predominantly focused their explorations of communication at two points in child development—the young child and the adolescent. Clearly, these are two important transitional times in the child's life. The first is when the child is just learning language and the parent has recently learned the child is deaf. The second is when the child is getting ready to become independent, but is still very reliant on the emotional support of parents.

Communication with Young Deaf Children

Touch, gaze, and voice are so embedded within the communication of mothers and infants that it is hard to imagine what would happen if one of these were missing. Although deaf parents replace voice with gesture, hearing parents have to consciously adapt their communication style once they learn that their child is deaf. Of course, voice is still important for many deaf children, but the saliency of voice is certainly diminished for the child with a hearing loss.

When we talk about the importance of communication between young deaf children and their parents, it is for two reasons. One reason is that communication is integral to the emotional bond between parents and children. Second, it is through the conversations between children and parents that children learn language. We call conversation the milieu of language acquisition. Children do not learn language from listening or watching others use language, person-to-person or on the television. They learn language by being engaged in conversations with others who are meaningful in their lives, who talk to them about things in their immediate environment that are important to them, from the time they are born.

The nature of the language between very young children and their parents is so unique and supportive of language acquisition that it has been given a special name—*motherese.* It is called motherese because mothers seem to be particularly attuned to the developmental levels of their children (McLaughlin, White, McDevitt, & Raskin, 1983). Mothers' language directed to their young children is generally simple, well formed, and clear. Mothers use higher pitch and more exaggerated stress and intonation than when they are communicating with their older children or with adults. And they typically ask more questions (DePaulo & Bonvillian, 1978; Garton & Pratt, 1998; Grieser & Kuhl, 1988; Snow, 1986).

Parents engage their babies in conversation long before the baby can participate. We have all seen mothers at the supermarket saying things like, "What do you think Dad would like for dinner?" Then she pauses. "Perhaps macaroni and cheese, with a nice salad. Is that a good idea?" She pauses again. Each pause is both an invitation to respond conversationally and a model of conversational turn-taking. Mom's gaze is equally significant to the conversation, signaling the child's turn to respond. When the child makes a sound during his or her "turn," Mom is typically very responsive. "Oh, you're right, Dad is on a diet. Instead of macaroni and cheese, how about a nice low-fat tuna casserole." Very young children let us know that they get the idea when they vocalize during the conversation between two adults, as if to say, "It's my turn now."

Several researchers have looked specifically at the characteristics of motherese used by mothers with their deaf children and found that they sign more slowly, use simpler sentence structures and exaggerated movements, and incorporate repetition (Masataka, 1992, 1996). There is also evidence to indicate that hearing mothers are more verbally controlling in conversational interactions with their deaf children, and they are less able to flexibly adapt their interactional strategies. However, some researchers have found that mothers of deaf children are just as likely to vary their communication style across diverse contexts as mothers of hearing children and that mothers become less controlling as their children's language becomes more sophisticated (Jamieson, 1994, 1995; Musselman & Churchill, 1991, 1992; Plapinger & Kretschmer, 1991; Power, Wood, Wood, & Macdougall, 1990).

Reilly and Bellugi (1996) videotaped deaf parents signing with their deaf infants and toddlers and found an intriguing difference in the importance of affect over grammar for these parents when compared to hearing parents. In American Sign Language (ASL), in order to ask a *wh*-question, the signer must use a furrowed brow as one of the grammatical markers. But this same furrowed brow affectively signals anger and puzzlement. The researchers found that 90 percent of the questions that the deaf parents asked of their deaf children under age 2 were ungrammatical in ASL because the parents did not use the furrowed brow. When the children reached their third birthday, the parents shifted to using the furrowed brow, which is the appropriate ASL grammatical marker. In an effort to provide unambiguous communication to their very young deaf children, these deaf parents eliminated a grammatical marker and did not use it until they intuitively felt their children could understand the seemingly contradictory information.

Parents are not the only members of the parent–child dyad who initiate interaction. The parents' response to child-initiated interaction is as important to the relationship as the child's response to parent-initiated interaction. In one study of mothers and infants, Koester (1995) found that the deaf infants used fewer typical initiating behaviors, such as smiling, greeting, or reaching toward the mother, but a greater number of less-typical behaviors, such repetitious motor activity, than hearing infants. Smith-Gray and Koester (1995) observed that these behaviors function as signals, and when they are integrated into the full picture of infant–mother interaction, few differences are found in eliciting behaviors between deaf infants and hearing infants. In another study, Spencer and Gutfreund (1990) found that the deaf infants produced fewer initiating behaviors such as gestures, physical contact with the mother, vocalizing, prolonged and pronounced gazing at an object, and large body movements than hearing infants, which seemed to promote greater initiating behaviors by the mothers of the deaf infants when compared to the mothers of the hearing infants.

Communication with School-Age Children and Adolescents

A common language is essential for connectedness between humans, and so the lack of a common language, or even a less-than-fluent common language, will affect the parent–child relationship (Kolod, 1994). Two assumptions have traditionally been made about the quality of language used between parents and their deaf children. The first assumption is that when the parents are hearing, they do not share a common language because the hearing parent uses speech and the deaf child uses sign. The second assumption is that they share a common language because either the deaf child is able to communicate orally or the parent uses sign.

In examining the first assumption, it seems straightforward that if the hearing parent communicates only in speech and the deaf child is not able to access speech via speechreading or amplification, then they will not communicate effectively with one another. They are simply using two different languages. If the parent uses spoken English, which the child does not understand, and the child uses sign, which the parent does not understand, there is no common language. There may have been points in history where this occurred, but increasingly this description does not apply to the complexity of communication between parents and their school-age deaf children and adolescents.

Meyers and Bartee (1992) found that greater numbers of parents are learning sign language, though their proficiency may not always be high. And from the alternative perspective of children being raised orally, Nohara, MacKay, and Trehub (1995) found that the conversational turn-taking behaviors of deaf adolescents and their mothers were just as sophisticated as those observed between hearing adolescents and their mothers. Bodner-Johnson (1991) examined the conversation of families around the dinner table, and she found a fairly balanced level of conversational control and invitation. The families in this study "set up relatively inviting conversational environments in which control did not function as a depressant on the child's willingness to participate" (p. 507). Indeed, the deaf children responded more loquaciously to questions than statements or expressions of ideas.

The second assumption about the commonality of language between parents and their deaf child is that they share a language because either the parents sign or the child is able to communicate in spoken English. There is considerable debate among educators regarding the importance of sign language use by parents and the role of a signing environment in the child's linguistic, social, and emotional development. Most of the research seems to be aimed at supporting one communication mode or language over the other. Therefore, it is difficult to find unbiased information about the quality of communication between older deaf children and their parents.

The actual amount of research versus opinion on the social–emotional consequences of using sign or speech is relatively small. Desselle found that greater sign proficiency by parents was positively related to higher self-esteem in their deaf children (Desselle, 1994; Desselle & Pearlmutter, 1997). Kluwin and Gaustad (1992) found that mothers generally make the decision about mode of communication, and mothers who sign tend to have more cohesive families than mothers who use speech or other means of communication. From the perspective of deaf youngsters who use speech, Niver and Schery (1994) found that the deaf children in their study actually spoke more frequently to their mothers than to their peers because these mothers encouraged conversation. Although much of the communication between parents and deaf children is conversational in nature, the nonverbal components are also meaningful.

NONVERBAL INTERACTION

Much of what we know about the nonverbal interaction between parents and their deaf child centers around the responsiveness of mothers. Earlier, some of the similarities and differences in the ways that deaf infants solicit their mothers' attention were discussed when compared to hearing infants. What happens when the deaf infant tries to solicit his or her mother's attention? Are there differences between the responses of deaf mothers and hearing mothers?

One of the differences in mothers' responses involves whether they wait for the child's attention. Hearing mothers and deaf mothers are both very responsive to their infants, but deaf mothers wait for their infants to spontaneously look back at them before responding. In addition, deaf mothers are much more likely to respond by using language that is consistent with the baby's focus of attention (Prendergast & McCollum, 1996; Robinshaw & Evans, 1995; Spencer, Bodner-Johnson, & Gutfreund, 1992). One group of researchers offered an interesting interpretation of how deaf infants respond to the vocalization of mothers who do not wait for the child's attention. Koester, Karkowski, and Traci (1998) postulated that the deaf infant actually perceives vocalizing as an instance of the mother observing and waiting, rather than a solicitation of attention, which the mother intends. In addition, they observed that hearing mothers often use vocalization quite effectively to regain eye contact with their infant as well as to simply comment on the child's new focus of attention rather than to call the infant's attention back to them.

Another difference is the mothers' style of interaction. Meadow-Orlans and Steinberg (1993) found that hearing mothers are less likely to use frequent and positive touch with their deaf infants. They are also less sensitive and more intrusive, less flexible, and less consistent in their responses to their deaf infants than mothers who are deaf. In a study by Waxman, Spencer, and Poisson (1996), the differing characteristics of interaction between hearing mothers and their deaf toddlers when compared to deaf mothers and deaf toddlers did not adversely affect the pleasure that the children took in the interaction. In addition, the hearing mothers facilitated their toddlers' play just as well as the deaf mothers did.

Much of the research on parent–child interaction has involved infants and toddlers. Tanksley (1993) looked at the interactions of deaf and hard of hearing children with receptive language ages between two and five. Their chronological ages were approximately 1 and a half to 5 and a half. When matched with hearing children with similar receptive language ages, Tanksley found no differences in interactional patterns between the mothers of the hearing children and the mothers of the deaf and hard of hearing children. Similarly, Fisiloglu and Fisiloglu (1996) found that the functioning of families with deaf and hard of hearing children did not differ from families with hearing children in areas such as problem solving, communication, roles, affective responses, affective involvement, and behavior control.

There is a complex relationship between the attitude of parents toward deafness, quality of communication, security of attachment between the parent and deaf child, and the coping strategies that parents use. Understanding the complexities of these factors is integral to understanding the linguistic, social, and emotional development of deaf children.

ATTITUDE, ATTACHMENT, AND COPING

It is perhaps not surprising that professionals involved in the lives of deaf children would be concerned about the attitude of parents toward deafness, the quality of the bond between parents and their deaf children, and whether parents can successfully cope with raising a deaf child. It is surprising, and somewhat disturbing, that there has been a fair amount of parent bashing in the history of deaf education, particularly related to hearing parents. From articles in the professional and popular press to conversations in the teacher's lounge, it is not unusual to hear about parents who can't communicate with their child, won't learn to sign, never show up for conferences, and only make their presence known when they have a complaint about the school. All professionals need to unpack whatever truths lie behind these views, understand the issues from the family's perspective, and find constructive ways to influence positive parent–child interactions if the relationship has gone awry.

Attitude and Attachment

We know that all infants become attached to their caregivers, and the quality of this relationship is integral to the child's psychological, social, and emotional development (Bowlby, 1969). Research on the attachment relationship between both hearing and deaf parents and their deaf children indicates no differences in the patterns of attachment than those found with hearing parents and hearing children (Greenberg & Marvin, 1979; Lederberg & Mobley, 1990; Meadow, Greenberg, & Erting, 1983). When parental attitudes are taken into account, there is some evidence to indicate that the more negative the parents' attitudes are toward the child's deafness, the more insecure the attachment relationship is with their deaf child (Hadadian, 1995). Also, negative attitudes of fathers toward deafness have been found to be related to lower language comprehension scores in their children (Hadadian & Rose, 1991).

Some researchers have viewed attitude toward sign language to be associated with attitude toward deafness. For example, Weisel, Dromi, and Dor (1990) found that mothers with higher social–economic status expressed more positive attitudes toward sign language, and that attitude toward sign language "should be considered representative of the mother's general level of acceptance of her child's hearing impairment and her orientation toward the sociocultural aspects of deafness" (p. 268).

Although there is relatively little information about the attitudes of families with diverse ethnicities, a couple of investigations have yielded some intriguing insights. Groups of African American hearing parents and Hispanic hearing parents were questioned by interview and survey (Jones & Kretschmer, 1988; Steinberg, Davila, Collazo, Loew, & Fischgrund, 1997). The parents reported a high degree of satisfaction with their children's educational programs and their access to services for the children. However, they also tended to be involved relatively little in their child's educational process, choosing to let the schools take care of this aspect of their child's development. The African American parents discussed the changes in their attitudes since their child was diagnosed and most reported a calm resolve. The Hispanic parents expressed either positive or neutral feelings about deafness and were most concerned about the stigmatization they felt toward their child from their extended families and communities.

Coping

All families must cope with the stresses of daily life. Families with a deaf child must also deal with learning about their child's hearing loss, figuring out how to communicate with their child, exploring educational options and working with educational programs, and interacting with the many professionals in their child's life. Teachers and psychologists have long been concerned about the stress these families experience and their ability to cope (Schlesinger & Meadow, 1972).

We have learned quite a bit about the factors that contribute to greater and lesser amounts of family stress, and we also have seen some important discrepancies among research findings.

1. Fathers experience less stress than mothers according to a 1990 study by Meadow-Orlans, similar degrees of parental stress according to her 1994 study, and greater degrees as occupational status and educational attainment of the father increased according to a 1989 study by Hagborg.

2. Parents of deaf children do not experience more stress than parents of hearing children, according to Meadow-Orlans's 1994 study, but mothers of deaf children in Quittner, Glueckauf, and Jackson's 1990 study reported higher levels of stress when compared to mothers of hearing children. In a 1995 study by Meadow-Orlans, she found that mothers report greater general life stress and depression than mothers of hearing children.

3. Parents of children with additional disabilities experience higher levels of stress and depression (Meadow-Orlans, 1990), and these families are more likely to be characterized as dysfunctional (Powers, Elliott, Patterson, Shaw, & Taylor, 1995).

4. Parents of profoundly deaf children do not experience greater or less stress than parents of hard of hearing children (Meadow-Orlans, 1994) or parents of hearing children with other disabilities (Hanson & Hanline, 1990).

5. Parents using oral/aural communication do not experience greater or less stress than parents using sign communication according to Meadow-Orlans (1990), but Hagborg (1989a) found parental use of sign language to be a moderator of stress.

6. Parental stress increases as the child becomes older according to Hagborg (1989), but decreases with age among Greek mothers according to Konstantareas and Lampropoulou (1995).

Meadow-Orlans suggested that the "findings confirm the wisdom of the current emphasis placed on social support by early intervention specialists. Furthermore, they may encourage professionals to increase their services to fathers and to help spouses develop effective support for each other" (1994, p. 99).

Indeed, marital conflict is often seen as a common occurrence in families with a child who is deaf. In one study of divorce rates, it was found that the rate among parents with hearing children was 15.3 percent, whereas the rate was 20.7 percent among parents with deaf children (Hodapp & Krasner, 1994–1995).

There is little available information that either confirms or disconfirms whether childhood deafness has a negative influence on marital relationships and, if this is true, why. Henggeler and his associates analyzed the marital satisfaction among the parents of 74 deaf youths and 57 hearing youths. In the families with deaf youths, 47 percent were headed by single parents compared to 35 percent of the families with hearing youths. Among the intact families of the deaf youths, high family cohesion and less severe hearing impairment were associated with high marital satisfaction. Marital adjustment was not found to be associated with how long it had been since the child's hearing loss was diagnosed (Henggeler, Watson, Whelan, & Malone, 1990).

When Meadow-Orlans (1990) conducted a study with 40 families, 20 with hearing children and 20 with deaf children, she found that the mothers were more likely than the fathers to report negative relationships with their spouses. These results and others have led many educators and researchers to focus their attention on the kinds of support that ameliorate stress and encourage healthy coping.

Social support has a powerful effect on parental coping. Calderon and Greenberg (1999) observed that social support is strongly related to maternal adjustment to having a child with a hearing loss because it appears to act as a buffer to current life stress. Similarly, MacTurk and his associates found that the amount of support that mothers receive from family, friends, and professionals is a significant factor in predicting the quality of mother–child interactions (MacTurk, Meadow-Orlans, Koester, & Spencer, 1993). But it is important to distinguish between social support and a social network. As Koester and Meadow-Orlans (1990) noted, "Some people in one's social network may not provide support, and may, in fact, add to the burden by demanding additional output of time and energy" as well as contribute to feelings of guilt or inadequacy (p. 304).

In Essay 2.1, a mother of a deaf child describes her family's response to learning that their child, grandchild, niece, and cousin was deaf.

One of the issues that all parents must cope with is their child's behavior. When the child is deaf and the parents are hearing, their ability to communicate becomes intertwined with their effectiveness in dealing with behavior.

CHILD BEHAVIOR AND DISCIPLINE

Much of what children learn about behavior does not come from the direct teaching of rules by their parents. And it does not come from the positive and negative consequences of their behavior, sometimes thought of as rewards and punishments. It comes from watching and listening to the consequences of other children's behaviors—siblings, friends, unknown children at another table in a restaurant, and all of the other children with whom they come into contact around multitudes of activities. They pay attention to the adults' words, tone of voice, and actions. They also overhear lots of conversations about "do's" and "don'ts" from other children who share stories about their parents. For the deaf child, the opportunity to overhear conversations and to understand the words that accompany the actions of other children's parents is limited. Their notions of appropriate behavior are molded almost exclusively by parents, and later teachers. For the parent who has difficulty communicating with their child, the message can be distorted, incomplete, and frustrating.

In a study of discipline strategies, Adams and Tidwell (1988) found that parents of deaf children who considered themselves successful at handling their child's misbehavior differed in two ways from parents who did not consider themselves successful. The successful parents perceived less misbehavior, which may be because they were good at disciplining their child or they simply overlooked more types of behavior than the parents who viewed themselves as unsuccessful. The successful parents also more often used discussion and explanation, whereas the unsuccessful parents more often used scolding as a disciplinary technique.

The perception of parents about their child's behavior was further investigated by Adams and Tidwell in a 1989 study. They found that high degrees of parental stress were associated with high perception of the child's misbehavior. They also made a surprising finding about the relationship between degree of hearing loss and misbehavior. The parents of children with greater degrees of hearing loss reported a lower incidence of child misbehavior than the parents of children with lesser degrees of hearing loss. On the surface, these results seem contrary to the popular belief that parents will have more difficulty communicating with children who have greater degrees of hearing loss, and this communication difficulty will result in more difficulty in disciplining the child. Adams and Tidwell suggested that the parents of children who are hard of hearing "may be of the belief that their children are more able to understand their world, therefore spend less time with explanations and interpretations during interactions. This may cause more confusion, frustration, and ultimately more behavior difficulties in their children over time" (p. 327).

Behavior is not all that parents teach their children. Indeed, we often say that parents are their children's first teachers. When the home environment is a positive learning environment, the deaf child comes to school with a wealth of knowledge and experiences.

EDUCATIONAL ACHIEVEMENT

A few critical dimensions of home environment are associated with positive educational achievement of deaf children (Bodner-Johnson, 1982, 1985, 1986; Kluwin & Gaustad, 1992).

1. *Family involvement and interaction.* When parents are involved in their children's lives and interact with them around important family and child activities, their deaf child is more likely to be successful in school. Interaction can take the form of being engaged in their child's educational activities and sports, discussing communication progress and understanding the child's communication abilities, discussing school performance and progress, understanding the child's current educational program and studies, making reading material available to the child through trips to the bookstore or library, planning and taking outings, being involved in the child's out-of-school activities and hobbies, and understanding the child's deafness. Powers and Saskiewicz (1998) compared the involvement of parents in their deaf and hearing children's school programs and found no differences. They did, however, find that the parents of deaf children tended to observe, whereas the parents of hearing children tended to participate and interact.

2. *Guidance and knowledge.* Parents who seek knowledge about their child so that they can provide guidance and direction are likely to see their child motivated to learn and succeed. The greater knowledge that a parent has about the child's language abilities, the more able the parent is to model and reinforce correct language usage, whether in ASL or English. Parents who pay attention to their child's school progress reports and meet regularly with the child's teachers are showing their child the importance of school. When parents and children watch television or videos together, jointly work on a hobby, and play together, they have an opportunity for much conversation around mutually interesting topics. And when parents read to their children, they bring them into the world of literature and demonstrate the value of literacy.

3. *Press for achievement.* Press for achievement has been found to be the factor most significant in reading and math achievement among deaf children. Parents who press for achievement are ones who have high expectations for their children's academic work. They show this by expecting their children to work hard and earn high grades. They talk to their children about their future after high school, they plan for college, and they hold high aspirations for their children's career. They read at home, and they expect their children to read for recreation and information. In one study of parental educational expectations, Masino and Hodapp

(1996) found that parents of deaf and hard of hearing children held similar expectations as parents of hearing children and parents of children with disabilities. However, expectations have clearly not been the only factor related to college attendance, given that 33.4 percent of deaf students attend college compared to the 53.7 percent rate found among high school graduates without disabilities (Fairweather & Shaver, 1991).

4. *Adaptation to deafness.* A home environment in which the family has adapted to the child's deafness enables the child to be viewed as a child, first and foremost. Parents who participate in the Deaf community with their child are able to provide a multicultural milieu that reflects the values of the many cultural identities that the family members hold. Parents who have adapted to their child's deafness are not inclined to focus on deafness as a handicap. And they are typically found to be more permissive than overprotective in their child rearing. Children in these home environments are more likely to succeed academically than children in families who have not adapted to their deafness.

No formulas exist that parents can follow for guaranteeing their child's academic success. It is incumbent on teachers and other school professionals to understand the factors that underlie positive accomplishment so that they can encourage and support parents. As Kluwin and Gaustad (1992) noted, "A school program that would encourage the achievement of its deaf children must work closely with families in promoting greater ease of communication within the family and in providing information on specific ways that parents can support the learning of their children" (pp. 81–82).

Thus far the discussion on the role of families has focused almost exclusively on the deaf child's parents. Siblings also play a significant role in the deaf child's life.

SIBLINGS

Brothers and sisters have special needs of their own. Their parents are immersed in fulfilling multiple roles including teacher, counselor, spouse, and advocate, as well as parent. They may experience a number of different emotions about their deaf sibling and the effect on the family (Meyer, Vadasy, & Fewell, 1985a; Schirmer, Busch, & Classen, 1988). It has been observed that brothers and sisters often experience anger about the effect the deaf child has on the family and jealousy because of the attention the deaf child receives from parents. It is common for siblings to feel embarrassment about the ways that the deaf sibling communicates. Siblings often feel guilt for being "normal," sorrow for their deaf sibling, and the sadness within the family. They often resent how much attention and time their deaf sibling receives. They can feel much pressure to achieve, yet also realize that others often downplay their accomplishments. They can be expected to be caregivers at the expense of their own needs. They sometimes are worried about the future because they wonder if they will have to take care of their sibling, if they will "catch" the hearing loss, or if their own children will be deaf or hard of hearing. They can feel a sense of isolation if they do not know anyone else in their situation and if they are not able to communicate easily with their sibling.

Yet, they also frequently have greater independence, patience, maturity, responsibility, and compassion than their peers. They are commonly more tolerant of differences and show more understanding of others. Sense of pride, acceptance of responsibility, family closeness, and unselfishness are also some of the very positive qualities found in brothers and sisters. And growing up with a deaf child in the family is a particularly nourishing environment for the development of empathy.

Israelite (1986) examined the psychological functioning of adolescent hearing sisters of younger deaf siblings and found that they were essentially well adjusted and had similar perceptions about their self-esteem as siblings of normally hearing children. She also found that these girls defined and viewed themselves in their social milieu as different from their peers, which might contribute to feelings of inadequacy in social situations. In Essay 2.2, one brother discusses what it was like to grow up with a deaf younger sister.

■ ■ ■ ■ ■ ▬▬

ESSAY 2.2

Elihu Hirsch

I'm an architect, and I live in a suburb of Washington, DC with my wife, Paige, and our two sons. I was born in Washington, but from the time I was a few months old until I was eight, we lived in Ceylon (Sri Lanka), India, Afghanistan, and the Philippines because my dad worked for the Foreign Service. My younger sister, Ruth, was born in Afghanistan. When she was four years old, we moved back to Washington. At that point, two events happened, though we didn't know the effects of one for several years. Ruth contracted strep throat, and the doctor prescribed streptomycin instead of penicillin because my mom didn't know if Ruth was allergic to penicillin. At about the same time as Ruth became sick, our parents separated, and later they were divorced. Ruth stopped talking.

(continued)

ESSAY 2.2   CONTINUED

I remember that she had spoken English very well for her age and even a little Tagalog in the Philippines. The specialists thought Ruth was autistic. For the next several years, she attended a special school and received psychological counseling.

I'm not sure what prompted someone to consider the possibility that Ruth had a hearing loss, but when she was ten years old, her hearing was tested. She had apparently suffered nerve damage from the streptomycin, which was a rare side effect. She was fitted with hearing aids, but they didn't seem to help. My mom looked for schools that could cater to someone like Ruth. She was, at the same time, concerned about the possibility of isolating Ruth from her peers should she go to a "deaf only" school. She opted instead to persuade educators to allow Ruth to enroll in a regular public school and committed herself to providing Ruth with tutors and as much home support as would be required to pursue a mainstream education. By this time, my older brother was living with our dad overseas, so I became kind of the dad in the family. The debate between sign versus oralism never went away, but at the same time, Ruth managed to hold her own academically. Ruth became more outgoing, and she started to talk. I remember how difficult it was to understand her and how slowly she learned new words. She expressed herself in sounds and gestures. One time really stands out in my mind. She said "shoe," and I was amazed because she said it so clearly. But people outside of the family couldn't understand Ruth at all.

When Ruth was in the fifth grade, my mom learned about the Helen Beebe Speech and Hearing Center in Easton, Pennsylvania. I was in the ninth grade and pretty happy living in Washington where I had very few restrictions on my comings and goings. We knew it was best for Ruth, so we uprooted and moved to Easton. We had a goal, which was to help Ruth communicate. The high school in Easton was much stricter than the one I had attended in Washington. Nonetheless, I feel I adapted well. When I look back on it now, I feel that the opportunity to move to Easton allowed me to better focus on my own education and think about my future. Additionally, living in Easton meant that I could go to Temple University or any other state college for far less than the cost of attending an out-of-state institution had I stayed in Washington.

When we were growing up, Ruth had always been a little bit of a shadow to me, but I didn't mind taking her with me when I went places with my friends. Before the Beebe clinic, I remember we did things that didn't require a lot of conversation such as playing board games and going to the Smithsonian museums or monuments in Washington. She would tag along to the playground or the pool, and it never seemed burdensome to me. And it didn't seem embarrassing, perhaps because we had a relatively closed group of friends and family who all knew Ruth.

Ruth changed a great deal at the Beebe clinic. Her speech improved so much that she was understandable to people outside of the family. In Easton, she attended Catholic school when she wasn't in speech therapy at the Beebe clinic. When Ruth was twelve, I helped her study for her Bat Mitzvah and just like other Jewish girls at age thirteen, Ruth had her Bat Mitzvah with our family and friends in attendance to share this milestone in her life.

Once she began communicating more clearly, I would try to let her know what people were saying. But as we got older and conversations became more complicated, keeping Ruth in the loop presented a huge challenge. I would provide snippets, but I simply didn't stop to translate everything that people said. It was hardest during holiday times when the family would gather. People would talk to Ruth one to one, but at the dinner table, she was often completely left out. It wasn't as if she was treated like an empty chair, but she also wasn't a full participant in the conversations. It was so painful that Ruth stopped going to family get-togethers and only recently started attending again.

When Ruth was ready for high school, I was heading off for Temple University, and she and my mom moved back to Washington, DC. She attended the Duke Ellington High School of the Arts and received a partial scholarship to attend Shenandoah College in Winchester, Virginia, an arts and music conservatory, where she received her degree in dance education. I have great admiration for Ruth's determination and sense of self. She started to learn sign in high school, and today, she communicates both orally and in sign. I have never learned to sign, not because I'm disinterested, but because I just haven't been able to devote the time. However, learning to sign may still be in my future because my wife, Paige, is becoming a sign language interpreter, in large part because of her relationship with Ruth.

Ruth and I are still close, though we don't see each other as often as we would like. Ruth lives with her husband and two little girls, ages two and four and a half, in Manassas, Virginia, about one and a half hours from Silver Spring, where I live. It's still something of a challenge to communicate with Ruth, although technology has made it easier. We talk on the TTY, but after working all day I can be really torn between wanting to talk with Ruth and wanting to spend time with my sons.

No one knows if the autistic tendencies that Ruth exhibited when she first lost her hearing were a reaction to my parents' separation or a response to the sudden loss of sound in her world. It was a turbulent time for our family, and I had to take on responsibility that was beyond most of my friends. When my dad sought custody, I was able to express my own wishes, but Ruth couldn't express hers. When decisions were being made, opportunities seized, and sacrifices considered, I was part of the discussion. But during the early years, Ruth was not able to participate in the decisions being made about her life. My mother's health was not good since suffering a heart attack shortly after giving birth to Ruth in Afghanistan, and she had to spend a lot of her physical time working with Ruth and on her behalf. I had to grow up fast, but I don't remember ever resenting the attention my mother gave Ruth. I always liked her and thought of her as a happy person, except during her quiet or autistic days when you couldn't tell what kind of person she was.

I think I had a normal childhood despite my parents' divorce. It made me more self-sufficient. I'm sure Paige appreciated my ability to cook and do laundry when we got married!

Reprinted by permission of the author.

The issues confronting siblings along with the increased emphasis in the past decade on understanding and involving the whole family in the education of children with special needs has resulted in the establishment of sibling support groups. Often, the groups are designed for brothers and sisters of children with a range of disabilities, such as the "We're Special, Too!" group in Portland, Oregon. The following are typical purposes for sibling support groups (Atkins, 1987; Meyer, Vadasy, & Fewell, 1985b; Summers, Bridge, & Summers, 1991):

- To meet other siblings in a relaxed and enjoyable setting
- To find out that other siblings have the same questions, feelings, and concerns
- To share problems, ways to solve them, and ways to cope with them
- To get information about hearing loss and other disabilities and to clear up confusions
- To find answers to questions without asking parents
- To be reassured and supported

In addition to support groups, Malcolm (1990) noted that school programs can sponsor activities that help hearing siblings to feel more comfortable with deafness and closer to their deaf brother or sister. The deaf child's school program can invite siblings to visit the classroom, tour the audiology booth, and meet with deaf adults. School programs can also sponsor activities that bring hearing siblings into meaningful activities with their deaf brothers and sisters. For example, it is not unusual for hearing siblings to join activities such as Girl Scout and Boy Scout troops or to participate in team sports at schools for the deaf. The hearing child's school program can start a sign language club, show deafness-related movies, include books in the school library with themes on deafness and deaf characters, celebrate International Hearing and Speech month, and implement sibling groups facilitated by the school counselor.

Parents and siblings of deaf children have been discussed but that certainly does not exhaust all of the family configurations. When deaf children grow up, they customarily become parents themselves, and often their children are hearing. The issues with which these children deal throughout their lives have been the subject of much interest.

DEAF PARENTS AND HEARING CHILDREN

When Joanne Greenberg wrote *In This Sign* in 1972, it was the first time that the general public learned about growing up in a family with deaf parents. Even among professionals, there had been little information about the dynamics of family life when one or both parents are deaf. (In this section, *deaf* with a lowercase *d* is used because it is not referring exclusively to culturally Deaf individuals.)

Until the 1970s, professionals tended to believe that deaf individuals intrinsically had serious limitations as parents. For example, Flaxbeard and Toomey (1987) noted that communication and parental attitudes are two areas of difficulty faced by hearing children of deaf parents. In their view, "Communication with parents, however warm and close, will have intellectual limitations particularly in relation to abstract concepts of social behavior" (p. 104). They also asserted that for deaf parents, attitudes to parenthood "will be ill defined and based on their own limited experience of the world" (p. 104).

The concerns about the parenting skills of deaf individuals emanated from several beliefs, according to Ford (1984). The first is the relationship between the deaf parent and his or her own parents, who were likely to be hearing. The parent–child relationship provides a model for parenting and if it was not a positive one, then the deaf parent would have a poor notion of how to parent his or her own children. The second belief involves the parenting models that deaf children received when they lived in dormitories at residential schools for the deaf, which was the primary educational setting until the late twentieth century. It seemed obvious to many professionals that caregivers could not possibly provide good parenting models to large groups of children in a dormitory setting. A third belief involves the deaf individual's awareness of the hearing culture. It was believed that Deaf adults growing up largely in institutionlike residential schools would have a lack of knowledge about the broader culture and would not be able to provide a link for their hearing children to the larger society. The result is that "a relatively bleak picture is painted of the family situation, and success of parenting, in families of deaf parents with hearing children" (p. 2).

Since the 1980s, a number of researchers have examined the reality of these beliefs. Their studies have tended to fall into two categories: (a) parenting skills of deaf adults and (b) development of hearing children of deaf parents.

Parenting Skills

The parenting skills of deaf mothers and fathers have been examined at two points in the child's development—infancy and later childhood.

Parenting Skills during Infancy

One aspect of parental skills involves the parents' sensitivity to their child's cues. Crittenden and Bonvillian (1984) examined the interactional patterns of mothers and fathers with their 9- to 18-month-old infants and found that the deaf parents and the socioeconomically stressed parents were almost as sensitive to their infants' cues as the parents who had been identified as middle class nonrisk. The parents who showed significantly lower sensitivity included those with mental retardation and parents identified as abusive and neglectful. The researchers pointed out, however, that assessing the deaf parents with the same observational techniques as the hearing parents might have been invalid. For example, one of the measures involved response to the infants' vocalizations. "As would be expected, the deaf parents were much less likely to respond to their infants' vocalizations than were parents with normal hearing. Whereas such failure to respond may usually be taken as an indicator of parental insensitivity, we have no basis on which to assume that it measures or predicts any such adverse trends in the development of children with deaf parents" (p. 260).

When Rea, Bonvillian, and Richards (1988) studied mother–child interactive behaviors, they found results comparable to the ones found earlier by Crittenden and Bonvillian. The deaf mothers and hearing mothers used eye gaze and facial expression similarly. The deaf mothers used fewer exaggerated expressions than the researchers had expected, and the hearing mothers used greater exaggerated expressions than expected. Both mothers tended to maintain a more constant gaze and the infant controlled eye contact by initiating and disengaging. The deaf mothers and hearing mothers used touch and vocalization somewhat differently. The deaf mothers used touch more often, though their use of touch decreased as the infant became older. They also tended to touch for less time than the hearing mothers, which may reflect their differing purposes. The authors suggested that deaf mothers use touch to gain the child's attention and to form the child's hands into a sign. Expectedly, the deaf mothers used considerably fewer vocalizations than the hearing mothers. The deaf and hearing infants vocalized similarly until the 16- to 17-month age level, at which time the hearing infants began to increase their vocal production and the deaf infants continued at the same level as when they were younger. The authors concluded that "this general pattern of similarity across groups in behavior lends support to those investigators who have tended to describe the interactions of deaf parents and their children in a positive manner" (p. 324).

Parenting Skills during Later Childhood

In studies of parent–infant interaction, the parenting skills of deaf mothers and fathers have been observed to be similar to the parenting skills of hearing mothers and fathers. The same is true during later childhood. No pervasive and detrimental effects of having a deaf parent have been found. Instead, researchers have consistently found style differences that seem largely the result of differential communication modalities.

Mattock and Crist (1989) explored the interactions of mothers and their 8- to 12-year-old hearing daughters during a work task and a play activity. They found that the deaf mothers interacted more nonverbally and the hearing mothers interacted more verbally, but the amount and quality of interaction between mothers and daughters were similar. Rienzi (1990) examined the interactions among mothers, fathers, and their oldest child while they were planning a meal. The children of deaf parents were similar to the children of hearing parents in the number of complete thoughts they communicated without interruption, questioning of others, expression of disagreements, and generation of ideas. However, more of their ideas were accepted when compared to the children of hearing parents. Interestingly, the deaf fathers had fewer ideas accepted than hearing fathers, but no differences were observed between deaf and hearing mothers. In hearing families, the father seemed to exert the greatest influence, whereas in the families with deaf parents, the hearing child exerted substantial influence.

The similarity of interactions between deaf parents and their hearing children was further documented by Jones and Dumas (1996). They investigated the communication between parents and their 7- to 11-year-old eldest children during a vacation planning task, and they found no differences between families with deaf parents and families with hearing parents.

When Mallory, Zingle, and Schein (1993) analyzed the communication within families, they were interested in the language used by the deaf parents with their hearing children. Although most of the parents used ASL with one another, they typically used a mixture of ASL and English, such as ASL signs in English word order, with their hearing children. In addition, some parents mouthed words, with and without voice.

In Essay 2.3, three hearing children describe their feelings about having deaf parents.

■ ■ ■ ■ ■ ▬▬▬▬▬▬▬▬▬▬▬▬▬▬▬▬▬▬▬▬▬▬▬▬▬▬▬▬▬▬▬▬▬▬▬▬▬▬

ESSAY 2.3

Sam, Dan, and Beth Owolabi

Sam is nine and a half, Dan is fourteen, and Beth is seventeen years old. Their parents are deaf, and they are hearing. Sam is going into the fourth grade, Dan is starting high school, and Beth will be a senior.

Barbara: Tell me what it's like to have deaf parents. What's different in your lives than if you had hearing parents?

Beth: We wouldn't be here being interviewed!

Barbara: That's true. I'm not interviewing hearing kids of hearing parents!

Beth: I don't think it's that different at all.

Sam: People ask you questions like, "Can your mom drive?"

(continued)

ESSAY 2.3   CONTINUED

Barbara: People ask you dumb questions like that?

Dan: If they actually thought about it for a second, maybe they'd get the answer. People go up to you and say, "Can you cuss out your parents behind their backs?"

Beth: Sure.

Dan: But what's the point?

Beth: They can't hear you anyway.

Dan: I think it's a lot different. With deaf parents, they can't be close to everybody in the community because not everyone knows sign language. But if you're in the hearing community and have hearing parents, it's easy because your parents can just go over and ask for sugar or something like that. Without having to say, "Can you go over and interpret?" Or they have to write it down. It doesn't make it as free, you know. People don't come over as often to chat. It's just too awkward. If you don't know sign, if you're not fluent and go real slow, it's awkward. We have to do a lot of the stuff. My parents do a lot, more than other deaf people do, but we have to go beyond the kid thing. Like at the hospital you have to interpret. Wherever you are, you have to help your parents out. It's not that they're illiterate or stupid, it's just that they can't do it themselves. The reason is that you're there, you're hearing, and you're the closest person they know, so they might as well ask you. It kind of takes away the little kid in you because you know stuff that you're not supposed to know and you know stuff that other kids don't know about their parents, like the bills. You have to know it to interpret. It's just how you deal with all that stuff.

Barbara: Beth, do you agree?

Beth: In some ways I don't agree. Yes, they can be quite dependent, but they prefer not using us much as interpreters. Like when we were little, they used pen and paper or other means of communication. Out where we live, we're not as free with the neighbors, but some of them come over and talk with paper. When I was little, in Oregon, we had neighbors who would always come over. My mom learned Spanish from our neighbor through writing. I remember she wasn't fluent, but she knew enough to make conversation.

Barbara: Your parents are really well educated. You were saying that some other deaf parents you know might be more dependent on their kids.

Dan: You look at the Deaf community, and you see the jobs they have. A friend of mine, he has a job, and it's not really high and he's a smart guy. He doesn't have a college education, and he's like forty-two and he doesn't have time to go back and get a college education. Other people work in factories, they cook, they clean, they work at McDonald's. I know deaf people are more capable. Other people see them and create the stereotype that deaf people can't do it.

Beth: Seemingly it's like the majority of deaf people have lower wage jobs. I probably know two or three other deaf people out of all the ones I've seen who have high paying jobs.

Barbara: What about your friends? Do you ever have to explain stuff to your friends, or do they know you now?

Beth: I don't know how it is with Daniel, but when I met my friends, at first I didn't tell them my parents were deaf. And then the closer I got to know them, depending on how many times I invited them over, eventually I taught them some sign language, so they could communicate with my parents. Coincidentally, when I was in fifth grade, we had a deaf girl at our school. My friends would learn from her, and then they would also learn from my parents and me, and they would know enough to have a conversation. My best friend knows enough to know what my mom and dad are saying. It's really interesting. I generally tell my friends that my parents are deaf. "Just so you know." If they have questions, I try to explain, like what a TTY is. Through them, their parents know about us. It's kind of like a relay thing.

Dan: I don't do that. It's like when you make a friend and your parents are divorced. Not my parents, but someone else's parents. I don't know that. They don't say, "Just so you know, my parents are divorced. In case you don't want to be my friend." I don't say that. They just go for my personality and who I am, just normal, then after a while, they say, "Your parents are deaf?" "Yeah." If they ask a question, I answer it. I don't dwell on it. I'm going to answer their questions, but it's not that big of a deal. I mean it is, but you don't treat it like a huge deal so they think, it's not that big of a deal, your parents are normal, I lead a normal life. My parents are deaf, and my life is normal. They think that deaf people aren't all freaked out, and I'm not some kind of homicidal maniac with deaf parents.

Barbara: What about you, Sam? Did you tell your friends right away, or did you let it wait?

Sam: I let it wait, but the results weren't that good.

Beth: He stopped being Sam's friend.

Barbara: Because he was being ignorant?

Sam: Yes.

Barbara: Do other kids ever want you to teach them sign language?

Dan: All the time. "My mom's best friend's cousin's uncle wants to know if you can teach them sign language." I guess they're having a conversation about handicaps, and someone says, "I know a kid who has deaf parents." "Oh really? Can you have him teach me sign language?" I'm not in it for money. I could make tons of money from everyone who asked me. It's a tool I use. I don't want to use it for money. That's why I wouldn't want to be an interpreter. I don't want to use my skills. I think of it as talking. If no one else could talk, you'd have to teach everyone how to talk. I don't want to make a living off of it.

Beth: I used to do it for fun. Like in class, none of the teachers knew sign language. So in fifth grade, sixth grade, we decided, let's use it in class. But then some of the teachers started learning sign language. When Mom taught in high school, she used to teach them cuss words, all the cool words. She refused to teach me. It was really frustrating because people my age wanted to learn all the cool words so that we could cuss

(continued)

ESSAY 2.3 CONTINUED

at everybody. Primarily, it's a lot of fun for me. It's convenient. People say it's serious stuff, but I don't take it as seriously as some people.

Dan: I always felt uncomfortable going up in front of the class and signing. Every couple of years, you run into something in the reading book about sign language, and the teacher gets the bright idea to have your parents come in. Your parents are walking in the hallway sometime, cause you're late for school or they have to sign a paper, and everyone is like, "It's Dan's dad." I'm downstairs in the bathroom, and he's way up on the third floor, and someone comes in, "Your dad's here!" It was really frustrating in first grade because seventy people would tell me, individually, "Your dad's here." They didn't do that for the other parents. They would stare, and my dad would smile.

Beth: Or wave.

Dan: I'd feel embarrassed, but I knew they were being ignorant.

Beth: For the longest time, probably until about third or fourth grade, I was actually embarrassed to talk to my parents in public. Mom used to tell me stories about how we would be in a store, and if I saw a friend of mine, I would refuse to talk to her. My hands to my sides, don't say anything, wave a little. I feel really bad about that now. I don't see what the big deal is. But I guess I just hated the fact that people would stare, like at a person with a disability. I understand. I have a friend whose neighbor is blind. And it's kind of like, what do I do? So I understand it from other people's standpoint. How they feel when they see my parents.

Barbara: Sam, what about your friends? Is it weird to be signing when your friends are around?

Sam: Yes, especially when they're staring at me.

Barbara: Have you had the same experience as Dan?

Sam: Like one time when I got sick. The next day, everybody was telling me that my dad was at the school.

Barbara: They wouldn't do that if it was a hearing parent?

Sam: No.

Barbara: Maybe they're in awe.

Dan: I think a lot of it is being Black and deaf.

Beth: Yes! The combination!

Dan: We're in the middle of White people central.

Beth: Where we used to live in Ohio, they had a whole bunch of deaf kids there. So people were used to it. But in Oregon, it was a much bigger deal. In second grade, I was told that I had to sign this whole program. My mom said to just do it. So I signed this children's program. And I had to teach a second grade class the alphabet, and I was in third grade. I was thinking, "Why are you making such a big deal out of this?" But I realized that some of them had never ever seen a deaf person. It depends on where you are.

Dan: A lot of times they ask you to do things. Like, you come to a program to enjoy it, and they ask you to interpret. Last year, my principal asked me to interpret the Recognition program. I was class president. And he wanted me to interpret my speech. When you do a speech, and you talk, and you don't really know your speech and you don't really know the signs to it, and you're trying to be kind of funny and kind of light, and you have to sign at the same time, it just messes it up. So I told him I wasn't going to do it. And he said, "Why not?" I said, "Can't you just find an interpreter?" I felt that he can't ask me to do that. I'm graduating from eighth grade here. I don't need all this stuff, like interpreting, stand up in front of everyone in a little corner by myself, in front of my parents. It wasn't my job. I wanted to enjoy myself. But it's easier for the school.

Beth: They don't have to pay.

Dan: Just go ask the son. But they don't think how he feels about it.

Beth: The worst part is when you get in trouble, with your grades or something, they automatically assume it's because your parents are deaf. Like if you're having family problems, they automatically assume it's because the parents are deaf. I try to say, no, we have fine communication, but we have a little difference of opinion. They think, no, it's because your parents are deaf.

Dan: You tell them it's not why. They say, "No, you don't know what you're talking about. It's because your parents are deaf. I know and you don't."

Barbara: It's hard to imagine for hearing people who don't grow up with a deaf person what that would be like.

Dan: Whenever something happens, like my dad was in two car accidents, they assumed he got into the accident because he couldn't hear the horn or couldn't hear the road under him or something like that. One of them was the other guy's fault, but they still assumed it was because he was deaf.

Barbara: Sam, what about you? Do your teachers ever ask you to interpret or teach the class signs?

Sam: No.

Dan: Not yet.

Sam: I don't want to.

Dan: Later on it gets kind of hard because in the middle of class, the teacher says, "Dan, would you like to have your parents come in and teach?" And everyone looks at you and says, "Hey Dan, yeah!" So you say, "Fine," because if you say no they say, "Why? What are you, embarrassed or something?" So you say, "Fine, I'll do it. They'll come."

Beth: The fun thing about having deaf parents is how people react around deaf people. My mom and I talk about this. I gave a speech in my speech class about that. Mom and I went to the bank one time, she stepped up to the cashier, and the cashier completely exaggerated her mouth movements asking, "Can I help you?" She stretched out each

(continued)

syllable. It's the funniest thing. My mom and I kind of make fun of them.

Dan: They do it so bad that even if you could lipread, you couldn't understand.

Sam: Sometimes people try to use their hands.

Dan: And they talk extra loud.

Beth: They're deaf, why are you talking extra loud?

Sam: She can't hear you.

Dan: I was baby-sitting two kids just a couple of days ago, and they're deaf. We were at McDonald's, and this guy comes up to them. They had just lost a baseball game. He didn't know that they were deaf. He said, "So, good game." The little kid is kind of shy, so he just nodded his head. I said, "He's deaf." He said, very exaggerated, "Sorry" and walked away. We talked about it later, and we laughed about it. I told him about my mom's experiences. It was really funny.

Sam: This lady at the store was talking to my dad extra slow. My brother came up, and she said, "Can … you … hear?" I said, "Yeah." She said, "Sorry, I didn't know."

Beth: One thing about being hearing with deaf parents is you can pretend you're deaf. You know sign language. I love to see the reactions of people. I went into a restaurant with my friend one time. I decided to pretend I was deaf. The waitress was, you know how they get all flustered? "Can … I … help … you?" In the middle when we were eating, I said, "Well, you know, I'm hearing." I apologized because I didn't mean to scare her like that.

Dan: We were at the fair once, and I didn't realize how good my dad was at talking to hearing people. It was amazing. This guy we knew from church came up to us. We couldn't find Sam. Immediately, in like four hand motions, my dad expressed the problem. I didn't know he could do that. The guy knew exactly what he wanted, like that.

Barbara: What other things would you like to tell people who don't know anything about deafness but are going to be working with deaf people?

Sam: Never use meaningless gestures. And never talk extra slow. Just use pen and paper.

Beth: Some people ask what my parents did when I was a baby. Well, I don't know how they did it, like when I cried. I didn't know how to talk till I was three.

Barbara: So your parents just signed to you. Your first language was sign.

Dan: Hers was, but mine was a combination.

Beth: Because I talked to Daniel. And then we both talked to Sam. Dad said people thought I was deaf. They didn't realize I was hearing till I was about two and a half.

Dan: Cause when you're little, if your parents are signing and you're signing too, you don't think, why are my parents signing? They can hear, I can hear, we can all hear, but we'll just sign.

Barbara: Do you have any memory of that?

Beth: I remember learning to talk from Sesame Street. I don't know what my first word was. But I remember my first sign word. It was "Dad." Mom could talk. But she doesn't talk right. And so, basically, we kind of talk wrong because we learned it from her. My kindergarten experience was probably the worst. I knew how to say some words, but I didn't know how to say all the words right.

Sam: Like "milk."

Beth: Mom says "meerik." We were learning how to say "please" and "thank you" and "please pass the milk." Milk time came around two o'clock. We all lined up. The teacher went to each kid and said, "Do you want this?" And each kid said, "May I have the milk please?" It came to my turn, and I said, "May I have the meerik please?" And she said, "What? You mean the milk?" I said, "No. The meerik. Mom taught me that!" I kind of threw a tantrum and went outside. I had to go to a speech therapist until third grade.

Sam: Oatmeal. Oyaytee.

Dan: Yes, o-a-t spelled oyaytee. Mom says, "Oyaytee." She says it the way it's spelled.

Beth: We thought it was oyaytee.

Dan: What do you eat for breakfast every morning? Oyaytee. They thought, well your parents are from Nigeria, oyaytee.

Barbara: They thought it was a Nigerian word?

Dan: Yes, oyaytee. They thought, oh yes, I saw that in National Geographic or something.

Beth: When we realized it, I said, Daniel, o-a-t, oyaytee! It was weird. I was like in fifth grade.

Dan: I was like in second grade. O-A-T! It just kind of connected for us. It was really weird.

Beth: So we started calling it "oatmeal."

Dan: It was funny. Another one of my mom's big pet peeves is when people are interpreting for a waitress. They come up and say, "Can I help you?" You say, "She's deaf." The waitress says, "Sorry, what can I help your mom with?" My mom says, "No. Look at me. Tell her to look at me." Then I say, "Look at her when you're talking to me." It can be confusing.

Beth: Sometimes the bad thing about having a deaf parent is if she wants us to interpret for her, and it's really bad when she's mad and she's saying a lot of rash things. Sometimes you have to be the filter. You have to express her anger but be nice about it.

Dan: And you have to see the reaction of the guy, and if it's someone you know, you'd like to cut some stuff out. I kind of felt bad because

(continued)

ESSAY 2.3   CONTINUED

this is what she's saying and this is who she is, and I can't change what she's saying because that's not nice. You'd be just changing everything, what she wants. Like if she wants to barter or haggle.

Barbara: How's your dad doing?

Dan: I say the same thing over and over again. He's doing fine, and he's in rehabilitation on the fourth floor.

Beth: The worst thing about my dad being in the hospital is the stories we hear from Mom. When he first went in there, she told me that they didn't have an interpreter. It's very frustrating because how is he going to talk to people? This is our dad, and they're not treating him right.

Dan: There was one interpreter who could have come in, but they didn't want her because she didn't have a certificate. She's only a couple of days away from her certificate, but they needed her right then. I'm saying, would you rather have no interpreter and face a liability, or have an interpreter and save a man's life and then have to face a liability?

Beth: Sometimes it's cool having deaf parents because you can understand how your parents feel and kind of relate to them. I remember one time we were at this Hallelujah Chorus thing, and it was a special Martin Luther King Day event. Mom was excited because they were honoring her. They brought in this interpreter who was not very good at all. We knew more than she did. And it was really frustrating. It made us very angry. She didn't know half the words they were saying. Mom told her, "We don't want to hurt your feelings but I'd rather have one of my kids go up there."

Dan: She was one of those ladies that has a deaf kid, and she learned a little sign language but thought, "Hey, I know sign language." She's willing to do it because she's really nice and she comes, but she really doesn't know. And she doesn't know that she doesn't know.

Beth: She doesn't realize.

Barbara: Sam, do you have any stories you want to share?

Sam: Every time we get on the phone, Mom always asks who it is.

Beth: The phone, the radio. The TV they can see. We never had a radio until I was in seventh grade. The only music we heard was at school. When we started listening to the radio, she just assumed we were listening to bad music.

Dan: When do you ever hear about the good music?

Barbara: Sure because she would have no way to screen it out.

Beth: We'd be listening to oldies, and she'd say, "You're listening to devil music." Another one is the telephone. She thinks we're talking to somebody bad.

Dan: I think when you're deaf, there's this extra paranoia.

Beth: It's just Mom.

Dan: I was in the car, talking to the mom of the kid I was baby-sitting. When they were in Jamaica, they met this guy, and he was deaf. He had a really bad rap sheet, like he was in for rape and blah blah blah blah blah. He went up to her husband who is deaf and she's hearing, and he told them to follow him to this restaurant or something. And they knew he had a rap sheet, but they followed him anyway. She was really uncomfortable with it, but her husband said, "It's OK. You can trust him. He's deaf." But like a guy came over to fix their heater when I was there, and I was the last one to leave. He said, "Before you leave, make sure you stay here and wait until the guy leaves." This is a company that's been in business for about a hundred years. They're not going to steal his chain saw or something. And that's what he was afraid of. I asked him why. He said, "Because you don't know what he's going to do." It's like, trust all deaf people but be wary of all hearing people.

Barbara: What brought you out to Ohio?

Dan: My dad got a job as a pastor.

Beth: You know how little kids can say things like, "Well my dad is so and so." And I say, "My dad teaches at a university."

Dan: I used to say, "My dad teaches at Akron University." Now I say, "My dad is a professor at a university" instead of a "teacher at a college."

Barbara: And your mom teaches here at Kent State.

Dan: She's a professor at Kent State.

Reprinted by permission of the authors.

Child Development

Three areas of concern about the development of hearing children with deaf parents have traditionally been raised—language development, self-concept, and social–emotional development.

Language Development

Evidence for normal, delayed, and deviant development of language has been found among hearing children of deaf parents (for example, Murphy & Slorach, 1983; Prinz & Prinz, 1979, 1981; Sachs, Bard, & Johnson, 1981; Schiff-Myers, 1982; Schiff-Myers & Ventry, 1976). Given the discrepancies found in studies of language acquisition, Seal and Hammett (1995) suggested that "determining whether a hearing child of deaf parents is at risk for delayed and possibly disordered language development is possible only on a case-by-case basis. Atypical language development may occur for some hearing children of deaf parents" but certainly not for all (p. 16).

Much of the research on language development has been focused specifically on the spoken English development of hearing children with deaf parents. Orlansky and Bonvillian (1985) examined the sign language acquisition of hearing children and found that they acquired their first signs considerably younger than hearing children acquired their first spoken words. The deaf children in their study acquired their first recognizable signs at an average age of 8.6 months, whereas the normal child's first words typically appeared between 11 and 14 months of age. The deaf children began to combine signs at an average age of 17.1 months, compared to hearing children who usually started using two-word utterances between 18 and 24 months of age.

Self-Concept

The psychoanalytic literature is replete with case studies of hearing offspring with poor self-concept that seemed to be the result of negative feelings toward their deaf parents and resentment of increased responsibility (Frank, 1979; Robinson, Olethia, & Weathers, 1974; Taska & Rhoads, 1981). These studies, however, appear to present a skewed picture of the self-concept of most hearing children of deaf parents.

Chan and Lui (1990) compared the self-concept among hearing Chinese children of deaf and hearing parents, and they found no differences. They concluded that deaf parenthood has no negative impact on the development of self-concept in hearing children; however, they did find that the self-concept of the deaf parents was significantly lower than the self-concept of the hearing parents. Similar to the Chan and Lui findings, Charlson (1990) examined the self-concept of hearing adolescents with deaf parents and found that they did not differ from their peers with hearing parents. In other words, adolescents' self-concept did not depend on whether they had deaf parents.

Social–Emotional Development

Much of what we know about the social–emotional development of hearing children with deaf parents centers around their response to having to take on the role of communication mediator with the hearing world. And, clearly, hearing children are frequently expected to assume this role. Mallory, Schein, and Zingle (1992) observed that deaf parents rely heavily on the oldest child in the family and less frequently expect younger children to mediate with the hearing world. They also observed that the resentment of the hearing child depends to a great extent on the demands of the situation. For example, they found "particular stress when the mediation task was to educate their parents, mediate communication at public events, seek intervention in family crisis, or assist in medical emergencies" (p. 205). On the other hand, routine communication tasks became boring, and hearing children often resisted them.

Buchino (1993) conducted an important study on the perceptions of the oldest hearing child of deaf parents. The most significant finding was the similarity between children of deaf and hearing parents in their overall perception of their relationship with their parents. Both groups of children felt able to communicate with their parents, expressed positive feelings toward their parents, and considered their parents as the decision makers. The only area of difference involved interpreting. These eldest children of deaf parents viewed themselves as their parents' primary interpreter, and there was no comparable role among hearing children of hearing parents. Because of this interpreting role, these children tended to see themselves as more integral to family decision making than the children of hearing parents. They reported being frustrated at times because of the difficulty in interpreting complex vocabulary, content they did not understand, and information their parents did not understand easily. But they also realized how much better they knew their parents than their friends typically did, and they felt that they were gaining valuable skills in communicating with a wide variety of people.

In the preface to Paul Preston's book about the lives of hearing children with deaf parents, *Mother Father Deaf*, he explains that he chose the title from the phrase that connects hearing children to the deaf world. "Although used for both hearing and deaf children, 'mother father deaf' remains a lifelong identifier for hearing children. Deaf children of deaf parents become known in the Deaf community in their own right as deaf persons. However, for hearing children and adult children of deaf parents, this phrase legitimizes their connection to an often separate and impenetrable land" (1994, p. x). Given the unique experiences of deaf children with deaf parents, and their connection to the Deaf community, it is not surprising that they have acquired their own group name—CODA, children of deaf adults.

The issues confronting parents in raising their children led to the establishment of parent support groups. These groups are designed almost exclusively for hearing parents of deaf children.

PARENT SUPPORT GROUPS

Each April, the *American Annals of the Deaf*, which is managed by the Convention of American Instructors of the Deaf and the Conference of Educational Administrators of Schools and Programs for the Deaf, publishes a reference issue. Included in the array of information about the schools and programs in the United States and Canada are the services that are available within each program. Parents and teachers can learn which schools include family support services, parent education programs, and programs for deaf infants and their families. They can also learn if boarding facilities are available or if they serve day students only, if they are public or if parents pay tuition, the enrollment, grade and age ranges, the type of communication used in the school, and other available services such as speech therapy, counseling, programs for students with multiple disabilities, vocational training, oral and/or sign interpreting, social workers, audiological evaluations and services, notetakers, sign language classes, and adaptive physical education.

In 1996, several researchers from Gallaudet University used information from the Annual Survey of Deaf and Hard of Hearing Children and Youth that is conducted by the Center for Assessment and Demographic Studies in order to investigate the support services received by parents of deaf and hard of hearing children (Meadow-Orlans, Mertens, Sass-Lehrer, & Scott-Olson, 1997). They specifically targeted families with 6- and 7-year-old children. They found that almost 75 percent of the parents had received relevant information, sign language instruction was available to 71 percent of all parents and 89 percent of the parents whose children were enrolled in Total Communication programs, and parent group meetings were available to 69 percent and individual counseling to 43 percent of the parents.

In the past, the relationship between parents and professionals was typically characterized as paternalistic. Professionals took responsibility for the educational needs of the child, and often their social and emotional needs as well, without expecting much more than cooperation from the parents. This view began to change during the last two decades of the twentieth century, prompted by the research on the family system and legislation that mandated increasing parental participation in educational decision making. The model of the professional as expert gave way, at least in principle, to the professional as partner (Dunst, Trivette, Boyd, & Brookfield, 1994; Roush, Harrison, & Palsha, 1991).

Families reflect many profiles, and family-centered support programs must be flexible in adapting to the needs expressed by parents. Mothers typically want and respond to different types of programs than fathers, and hearing parents have different needs than deaf parents. Parents' age, education, marital status, socioeconomic status, culture, ethnicity, and home language are all factors that play a role in the types of support program that will be effective for any given parent. The needs of parents change as their children become older, parents of profoundly deaf children have different needs than parents of hard of hearing children, and parents of deaf children with a disability benefit from different programs than parents of children who have no concomitant disability. As Meadow-Orlans and Sass-Lehrer (1995, p. 328) wrote:

> Professionals need to assess their views and practices in designing and implementing support to families. Family-centered professionals encourage active involvement of families in all aspects of a program, recognizing that families with different interests and resources will participate in different ways at different times. Those who work with children who are deaf and hard of hearing come from a field with a long tradition of professional rather than parent-centered decision making. This tradition is reflected in parent meetings with topics selected by professionals who present information and provide limited opportunities for discussion or interaction. Effective parent support encourages families to bring their own agenda—to identify their issues, concerns, and questions.

Parent education and support programs are more of a challenge when families live in rural areas than when they live in urban and suburban areas. Not only do rural areas have fewer educational programs, but the programs are also limited in scope and, by necessity, offer fewer support services. When McKellin (1995) examined the options available to families in rural areas of British Columbia, he found that parents had limited options for their children and themselves. For example, some families chose to have their children live at the school for the deaf, which then impacted the child's relationship with family members and the family dynamic. Clapham and Teller (1997) suggested that when the child's parents live in a rural area, educational programs could help bridge the communication gap through the use of video. At one school in Louisiana, for example, the deaf children communicated with their parents, the teachers modeled strategies that the parents could carry out at home, and the teachers and interpreters taught parents new sign vocabulary on videos that were sent home.

SUMMARY AND CONCLUDING THOUGHTS

This chapter discussed the issues involved in families with deaf children and adolescents and in families with hearing children and deaf parents. Professionals are typically involved in the lives of children for brief moments when compared to the time that children spend in their homes with their parents. Understanding the preeminent role of parents and respecting their position in their children's lives is critical to the healthy development of each deaf child.

This chapter began with a quotation from David Luterman's book, *Deafness in the Family,* and ends with a quotation from the same book (1987):

> Many parents come through the experience of having a deaf child with a clearer sense of themselves than they had before their child was diagnosed as hearing impaired. Many parents find that their child's deafness gives their lives meaning and direction. Their joy stems from actively participating in their child's growth. They take nothing for granted. They can see what needs to be done and they can rejoice when a milestone is reached. They also know that they had a direct hand in reaching that milestone. (p. 116)

CHAPTER THREE

LANGUAGE, COMMUNICATION, AND CULTURE

FOCUS QUESTIONS

- What are the challenges that deaf children face in learning English and ASL?
- Why were manually coded English systems developed?
- In what ways can hearing loss influence the child's reading and writing ability?
- How will advances in technology change communication for deaf individuals?
- Why is *deaf* written with a lowercase *d* sometimes and other times written as *Deaf* with an uppercase *D*?

Language is central to the lives of all individuals because it is the means for communicating with others and for thinking and learning. Language is a shared code. It can be spoken, signed, and written, but whatever its form, it must be shared to be language. The communication issue for deaf individuals has never been the degree of hearing loss but rather the ability of the deaf person to communicate in a language that others share. For some individuals, this shared language is English or other home language. For others, it is ASL or the sign language of the country in which they live. And for yet others, it is a mixture of languages, dialects, and pidgins.

This chapter discusses the languages of deaf individuals, the link between language and communication, and the relationship between language and culture. The first step in this discussion is to understand how deaf children learn their first language.

LANGUAGE ACQUISITION

Children who are deaf have the same cognitive ability to learn language as children with hearing. The child's cognitive ability has been likened to a language seed (Rice & Kemper, 1984). Just as a plant seed seeks nourishment in the form of light and water, the language seed seeks nourishment in the form of interaction with parents and others who communicate in meaningful ways. When the nourishment is rich, the language grows and matures.

Children learn language from the individuals who talk or sign with them from virtually the moment they are born. No language is universal or innate. In the days of Sophocles, we learned that if a child is left on a mountainside and no one uses language for interaction, the child will develop no language. If someone interacts in Swahili with the child, then the child will learn Swahili. If someone interacts in British Sign Language, then the child will learn BSL. One language is not easier or more difficult for the child to learn as a first language. However, it is easier to learn language when the language is used consistently by significant adults and older children in conversation with the child; it is more difficult to learn when the language is used inconsistently by adults and older children and conversation is infrequent. Language is also easier to learn when the child has full access to the language and more difficult when obstacles prevent full access.

Language Development

The order of progression in knowledge of a first language is approximately invariant across children learning any language. The earliest research into these universals of language development was conducted with hearing children (Brown, 1973). Subsequently, a number of researchers examined the language development of deaf children and found stages and sequences of acquisition in oral and signing deaf children that paralleled those found in hearing children (Caselli, 1983; Crowson, 1994; Curtiss, Prutting, & Lowell, 1979; Petitto, 1987; Prinz & Prinz, 1985; Robinshaw, 1996; Schirmer, 1985).

The four interrelated components of language are syntax, semantics, pragmatics, and phonology. *Syntax* is the structure of language and involves the rules that govern how *morphemes* (the smallest meaningful unit of grammatical form) are combined into words (morphology) as well as how words are combined into sentences (syntax). *Semantics* is defined as the meaning or content of language. As children learn the content of language, they are discovering the rules that govern the meaning of words, phrases, and sentences. *Pragmatics* involves the ways that individuals use language for interacting with others. *Phonology* involves the sound patterns of language. When describing ASL, phonology refers to the smallest contrastive parts of holds and movements of the sign (Liddell & Johnson, 1989).

For children to learn language, they need a considerable amount of experience in conversation with adults. Through these interactions, children discern the underlying rules of the language used by adults. Children are cognitively endowed to learn language through this process. At any given point in their linguistic development, deaf children show us their current hypothesis of the rules by the ways they use language. For example, if oral deaf children say, "I have two foots," it is because they have overgeneralized a pluralization rule that they are still figuring out. Similar issues show up with deaf children learning ASL. If they are engaged in conversations with adults who are using the rules of the language consistently, they will ultimately figure out these rules and use them expressively in their own language. However, if they are exposed to inconsistent and incomplete language models, their own language will be a mix of forms that matches neither English nor ASL because they have never been exposed to language that follows the rules from either language. It is not uncommon for deaf children to use a mix of English, ASL, pidgin sign, and gesture.

When teachers assess the language abilities of the deaf children they teach, their objective is to determine the child's syntactic, semantic, pragmatic, and phonologic abilities in order to plan instruction that enables the child to continue developing in all of these areas. In the past, teaching methods developed for use with deaf children relied heavily on the notion that their language needed to be straightened out. Teachers were therefore advised to use strategies that focused almost exclusively on English syntax and morphology (McAnally, Rose, & Quigley, 1998). Current knowledge of language acquisition has led to dramatic changes in the way language instruction in the classroom is viewed. It is widely recognized that drilling the deaf child on grammatical structures has no lasting or significant influence on the child's internalization of the language itself, whether that language is English or ASL. Instead, teachers are now advised to create a classroom environment that is replete with opportunities to interact with others using the language for meaningful communication. As Harrison, Layton, and Taylor (1987) noted, "Developmental language programs for deaf children must be constructed around the notion that the acquisition of language and the concurrent understanding of the function of language occur through topical communicative exchanges which are the product of shared activities" (p. 230).

The next section presents the languages and modes of communication used by deaf individuals and discusses how the languages and modes used by hearing parents with their deaf children and teachers with their deaf students can enhance or impede language acquisition.

Languages and Modes of Communication

The languages and modes of communication used by deaf individuals are essentially native sign languages at one end of the continuum and spoken languages at the other end. In the United States and Canada, American Sign Language is the native sign language, and English is the spoken language. Along the continuum between these two languages are pidgin sign language and manually coded English.

American Sign Language

American Sign Language is a visual–gestural language with a rule structure that is distinct from other languages, including English. The rules of syntax, morphology, semantics, pragmatics, and phonology are as complex and rich as other languages (for example, Klima & Bellugi, 1979; Stokoe, 1971; Wilbur, 1987). In ASL, the shape, location, orientation, and movement of the hands, the intensity of the motions, facial expression, and body movement all communicate meaning. Because of the different rule structures for each language, it is not possible to sign ASL and speak English at the same time.

All languages develop over time. English developed from Germanic and Germanic developed from Indo-European (Fromkin & Rodman, 1998). Because of this historical development, English shares many linguistic features with other languages that developed from Germanic including German, Yiddish, Flemish, and Dutch. ASL also developed over time through communication between deaf individuals. It has its roots in French Sign Language, which was brought to the United States by Thomas Gallaudet and Laurent Clerc. The reason that ASL is different from other sign languages worldwide is because the Deaf communities did not interact with one another until quite recently. As they interact more often, it is likely that the languages will begin to share linguistic features, just as English currently shares features with languages from different linguistic trees such as Spanish. Indeed, ASL shares some features with English because of the degree of interaction between deaf and hearing individuals.

ASL, like all languages, is constantly changing. The rule structure of ASL looks somewhat different than it did fifty years ago, and it will look different fifty years from now. Educators, parents, and members of the Deaf community cannot prescribe the rules of ASL, mandate that they be used the same throughout the United States and Canada, or keep them static. In spite of this, many individuals have tried to create descriptions of ASL that try to accomplish a uniformity of definition and use (Moores, 1996).

In order for deaf children to learn ASL, they must have communicative interaction with individuals using ASL. Just as hearing children are not cognitively programmed to learn English or any other spoken language in the absence of communication with native speakers, deaf children are not cognitively programmed to learn ASL in the absence of communication with native signers. Although aspects of gestural communication may be universal, the rule structure of ASL is not universal.

It is important to note that the recognition of ASL as a legitimate language occurred relatively recently in the history of deaf education. Research into ASL did not begin in earnest until the early 1970s, although Stokoe had begun his research in the early 1960s. Much of the early research was ignored until the 1970s when English sign systems were being developed. Prior to this point, sign languages were considered primitive and incomplete versions of English (Stewart & Akamatsu, 1988).

Fingerspelling. Fingerspelling is the hand configurations that represent the letters of the alphabet. Fingerspelling is generally used for spelling words and proper names that have no known sign. When fingerspelling, an individual uses the manual alphabet to spell words letter by letter. A chart of the manual alphabet used in the United States and Canada is presented in Figure 3.1.

ASL Literacy. No written form of ASL currently exists, though some efforts are under way. The link between ASL proficiency and English literacy has been debated extensively by educators. Since the late 1960s, research has indicated that children from deaf families demonstrate higher academic achievement than children from hearing families (Charrow & Fletcher, 1974; Geers & Schick, 1988; Stuckless & Birch, 1966; Vernon & Koh, 1970). Some individuals have suggested that there must be a relationship between ASL proficiency and English literacy if the achievement of students with deaf parents is consistently higher. Mayer and Wells (1996) proposed that linguistic transfer between the two languages is unlikely, though cognitive and conceptual transfer is quite likely. In other words, although ASL can develop cognitive power that provides a bridge between external language and inner language, it cannot provide a bridge from inner language to written English. Drasgow (1998) suggested that successful early language acquisition of ASL results in real-world knowledge. Though "ASL alone will not result in a bridge between inner 'sign' and written English for deaf children, perhaps mastery of the conversational form of ASL, and its subsequent internalization, can serve as the foundation upon which a bridge can be built" (p. 337).

Spoken English

In 1968, van Uden began his book, *A World of Language for Deaf Children*, with the comment, "The paradoxical combination of 'teaching' and 'mother tongue' is the central and perhaps most difficult problem in the

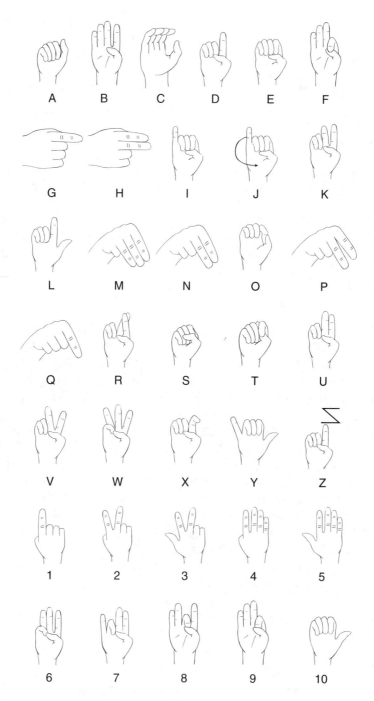

FIGURE 3.1   Manual Alphabet

education of deaf children" and ended his book with the observation, "There are actually many deaf children who have a better command of English than some hearing children" (p. 122). Deaf children learning English as their first language are faced with a daunting challenge. Through amplification, they may hear some sounds but certainly not clearly and without distortion, as discussed in Chapter 1. Their ability to read others' speech, sometimes called *lipreading* but more recently called *speechreading*, can be enhanced through training, but given the sounds that are not overtly formed on the lips, they have to fill in a substantial amount of missing information. Along with gestures, facial expressions, and body language, the deaf child learning spoken English is exposed to a language used consistently by hearing adults, for whom it is their mother tongue or native language, but the features of the language that the child receives will not always be consistent or understandable. Yet, as van Uden noted, many deaf children are able to develop a deep level knowledge of English through its spoken form.

One of the benefits of being immersed in a linguistic environment in which English is used exclusively is that for the approximately 90 percent of deaf children whose parents are hearing, the parents do not have to learn another language or language system to communicate with their own children. The language they use for conversation is the one in which they are fluent and knowledgeable. Another benefit is that being able to use spoken English for communication enables the deaf child, and later the deaf adult, to function in the hearing world. Yet another benefit is the relationship between spoken and written English. The deaf child who is able to attain fluency in spoken English can use this knowledge in becoming literate in English, just as hearing children do, though fluency in spoken English is no guarantee that the deaf child will be able to become a proficient reader and writer.

A spoken English environment also presents serious drawbacks. Many deaf children cannot learn English through the spoken form, and the time spent in trying and failing results in lost time for learning language, which concomitantly affects cognitive development. Another drawback is the loss of participation in the Deaf community, whose language is ASL. Chapter 7 discusses the teaching approaches used with children learning spoken English.

Manually Coded English

Manually coded English is a sign system developed to represent English in a visual–gestural modality. Sometimes referred to as *manual English*, manually coded English is actually a group of systems, many of which were developed in the early 1970s. Manually coded English systems were designed to provide deaf children with access to English by making it visible. Each manually coded English system adheres to English syntax and morphology; the sign vocabulary is a combination of ASL signs and invented signs used to represent concepts.

The three most popular manually coded English systems in educational programs for deaf children are Seeing Essential English (Anthony, 1971), Signing Exact English (Gustason, Pfetzing, & Zawolkow, 1972), and Signed English (Bornstein, Hamilton, & Saulnier, 1975). Seeing Essential English is typically referred to as SEE I and Signing Exact English as SEE II. Both follow the two-out-of-three principle for determining the match between an English word and sign. According to this principle, the three determinants are spelling, pronunciation, and meaning. If two words in English share two of these three, both words share the same sign. For example, the word *cross* has one sign in SEE I and SEE II because each meaning shares the same spelling and pronunciation; however, it has multiple signs in ASL to represent the multiple meanings of "cross the street," "cross your fingers," "cross out the wrong answer," or "the teacher is cross with you." All three of these manually coded English systems consist of a set of invented signs to represent English structures such as pronouns, verb tenses, plurality, adverbs, possessives, comparatives, and articles.

Manually coded English systems are often called artificial or contrived because they derived from no language community. Indeed, Bornstein, Saulnier, and Hamilton (1980) stated that "Signed English is not a language. It is not a substitute for the American Sign Language. It was designed for a different purpose" (p. 469). Manually coded English systems are meant to be used in educational programs to provide deaf children with access to English.

Proponents of manually coded English systems offer the following benefits to using one of these systems with deaf children (Luetke-Stahlman & Luckner, 1991):

- Manually coded English enables deaf children to learn the English language and use it for face-to-face communication.
- Parents are more able to learn a manually coded English system and, therefore, are more likely to provide a consistent language model in communicating with their deaf children.

Opponents of manually coded English systems offer the following concerns about the use of any one of these systems with deaf children (Allen & Woodward, 1987; Johnson, Liddell, & Erting, 1989; Kluwin, 1981; Marmor & Petitto, 1979):

- It is inappropriate to take features from a bona fide language in creating an artificial one.

- They are cumbersome to use and, therefore, individuals using a manually coded English system typically leave out significant linguistic information.
- It is not possible to speak and sign fluidly and at an appropriate rate.

The question of whether signers using one of these systems can represent English manually has been studied and debated. Some researchers have found that signers using manually coded English do not accurately represent English, whereas others have found that some teachers are quite proficient at encoding spoken English into sign (Hyde, Power, & Cliffe, 1992; Luetke-Stahlman, 1988; Mayer & Lowenbraun, 1990; Woodward & Allen, 1988).

Pidgin Sign Language

Pidgin sign language is sometimes referred to as *Pidgin Sign English.* Pidgin sign is generally used to describe an individual's use of ASL signs in English word order and with some inclusion of English morphemes. It is often used simultaneously with speech or a mouthing of words with no voice. Instead of pidgin sign, some individuals use the term *contact signing*. Valli and Lucas (1995) define contact signing as "a kind of signing that results from the contact between American Sign Language and English and exhibits features of both languages" (p. 409).

Pidgin sign provides a way for individuals who are fluent in ASL and individuals who are fluent in English to communicate with one another. It also allows teachers to present information in sign to their students when the manually coded English system they are using becomes awkward. Nonetheless, pidgin sign is not a language in itself. It is an incomplete version of ASL and an incomplete version of English, providing none of the grammatical complexity of either language.

As a contact language, pidgin sign facilitates communication between deaf people using ASL and hearing people who are not fluent in ASL. As Coryell and Holcomb (1997) noted, pidgin sign is widely variable due to differences in the language abilities of the individuals involved, their bilingual proficiency, and the communication setting. For example, how an individual uses pidgin sign in an informal conversation may look quite different from how this same individual expresses him or herself when instructing students.

Gesture

One mode of communication is gesture. Although not a language, gesture provides additional meaning when individuals share a language, such as ASL or English. Gesture can also provide meaningful information when individuals do not share a language. Marschark (1994) found that the gestures produced by deaf and hearing individuals have notable similarities, although the gestures of deaf individuals are more difficult to distinguish from sign language because both the gestures and sign language use a manual modality.

Much of the research on gesture has focused on how gesture is used by prelinguistic children to express meanings and functions. The following are tentative conclusions from this body of research (Acredolo & Goodwyn, 1988; Bates, Thal, Whitesell, Fenson, & Oakes, 1989; Carroll & Gibson, 1986; Goldin-Meadow & Morford, 1985; Volterra & Erting, 1990; Yoshinaga-Itano & Stredler-Brown, 1992):

- Both infants who are hearing and infants who are deaf use symbolic gestures to communicate.
- Symbolic gestures appear approximately at the same time as spoken words in hearing children.
- Symbolic gestures seem to be used for requesting before they are used for labeling.
- Gestures and words are both used first in routinized activities such as bath time and mealtime.
- Gestural communication is an important stage in the acquisition of language.

Gesture has also been an important area of study for researchers focusing on deaf children who do not have either a spoken or sign language. This type of communication is sometimes called *homesign systems*. Across cultures around the world, deaf individuals with no spoken or sign language have been found to communicate with gestures, and deaf children who use homesign exhibit regularities in their communication development that are similar to children learning a conventional language (Goldin-Meadow, Butcher, Mylander, & Dodge, 1994; Goldin-Meadow, Mylander, & Butcher, 1995; Morford, 1996; Morford & Goldin-Meadow, 1997).

Chapter 7 describes how these languages and language systems are used in educational settings. The next section discusses the role of written language.

READING AND WRITING

Individuals communicate through face-to-face interaction and through reading and writing. Although individuals can use ASL or English for face-to-face interaction, currently they can only use English for reading and writing because there is no generally accepted written medium for ASL.

The Reading Process

The reading process has been described as an interaction between the reader and the written material. The reader brings knowledge and skills to each new piece of reading material. The greater the match between the reader and the material, the more comprehensible the material will be to the reader. The factors involved in this match include prior knowledge, experiences, vocabulary, word recognition, and sentence structure complexity.

Prior Knowledge and Experience

The reader brings prior knowledge and experiences that shape his or her expectations for the material. As these expectations are confirmed, or not confirmed, the reader develops understanding. In this view of reading, meaning is not fixed by the author but is constructed by the reader (Dreher & Singer, 1989; Strickland, 1982; Wittrock, 1982).

The reader's prior knowledge and experiences include the following (Beck, 1989; Blachowicz, 1984):

- General world knowledge
- Specific knowledge of the topic
- Past experience with the written genre

The reason that individuals can read the same material and construct different meanings is because each person has different general world knowledge, specific knowledge of the topic, and experience with the genre. If individuals have weak general world knowledge, slight knowledge of the topic, and little experience with the genre, it is unlikely that they will understand the material very well. The greater their prior knowledge and experiences are, the better their comprehension will be.

Studies with deaf children on the influence of prior knowledge and experience have found the following (Akamatsu, 1988; Andrews, Winograd, & DeVille, 1994, 1996; Donin, Doehring, & Browns, 1991; Jackson, Paul, & Smith, 1997; Luetke-Stahlman, Griffith, & Montgomery, 1998; Schirmer, 1993; Schirmer & Bond, 1990; Schirmer & Winter, 1993; Yoshinaga-Itano & Downey, 1986).

- General world knowledge, particular information about a topic, and personal experience of a topic have a positive influence on reading comprehension.
- Improvement in comprehension can be obtained by building background knowledge.
- Knowledge of a genre enhances reading comprehension and improves writing.

- Deaf students typically demonstrate a less well-developed understanding of genre than hearing students.
- Deaf children with deaf parents demonstrate a better understanding of genre than deaf students with hearing parents.

Vocabulary

Vocabulary knowledge is critical to reading comprehension. It is important to distinguish between levels of vocabulary knowledge because "knowing" a word depends on how the word is being used by the author (Graves, 1986). When children learn new vocabulary, one level is learning new meanings for known words. A deaf child who knows the word *ball* in the context of *throw the ball* may not know the meaning of *she bawled her eyes out* and *Cinderella had a wonderful time at the ball*. Another level is clarifying and enriching the meanings of known words. A deaf child who knows the meaning of *open* when used in contexts of *open the door* and *open your mouth* may not quite understand the concept of *she is a very open person*. A further level is learning new labels for known concepts. A deaf child who understands *mistake* also needs to know *wrong, error, blunder, slipup, gaffe, inaccuracy,* and *misstep*. A different level is learning words that represent new and difficult concepts. Deaf students who are studying government may not know the concepts of *democracy, monarchy, fascism, communism, socialism,* and *authoritarianism*. Yet another level is learning to use words expressively. Children have far more words in their receptive than expressive vocabularies.

Studies of deaf children have shown the following about their vocabulary knowledge (Conway, 1990; Davey & King, 1990; deVilliers & Pomerantz, 1992; Garrison, Long, & Dowaliby, 1997; Gilbertson & Kamhi, 1995; Kelly, 1996; LaSasso & Davey, 1987; Nolen & Wilbur, 1985; Paul, 1996):

- Vocabulary knowledge is positively related to reading comprehension.
- Deaf students demonstrate better understanding of the semantic properties and relationships of words than word definitions.
- Students who are deaf do not have greater difficulty learning novel words than hearing children.
- Direct instruction in word definitions is not effective in improving comprehension.
- Deaf students are able to derive some word meanings through the context of the word in reading material.

Word Recognition and Sentence Understanding

In addition to prior knowledge and experiences, readers bring other skills to reading situations that influence how well they will be able to read and comprehend the material. These skills include the ability to recognize the words and understand the sentences.

Word Recognition.   Readers have essentially four strategies for recognizing words in print. The first is *lexical cues,* which are cues that signal an immediate recognition of the word as a whole. Teachers sometimes refer to these cues as *sight vocabulary.* Skilled readers have virtually hundreds of words in their sight vocabulary. The second strategy is *graphophonic cues,* which are cues that involve predictable letter–sound relationships. Teachers sometimes refer to these cues simply as *phonics.* The third strategy is *structural cues,* which are cues that involve the meaningful parts of a word such as the root, prefix, suffix, and compound parts. The fourth strategy is *context cues,* which are the cues from the sentence structure and the meaning of known words. The more attention readers give to word recognition beyond the first strategy of lexical cues, the less attention they can give to comprehension.

Research on word recognition with deaf readers has found the following (Bebko, 1998; Brown & Brewer, 1996; Fischler, 1985; Hanson, 1989; Hirsch-Pasek, 1987; Kelly, 1995; Leybaert, 1993; Schaper & Reitsma, 1993; Siedlecki, Votaw, Bonvillian, & Jordan, 1990):

- Some deaf students, oral and ASL, effectively use phonological-based codes, or cues based on letter–sound relationships, to identify words in print.
- Some deaf students use fingerspelling, and others use signs for word recognition.
- Rapid identification of known words in print is an important factor in fluent reading and is no different for deaf and hearing readers.
- Less-skilled deaf readers may be slower and make more errors in word recognition than more highly skilled deaf readers.

Sentence Understanding.   In order to understand written material, students must also understand the sentence structures that the author uses. Simple sentences that follow subject–verb–object structure are considerably easier for deaf readers to understand than sentences that involve more complex structures. For example, *Carlos crossed the street* is less complicated than *The street was crossed by Carlos,* which is less complicated than *Carlos decided to cross the street before waiting for the light to change.* The task for the deaf reader becomes even more difficult when the author uses figurative language, such as *Carlos crossed the street like a baseball player coming into home plate just ahead of the ball.*

Investigations of sentence understanding by deaf readers have found support for the following (Hanson & Wilkenfeld, 1985; Israelite &

Helfrich, 1988; Kelly, 1996; Lillo-Martin, Hanson, & Smith, 1992; McKnight, 1989; Stoefen-Fischer, 1987–1988; Wilbur & Goodhart, 1985; Wilbur, Goodhart, & Montandon, 1983):

- Although specific syntactic structures are particularly difficult for deaf children to comprehend, difficulties with syntax may be less of a factor in comprehension than word recognition skill.
- Syntactic difficulties may depress the deaf child's ability to apply knowledge of vocabulary while reading.
- Deaf readers, like hearing readers, are sensitive to the meaningful units within words including phonemes and morphemes.
- Limited context inhibits the deaf child's comprehension, and greater context facilitates comprehension. Therefore, the deaf child is more likely to exhibit greater comprehension difficulties with brief stories than with longer stories or novels.
- Material that is rewritten to control for sentence length and complexity may be more difficult for deaf students to understand because of the lack of text coherence.

Reading Achievement

Children who are deaf begin to develop as readers and writers from the point in early childhood when they become aware of print in their environment and the uses of print by significant individuals in their lives, just as hearing children do. Preschool deaf children have been found to demonstrate developmentally appropriate knowledge and understanding of written language and uses of literacy even when language acquisition is delayed in comparison to hearing children (Rottenberg & Searfoss, 1992; Williams, 1994; Williams & McLean, 1997). However, as children who are deaf are engaged in formal reading and writing instruction in school, literacy development typically does not proceed at a pace considered average for hearing students (Holt, 1993; LaSasso & Mobley, 1997; Wolk & Allen, 1984). Wolk and Allen conducted their study with 1,664 students enrolled in special education programs and found that the average deaf student gained one-third of a grade equivalent change each school year. If it takes three years to progress one level in reading, this observation seems to mathematically explain why many deaf students graduate from high school with a fourth-grade reading level.

Achievement of the average deaf student tells us very little, though, about the potential of any single child. Many children who are deaf achieve at reading levels commensurate with hearing children, and many deaf adults read proficiently (Erickson, 1987; Geers & Moog, 1989; Livingston, 1997; Paul, 1998). Several researchers have suggested that the problem lies not with the deaf reader but with the quality of reading instruction provided to deaf children (Limbrick, 1991; Livingston, 1997; Truax, 1992).

An important factor in reading ability is metacognition. *Metacognition* refers to thinking about thinking or reflecting on one's own cognitive processes. When applied to reading, metacognition has four aspects. First, metacognition enables readers to know when they do understand and when they do not understand what they have read. For the reader, it is that moment during reading when he or she realizes that the material makes sense or does not make sense. Second, metacognition allows readers to figure out what they understand and what they do not understand. At this point, the reader is not only aware of understanding or lack of understanding, but he or she has also figured out the part of the material that does not make sense in contrast to the parts that do make sense. The third aspect enables readers to figure out what they need to know. Once the reader has determined the part of the material that does not make sense, if the reader is able to metacognitively reach this third point, he or she can identify what information will bring sense to the material. The fourth aspect enables readers to invoke strategies for obtaining the needed information. For example, readers can reread the section, read on, look up information in a reference source, suspend judgment until later in the material, or make an inference.

Strassman (1997) conducted a review of the research on the linkages between metacognition and reading in children who are deaf. Three issues emerged from this body of research.

1. Instructional practices that emphasize skills and activities such as completing worksheets, answering teacher questions, and memorizing vocabulary words may hinder metacognition and reading ability.

2. Reading material that is typically given to deaf students because it matches their assessed reading levels may actually be low level and may not provide them with an opportunity to develop and practice metacognitive strategies.

3. Deaf learners benefit from instruction on metacognitive strategies.

The Writing Process

Writing is conceptualized as a problem-solving process. Authors plan, compose, and revise, constantly moving back and forth between these three interrelated activities. Authors have many problems to solve. They must figure out their audience and the style they want to use. As they write, they have to assess how well they are expressing themselves and whether they are accomplishing their intended purpose. They have to take the reader's perspective and consider issues that might be unclear.

We know that deaf writers engage in the writing process just as hearing writers do. However, we know considerably less about how deaf individuals develop as authors than we know about how they develop as readers. And we also know considerably less about effective instructional approaches for teaching writing to deaf students than we know about effective approaches with hearing students.

A few researchers and educators have written about classroom writing programs that they believe have a positive influence on writing development (Kluwin & Kelly, 1992b; Luckner & Isaacson, 1990; Pogoda-Ciccone, 1994; Schleper, 1996). Others have conducted studies on strategies that they found to be positively related to improved writing (Akamatsu, 1988; Cambra, 1994; Lieberth, 1991). One strategy involves teaching the characteristics of genre, which appears to assist deaf students in writing a particular genre as well as comprehending the genre. Another strategy is the use of *dialogue journals,* which are written conversations between the deaf student and teacher, between deaf students, or between deaf and hearing students. Further discussion of these and other strategies will be provided in Chapter 7.

Writing Development

Children write long before they begin to use conventional print symbols. Their writing development is linked to their spoken and sign language development and to their reading development. Sulzby (1992) identified seven categories of emergent writing. She found that children move back and forth between these categories and sometimes combine several categories within the same composition.

- *Drawing as writing.* The child uses pictures to represent writing.
- *Scribble writing.* The child uses continuous lines to represent writing.
- *Letterlike units.* The child makes separate marks, often in a series, that have some characteristics of letters.
- *Nonphonetic letter strings.* The child writes strings of letters that do not reflect letter–sound relationships.
- *Copying from environmental print.* The child copies print from the environment.
- *Invented spelling.* The child writes words based on letter–sound relationships.
- *Conventional writing.* The child writes most words based on correct spelling.

Williams (1994) examined the literacy environments and activities of three profoundly deaf preschool children, one oral and two who signed, and found that despite the children's language delays, they demonstrated knowledge and understanding of written language that were developmentally appropriate. Johnson, Padak, and Barton (1994) examined the developmental spelling strategies of 86 children with hearing loss, who primarily used oral/aural modes of communication, and found that the strategies they used to invent spellings were developmentally and phonologically similar to those used by hearing children.

The writing achievement of deaf students has simply not been documented. Educators typically consider deaf children to have more difficulty with writing than with reading. However, this observation is based largely on assessment of their writing along one criterion only—correct usage of English sentence structures. When they are taught the qualities of good writing and their writing is analyzed along more than one dimension, deaf students demonstrate abilities in areas such as making ideas clear, using relevant descriptions, and providing a logical organizational structure (Heefner & Shaw, 1996; Schirmer, Bailey, & Fitzgerald, 1999). It is clear from the literature that deaf children can become skillful writers who use writing for thinking, learning, and communicating (Cambra, 1994; Conway, 1985; Nower, 1985; Staton, 1985; Truax, 1985, 1987).

Literacy development involves reading development and writing development. The relationship between the development of face-to-face language and the development of literacy in children who are deaf is not completely clear, but we do know that deaf children have the cognitive ability to become proficient readers and expressive writers, and that we do not have to wait for some arbitrary stage of language development prior to initiating reading and writing instruction. Indeed, we know that literacy and language are interrelated and that classrooms and homes that encourage the development of literacy also encourage the development of face-to-face language, and vice versa. We also know that deaf children do not wait for teachers to instruct them in reading and writing. They start to understand and use written symbols long before they come to school.

COMMUNICATION WITH TECHNOLOGY

Technological advances have enabled deaf individuals to easily and readily access information and to communicate with others. When deaf individuals communicate with hearing individuals, they often rely on the services of sign language interpreters. In large group settings, deaf individuals using spoken English often use oral interpreters. Although the use of interpreters is invaluable, technology can allow deaf individuals to communicate directly with hearing individuals who do not know sign or with deaf individuals across time and distances. As Lynn Woolsey described in her essay in Chapter 1, interpreters insert a layer between the source of the information and the deaf person, and the interpreter's decisions about how to capture the information may not always be the best or most accurate representation.

In essence, technology enhances the deaf individual's ability to function independently. Some of the most common forms of technology include text telephones, telephone amplifiers, captioning and real-time graphic display, the Internet, and alerting devices.

Special Telephones

Telecommunication devices for the deaf were originally referred to as *TTYs*, for *teletypes*, the name was then changed to *TDDs*, for *telecommunication devices for the deaf*, and recently has been renamed *TTs*, for *text telephones*. Text telephones, which look like a computer keyboard with a cradle for the telephone handset, enable individuals to send a typed message over telephone lines to anyone else who has a TT. With the implementation of the Americans with Disabilities Act (ADA), all states have relay services to connect callers who use text telephones to people who do not. The relay operator, who has a TT, relays the message between the person using a TT and the person using a conventional phone. Relay numbers are published in every phone directory, usually in the front of the white pages. Also, many public places make TTs available as special pay phones.

Telephone amplifiers are used by individuals who are hard of hearing. Amplifiers can be built into phones or added to phones, and some phones are hearing aid compatible. Hard of hearing individuals can use these telephone amplifiers to carry on spoken conversations.

Telecommunications companies have developed pagers that use a vibrating beeper to notify the customer that a message has been received. Not only can these pagers hold dozens of messages, but as the technology has improved, the maximum length of messages has also increased. In addition, some pagers have small keyboards that can be used to send messages.

Captioning and Real-Time
Graphic Display

Captioning is the appearance of printed text that is designed to capture the dialogue and action of a television program, movie, newscast, sporting event, or advertisement. Most prerecorded programs, and many live broadcasts, are closed-captioned. Since 1993, a federal law has required all new television sets with screens larger than 13 inches sold in the United States to be equipped with an internal decoder that can receive captions. The captions are typically scrolled across the bottom like a film with subtitles, though some televisions allow the user to position the captions anywhere on the screen. Individuals with older television sets must use an external decoder that attaches to the television.

Television shows, such as sports, news, and awards, are captioned as they occur. This is referred to as real-time captioning. The technology used in real-time captioning is also used in real-time graphic display. Individuals who attend lecture-type events will more and more frequently see presentations captured on real-time graphic display. An individual trained as a stenotypist or court reporter types into a device with phonetic shorthand symbols, the device is connected to a computer that translates these codes into English, and the English is displayed on a screen that the audience can view. Many classrooms use real-time graphic display for deaf students. Some college and university classrooms use remote captioning services. In this type of service, the lecture is sent by audio to a remote site where a captionist transcribes the lecture, sending it back over the phone line to the student's laptop computer. The transfer from audio to text takes just a few seconds.

The Internet

The Internet has opened up a metaphorical world of communication possibilities for everyone, and it is a perfect medium for deaf individuals. Through e-mail, they can communicate rapidly and clearly to anyone else who has e-mail. The World Wide Web offers entertainment and information to anyone with a computer, modem, and Internet software.

Linkages between computers and telephone lines have resulted in computer software that enables deaf individuals to use their computers as a TT. Advances in the technology have added video capability so that senders and receivers can see one another, as well as read their messages. Many deaf individuals also use fax machines for sending and receiving messages.

Speech recognition software offers several possibilities as the technology improves. Jensema (1994) suggested four applications:

1. Current technology is available that can recognize words spoken by one person. "It is possible to develop a speech recognition system that could be programmed to understand a limited vocabulary spoken over a telephone by a friend or relative" (p. 26).

2. Technology should soon enable deaf individuals to use simple voice mail systems. One particularly valuable feature will be a speech recognition system that enables the deaf person to follow directions regarding which telephone button to press to route their call.

3. When technology can be used for recognizing the continuous speech of a person, hearing individuals will be able to speak directly to the deaf person face-to-face or through the phone system without the intermediary step of a relay operator.

4. In the future, technology will provide all translation from text-to-voice and voice-to-text.

Alerting Devices

Alerting devices use vibratory or visual signals to alert the deaf individual. Examples include vibrators connected to alarm clocks and the cribs of crying babies, and flashing lights connected to smoke alarms, doorbells, and telephones. Some deaf individuals own hearing ear dogs that alert their owners to important sounds in the environment.

Koenigsfeld, Beukelman, and Stoefen-Fisher (1993) examined the attitudes of deaf individuals toward technology for augmenting communication with hearing individuals who do not sign. The majority of the deaf individuals in their study interacted 16 or more times each month with nonsigning hearing individuals at work, church, home, and while shopping. They used speech, gesture, pointing, mouthing, and writing, with writing being the most successful in their view. They felt they would use a portable, electronic communication device if it were available, but currently used little technology beyond TTs and alerting devices for communication.

Language and communication are connected inextricably to culture. Indeed, ASL is the foremost identifying feature of Deaf culture. In discussing culture, it is recognized that virtually all Deaf individuals maintain multiple cultural identities. For this reason, discussion of culture must be cast within the context of biculturalism or multiculturalism.

CULTURE

Culture is a pattern of beliefs, values, behaviors, arts, customs, institutions, social forms, and knowledge that are characteristic of a community. The patterns of beliefs and values are used by the community to interpret their individual and collective experience, past and present. Culture is transmitted to succeeding generations through material products, physical interaction with members of the community, and language. When children learn the language of their parents, they are learning their own culture and when children learn a second language, they learn a second culture (Saville-Troike, 1979). The experience of deaf children in learning their first language and their first culture does not neatly parallel the hearing child's experience. Many deaf children are exposed to two languages and two cultures, and sometimes the first language and culture are not the parents'.

One of the clearest symbols of Deaf culture is the use of capital *D* to refer to culturally deaf individuals as well as the particular set of beliefs and practices shared by Deaf individuals. Originally proposed by Woodward in 1972, the difference between *Deaf* and *deaf* can be best explained by the dichotomy of sociocultural and medical views of deafness. The medical view of deafness focuses on the hearing loss itself. In this view, attention is directed toward the impact of deafness on education, communication, intelligence, socialization, development, socioeconomic status, and other such issues. Deafness is seen as a disability. The sociocultural view of deafness focuses on the social and cultural experience of being deaf in a society in which the majority of individuals are hearing. Deafness is seen as a linguistic and ethnic minority culture.

Membership in the Deaf Community

Much controversy has surrounded the question of membership in the Deaf community. Who is authentically Deaf? Certainly, ASL is the sine qua non of membership in the Deaf community. The numbers of preceding generations of deafness give individuals greater credibility in being identified as Deaf. Individuals who mouth or use spoken English have less credibility. Those born deaf have greater credibility than those who lose their hearing. Hard of hearing individuals have little credibility unless they reject amplification and use ASL exclusively. Individuals who attended residential schools for the deaf have greater credibility than those who attended public schools. One other group of individuals has connection to the Deaf community, though not equal membership—the hearing children of deaf parents. Sometimes referred to as CODA, children of Deaf adults who grow up using ASL are considered a part of the Deaf community. Dolby (1992) conducted a survey with Deaf adults in England and Canada to see what they considered to be criteria for membership in the Deaf community. Shared language, British Sign Language among the English Deaf and ASL among the Canadian Deaf, and a positive attitude toward the community were the only agreed-upon criteria. In Essay 3.1, students at The Learning Center for Deaf Children describe their understanding of Deaf culture and the Deaf community.

■ ■ ■ ■ ■ ▬▬

ESSAY 3.1

Students of Dynnelle Fields at The Learning Center for Deaf Children

ALEXANDRA LING

The generic definition for *deaf* is "partially or completely lacking in the sense of hearing." Little do people know that there's a second definition. In the third edition of the *American Heritage College Dictionary*, another definition is included.

(continued)

ESSAY 3.1   CONTINUED

This one, for *Deaf,* is "the community of deaf people who use American Sign Language as a primary means of communication." The differences in meanings between *deaf* and *Deaf* are important to the Deaf community.

Being born into a family of hearing people, my exposure to the Deaf community was minimal. I grew up with a small group of deaf friends, no more than ten of us. We saw each other during the week and on weekends. Our socialization with the outer world was limited. We were happy with each other, content to see each other every day. My childhood school was only for deaf children from preschool to sixth grade. After I graduated, I transferred to a middle school with a deaf program in a distant town. There I met many new deaf kids, and I realized that the Deaf community wasn't confined to such a small number. But I still wasn't able to go out very much and explore. The deaf kids there were like any middle-school kids. Everybody pestered each other, including me. At that time, deafness seemed so limited and boring. I started wishing that I were hearing so that my choice of friends could be broadened. High school was much better. I met more new people and made more friends. Some of these new friends were part of the Deaf community.

One summer, I made the decision to go to Youth Leadership Camp for deaf high school students. At first, I had some aversion to going to the camp because it was outside the safe circle of my friends. Upon arriving, the magnitude of new and different people was overwhelming. Some fit my personality, and some were as opposite to me as the north and south magnets. But I learned very much about friendships, teamwork, and unity. When I returned to school, I felt more involved and closer to many deaf people. We were all the same, deaf. We were a minority in America, so we had to stick together for support and unity. I realized that this is what Deaf community means. The unity of the deaf people, a group of people together, knowing each other and having a connection despite any distance.

JONATHAN LANGONE

Deafness is boiling blood flowing through my veins. It's my whole life. Deaf culture is my soul. American Sign Language is my "voice" and "ears" because I hear with my precious eyes and I speak with my hands. Staring through my green eyes I see my Deaf friends smiling, laughing, and chatting. Everyday, I sense pure happiness and pride in them for being Deaf.

I was a premature baby who was born two months early. How I lost my hearing is a mystery. It may be due to the medications that the doctors used to keep me alive. I'm not looking for the answer to why I'm deaf. I'm very happy with the way I am. My parents discovered that I was deaf when I was about eight months old. They wanted the best for me, so they chose The Learning Center for Deaf Children. I feel that they picked the best school in the world for my needs. I'm thankful because I have the tools to be successful in life. I led a normal childhood, and I have a Deaf identity. I communicate with my parents through sign language. I'm thankful for that. I know many deaf people whose hearing parents can't sign at all. I would find that very difficult. Many deaf adults have told me that I'm lucky my parents use sign language.

I never really think about being deaf. I have played on a hearing sports team, and my teammates used hand signals with me. I was the best hitter on my little league baseball team, and my teammates depended on me. They accepted me as a person, not as someone who is deaf. I am a resident at my school, so I don't see my old teammates very often but when I do, I give them a wave. My best friend is hearing. We grew up together and communicated through American Sign Language. We hang out together on weekends. He's the nicest kid I'll ever know.

As I write this essay, I'm in the computer lab, in a Deaf world. We have all types of people with various interests and personalities, just like in the hearing world. I glance over at Kristin, who is like a sister to me because I've known her all my life. She's the athlete in the group. I'm saddened that she is a senior now, and it means that soon I won't be seeing her sitting next to me for the first time in my life. Typing right across from me is Joey, who is my roommate in the dorm. We can talk about anything. He has been here for five years, and we have grown as close as brothers. Sitting next to Joey is Alla, a good friend of mine and a great debater. I have known her for two years. We're growing closer as time goes by. Randy sits across the room, typing an essay. He's a great kid and my Trekkie buddy. We share a common interest in science fiction. Finally, sitting on my other side is Erin, chatting with Kristin. I have known her for six years, and we have grown as close as siblings.

That's how The Learning Center is; everyone is family, including the teachers and staff. I live in a world where I can communicate freely and go about my daily life with a complex group of people who see me as Jonathan and don't think about my deafness. We are just people living and growing together.

KRISTIN FELDMAN

My parents didn't find out that I was deaf until I was about one year old. They had a hard time accepting my deafness. They went through a difficult time. The doctors thought I should have a cochlear implant, but my parents were too confused at that time to go ahead with it. They sent me to The Learning Center for Deaf Children in Framingham, Massachusetts, which was five miles from my home. I learned how to sign there. My parents could see my eyes getting brighter as I learned how to sign and communicate with other people. I remember when I was finally able to communicate with my parents by asking for milk without crying. They finally didn't have to struggle to figure out what I needed or wanted.

Being Deaf is who I am. I can do everything but hear. Deaf people don't need to hear!

ERIN MCMANUS

The deaf population is unevenly distributed. In some areas, many deaf people reside, and in other areas, there are only a few deaf people. I feel very lucky because although I live in an area where only a few deaf people live, I have a deaf person living in my house, my fourteen-year-old sister. My sister and I are very close because we can understand each other with no problem. Communication is the most important thing to us. We use American Sign Language to communicate, to tell each other stories, news, events, concerns, and memories. As we sign, we use gestures, facial expressions, and body language to express what we feel. It's important to have communication so that we can share and express with each other.

Teaching is another reason having a deaf sister is important. The saying, "We learn something new every day" is true for everyone, including my deaf

(continued)

ESSAY 3.1 CONTINUED

sister and me. She and I go our separate ways with friends, students, teachers, and family members. We always come back and tell each other what we saw and experienced. For example, we were unaware of many opportunities for deaf people such as deaf summer camps. Once we found out about them, we told each other, and the following summer, we went to a deaf camp in Connecticut. We met deaf people from different places, and it was a rich experience. Although I can learn from a hearing person, I can learn a lot more from a deaf person. Making these connections and learning from them was very important to us.

My sister and I value each other strongly. We keep our relationship strong. We support each other through the hard, sad, and happy times. I feel lucky to have a deaf sister because there will always be someone there who totally understands and supports me. My sister and I have seen some deaf brothers and sisters who don't get along well because the Deaf community is small, and they share the same group of friends. However, my sister and I realize how special the Deaf community is and how important it is to keep our relationship special as well.

JOEY CUMMINGS

I had just transferred to a deaf school for the first time after years of being mainstreamed in public schools. I joined the soccer team although I thought that I could not make it on the team. So I tried my best in the practice. I exhausted myself. I found out that I could play well. It was a great opportunity for me. I had always played on a hearing team, and my experiences had been negative. Being on the deaf team was not only a positive experience but taught me a lot about myself. The main advantage was increased communication and social skills.

When I went to my first soccer practice with a deaf team, I did not talk to anyone. I was used to being quiet at practices with my hearing teammates and just doing what I was told. Many practices later, I started to have a problem with the team. They said I did not socialize with the other kids in the practices or the games. I was used to holding in my thoughts. I realized that it was not only possible for me to socialize during practice, but it was also very important. My teammates helped me to regain my confidence. I developed my communication skills, and I became less frustrated. I learned to socialize, and I thank my teammates for helping me.

RANDY DEWITT

I have Usher's syndrome, which is a degeneration of my retinas. Gradual blackness creeps into your vision until you become blind over a period of many years. My vision is deteriorating at a very slow pace. I can't see downwards, but my horizontal visual range is much like others. In addition, I have difficulty following rapid movement, such as deaf people signing and small balls in the air. I went through many difficult times coping with Usher's syndrome. At times, I didn't know what to do. Thanks to a few people who supported me, I finally realized that I had to accept the challenges as they presented themselves. Although I have often longed to hide from Usher's syndrome, there were a few turning points in my life that helped me realize that it isn't the end of the world.

I played baseball with young hearing kids when I was seven or eight years old. When I was nine, I found out that I had Usher's syndrome, and I was crushed with feelings of immense despair. I was in complete denial because I was so young and unprepared to deal with being blind. Imagine a child not being able to see the world or hear words spoken to him or her? That child would ask everyone, Santa Claus, God, and the Easter Bunny, for help finding a cure. When I was twelve, I joined my mother's baseball club. I played with hearing adults simply because I wanted to have fun. I still fondly remember those good times when Usher's syndrome didn't matter to the people in the club. Unfortunately, when I entered high school, my eyes began to worsen slightly. But I have hope because technology might be able to cure my Usher's syndrome in the future.

Reprinted by permission of the authors.

Community Cohesion

The levels of status within the Deaf community are undoubtedly the result of the community's need to define itself separately from the hearing community. Deaf individuals are often described as sharing a heritage of oppression (Lane, 1992). Lacking meaningful representation and leadership in educational, professional, and political institutions that affected their lives, until recently Deaf people saw themselves as powerless (Kyle & Pullen, 1988). The creation of manually coded English systems have been portrayed as attempts to maintain subservience to the hearing community and cochlear implants as an attempt to annihilate the Deaf community (Dolnick, 1993; Reagan, 1985, 1995).

Negative attitudes toward hearing individuals reflect a tension within the Deaf community and are based on the belief by some that hearing people have been their oppressors. One of the most derogatory signs is the sign for a hearing person, the index finger, placed parallel to the lips, making a continuous circle in front of the mouth, used to identify a deaf person by placing the sign at the forehead as in, "thinks like a hearing person" or "has a hearing center." It is akin to calling an African American person an "Uncle Tom" or an Oreo, black on the outside and white on the inside. Some Deaf individuals express open prejudice and hostility toward hearing people (Cumming & Rodda, 1989; Masters, 1994). This attitude marginalizes hard of hearing individuals who choose to use spoken English and amplification (Ross, 1994) and deaf individuals who choose cochlear implants, regardless of their former Deaf or deaf status.

The Deaf President Now movement at Gallaudet University was triggered by the hiring of a hearing person as the President. Elisabeth Zinser, who was President-in-exile for four days in March of 1988, wrote, "A major firestorm of protest erupted from the deaf community, since I, the new president, was not deaf. I learned quickly—by surprise—that it was their moment in time to be recognized for who they are and can be.

What was done with that surprise quickened the resolution of conflict and made legitimate a historic social movement. It was a unique revolutionary moment" (p. 23). Details of the protest are presented in Christiansen and Barnartt's book, *Deaf President Now: The 1988 Revolution at Gallaudet University* (1995). The authors observed that while the long-lasting effects of the protest are still uncertain, it surely influenced the passage of the Americans with Disabilities Act and continues to serve as a beacon for future generations of Deaf individuals.

> During one week in March 1988, protesters at Gallaudet University in Washington, D.C. captured the attention and imagination of millions of people in the United States and, indeed, throughout the world. It is quite likely that most of those people had never heard of Gallaudet before and were perhaps unaware that there even was a college geared toward meeting the special needs of deaf students. But after a week of protest, which came to be called "Deaf President Now" (or DPN) and which culminated in the selection of I. King Jordan as the first deaf president of the then 124-year-old university, the name Gallaudet, if not yet a household word, attained recognition undreamed of only a few weeks earlier. (p. vii)

Not only was Dr. Zinser a hearing person, but she was a nonsigning hearing person. Orlans (1989) observed that Gallaudet's Board of Trustees felt that it was more important that the new president be able to communicate with them, most of whom were nonsigners, the hearing world, and the Congress than with Gallaudet's students and alumni. What became apparent after the revolution at Gallaudet was the unique and important role of the university in the lives of its students and alumni.

> It is a place where, sometimes for the first and often the last time in their adult lives, deaf people are in a large, thriving community where deafness is normal, where everyone signs and the few hearing people who do not are as lost as a cat in a dog pound.... During most of their lives most deaf people do not live together in communities. They are scattered across the nation, isolated in hearing families, hearing neighborhoods and cities, in a world made by and for hearing people who do not sign.... Gallaudet is the largest, grandest, most important residential community of deaf people in the nation and the world. (Orlans, 1989, p. 16)

It is important to recognize that although we often use the term *Deaf community*, in reality Deaf communities are heterogeneous and international. The common denominator is that sign languages throughout the world are the most identifiable features of these communities. For example, although most Deaf Canadians use ASL, those in Quebec use Quebec Sign Language and those in Nova Scotia use British Sign Language (Janesick, 1990). These sign languages, along with others such as French Sign

Language, Spanish Sign Language, and Chinese Sign Language, are no more mutually intelligible than respective spoken languages (Reagan, 1995).

In Essay 3.2, Sheila Owolabi, an African Deaf woman, describes her experiences growing up in Nigeria and coming to the United States.

■■■■■ ▬▬▬▬▬▬▬▬▬▬▬▬▬▬▬▬▬▬▬▬▬

ESSAY 3.2

Sheila Owolabi

There were no deaf people in our family until I was born. My parents had eleven children. Seven actually lived. I was the fourth born out of the eleven. When I was five, I got smallpox. My parents didn't know at first that my hearing was affected. But as a result of the smallpox, I was completely deaf. My mother remembers calling my name, and I kept walking and didn't respond. When she dropped things or made noises, she noticed that I didn't hear what was happening. So my mother took me to a doctor. He told my mother that I was deaf.

My parents were hoping that I'd be able to talk really well in spite of losing my hearing. They took me to the doctor quite often, and each time, the doctor tested my hearing and my ears, nose, and throat. He would turn me around and make noises in back of my head. He'd move to different sides behind my back. Every time it was the same thing. He gave me medication, but nothing worked. Finally, my mother was tired of all that. One morning she told me that when I went to the doctor and he called my name, I should raise my hand. We practiced at home. The doctor did the same tests again, ear, nose, throat, heart beat, that sort of thing. Then the doctor said, "Turn around" to me. First, the doctor clapped. I saw him in my peripheral vision and I raised my hand. Each time he clapped, I tried to see if he was clapping out of my peripheral vision, and when I did, I raised my hand. The doctor was so delighted. He said that I could hear now. I didn't know what the big deal was. But the next day, when I asked my mom if we were going back to the doctor, she said, "No, we're done. We convinced that doctor that you're all right." I was so happy that I never had to go there any more. It was a really long walk, and I could play again with my friends.

My dad was still very concerned that I couldn't hear. My parents discovered that I could hear some music and dance really well. This was when I was five or six years old. Actually, I could feel the vibration and so they thought I could hear the music. When the music stopped, I kept dancing. You know how music gets louder and softer? I didn't realize the music had stopped. I just thought it had gotten softer. People would laugh at me. My friends would also laugh at me because of the way I pronounced things.

My dad decided he wanted to take me to an herbist. He asked the herbist what they could do for me because I couldn't hear. The herbist recommended all these different leaves and herbs, showed my dad how to mix them with other foods, and explained how I should take them. My dad would mix all these

(continued)

herbs up, put them into this horn-shaped object, and have me drink it. Every morning, my dad told me to go into this dark quiet place, and he mixed up these herbs for me. I would drink it all because he told me to. And then he'd make these different noises. I could hear these little drumbeats that he was making. Then he would do them more quietly because he was experimenting with my hearing. And he would tell me that I could hear better. But the herbs never really helped. My hearing was the same, my lack of hearing, rather.

I had a hard time with different things in my childhood. I had a great family. My parents worked with me. When I was ready to go to school, they sent me to a public school. I remember being so excited to be in first grade. Everyone was like me, and we played. Outside there were no problems, during recess and that sort of thing. But sometimes the kids would laugh at me, just like in my neighborhood. I was familiar with that. Everyone would say that I was deaf and talk to one another. They would blow paper between their lips to make fun of me. It hurt my feelings. They made fun of me because I was deaf and couldn't talk. I had two really close friends who fought for me.

In the classroom it was different. The teacher knew nothing about deaf people or how to teach a deaf person. The principal knew that I was deaf. In the classroom, the teacher would say something like, "Two plus two is four" or the alphabet, "a-b-c-d-e-f-g." I would read her lips. No one taught me to lipread. I just learned that on my own. I would see her saying "a-b-c-d-e-f-g," and I would try to lipread her and write down what she had said. When the teacher actually started teaching other things, like in my home language, I didn't understand the form of the language. We were supposed to copy what she had said. I would struggle and struggle, trying to understand, while everyone in the class who could hear understood her. So what I did was to copy someone else's paper to get the right answer. And that's how I got through. Sometimes my answers were right, and sometimes they were wrong.

Every morning you had to get in line, and the teacher would talk to us. I had no idea what she was saying. The teacher would make sure our fingernails were clean and cut, and make sure we were groomed well. If there was something out of place, she told the students to get out of line and go clean their faces, brush their teeth, or brush their hair. I remember the teacher saying something to me, but I had no idea what it was. One day the principal gave me a letter and told me to give it to my parents. My parents read it, and I made the changes to my grooming that the teacher had been telling me.

In class, the teacher called everybody's name. Sometimes I forgot to watch her. She would call my name over and over while I'd be looking in my desk. I'd feel all eyes on me. I'd close my desk and feel mortified and embarrassed. The teacher just didn't understand what it meant to be deaf. When the school year was done and the grades were handed out, I didn't understand what my grades meant. I brought my report card home and my parents looked at it, put it away, and didn't talk to me about it.

School started again in the fall. I was so happy. I didn't know what grade I was in but I knew some of the children who were in the same class as me. The British system is different from the American grade system. I remember being in line two, seeing people I recognized going into the two classroom, and going into the classroom and finding my seat. I watched the teacher as she pronounced everyone's name. When she finished roll call, I told her I didn't hear my name. The teacher said something to me but I didn't understand what she was saying. She then asked me to come with her. We went to the principal's office. I watched the teacher and principal talking. They told me to stay seated. So I stayed all morning in this one room. There was nothing to do. When it was time to go to recess, they told me to go outside. After recess, the teacher told me to come back into this room again and just sit there. I thought I was a troublemaker. The next day, I went in the same line as the previous day and into the same classroom. The teacher told me to go to the principal's office. This happened for a week. Finally the principal said, "Come with me." I went with the principal to the outside of the school building. There was another principal there and the two principals started talking.

There was another school next door and we went over to that building, which I learned was a really small deaf school. My parents didn't even know about it. They told me that I'd be going to this new school every day. The principal wrote a letter to my parents. My parents read the letter, and the next day they went with me to this new school. I looked around and saw people gesturing and pointing to one another. I seemed to understand them better. And then I met my best friend. She never made fun of me. She was the first kid I'd ever met who never made fun of me. The teacher in the classroom started to teach math and figures, such as the numbers and addition my other teacher had taught. It was the first time I understood clearly what the teacher was trying to teach. I began to understand addition problems very quickly.

The teacher talked with the principal and the teachers at the other school, and they were shocked that I could learn. She told them that I was very smart, and she was very glad to have me in her class. The principal started to respect me and understand that I was capable of learning. Time progressed. It was the British system of education, and they were really into the oral track of learning, such as how to lipread. They always taught two subjects together. For example, if they were teaching math, it was math and speech. Speech was highly emphasized. Writing wasn't emphasized that much. We had handwriting practice, but language development was not emphasized.

I must have been eleven when I moved to a new school. The first school for the deaf was a day school, and I went home every day. The new school was a residential school. It was beautiful. We stayed at the school during the week and came home on the weekends.

After Primary Six in the English system, there was a proficiency test. When we took the test, the students sat together. We took the same test as the public school kids took. Our teacher supervised us, but in the public school, teachers were not allowed to be in the room supervising their own students during the test. While we were working on our proficiency test, if someone didn't understand something, the teacher figured it out and provided the answer. No one said anything. When we received our results, everyone was so happy that we had passed the proficiency test and had even done better than the students in the public school. They were really proud and happy for us. But in my heart, I was sad about that. The teachers didn't understand that someone who wants to learn for themselves wouldn't really want to pass the test with help. We don't feel good when someone gives us the answers.

(continued)

ESSAY 3.2 CONTINUED

When we got into high school and were mainstreamed, we faced the same problems as we did in the younger grades. The teachers didn't understand how to work with deaf students. There were five students in my school who were deaf, and we all struggled. There were no interpreters because it was oral education. We had to sit and watch the teacher. When the teacher turned around, we'd watch the back of the teacher's head. We'd ask friends if we could copy their notes. It was twice as much work, first sitting in class and then copying the notes at home.

A deaf person told me that I should go to a deaf church. I was so impressed with the self-esteem of the people there. There were deaf leaders and deaf singers. They did everything themselves. All my life I had seen hearing people do everything for deaf people. I always thought that deaf people couldn't do anything. Even though I had tried to act like a hearing person as much as possible, I knew I wasn't. So when I went into this church and I saw deaf people freely communicating with one another using sign language, I realized that they were no different than a group of hearing people talking to each other. They discussed politics and shared information. I felt that everything I had missed growing up was there at that church.

At church, I had the fortunate opportunity to meet Andrew Foster, a Black gentleman from America. He was establishing deaf schools in Africa and bringing American Sign Language into our country. I couldn't believe how smart he was. My own father wasn't a role model for me like this man was. I really looked up to my father, but he was hearing and it was hard to communicate with him. All my brothers were hearing, and they all went to the university. None of them really impressed me. But here was this deaf man who signs and lipreads. When I asked him questions, he could answer me. I was never able to ask questions of my father. So I asked Mr. Foster many questions. At the church, he told us about universities and what was available to us. He told me that I was very smart, and I should go to the seminary. I thought how wonderful that would be. When I asked him how I would pay for it, he said that he would pay for my education. My dad had told me that when I graduated from high school, I should learn how to type. But I didn't want to do that sort of thing. I saw that other people had academic degrees, and that's what I wanted.

Some of my friends said that I should go to college and not to the seminary. Being polite, I didn't know how to tell Mr. Foster that I preferred going to a college like Gallaudet. He urged me to go to the seminary and so I didn't know what to do. I had to take a test to get into the seminary, and I failed it. I was so happy. I told him that I didn't pass the test so I couldn't go to the seminary. At that time, there were a lot of deaf people in Nigeria who were planning to go to a college or university in America. I talked to them and asked if they would help me with school preparation. I didn't know how I was going to afford it. I made an application to the government and explained why I needed my education to be financed. The special education department had a scholarship available. I applied for it, and my family didn't even know what I was doing. They thought that I was deaf and didn't know anything. I thought of myself very differently. I was very assertive, so I looked at different avenues to try to find financing. Ultimately, I received two scholarships. One of them was for federal aid and the other was a state scholarship.

I told my family that I wanted to go to America. My mother was happy. She was so proud, she told everyone she knew. No one could believe that I was deaf and going to America. Also, males were considered upper class in our society and women were not. The process of actually getting the scholarship was very difficult. The way the system works is unbelievable. Once you apply, you must have an interview, and after you interview, you wait several weeks. Every time I went back to the office to ask about the scholarship, they would tell me to come back in a week. I was continually going to their office. The College of South Idaho accepted my application and wanted me to come on a certain semester. I had a boyfriend, who happens to be my husband now, and he was trying to help me with the application process. I needed my scholarship money in order to go. The whole process took almost two years. I felt like giving up. I talked to so many different people in the government and tried so many different avenues. They kept saying I would get it, but there was always someone else I needed to talk to. Often, they would make me talk to the secretary once they realized I was deaf. It made me very angry to be treated this way. Each time I had to see a man who was the head secretary for the state scholarship department. He did not like deaf people. When this man transferred to a different position, a woman was put in his position. She asked if she could help me, and I just started to bawl. I told her what had happened during the last two years. I showed her my acceptance letter from the university. In two days, I had my scholarship. I couldn't believe it. Everyone had lost hope in me.

I got my passport and showed it to my mother. I said to her, "This week I'm going to America." My mother could not believe it. I ran around getting everything arranged. I needed money and clothes. My mother told me to open her closet and pick whatever I wanted. She had never said that to me before. I didn't even know what I wanted. I picked a few things but, really, all I had on my brain was America. I packed it all up. My mother and sister told everyone, so everywhere I went in town, people said, "There goes Sheila, the American girl." If I were hearing, they probably would have killed me over jealousy, but because I was deaf, they thought it was no big deal. The next day, my father came to my sister's house. I knew it would be the last day I would see him. My mother was crying because I was leaving the next day. My mother wanted to know how I had achieved everything that I had achieved. I told her that I did it myself. By this time, I was 22 years old. My mother told me not to get into any fights in America because there are guns in America. They only knew what they saw on tv, like the cowboy movies. They thought that a lot of killing happened in America.

When I got to Idaho, it was snowing because it was wintertime. I had no coat. I remember, though, that I wasn't feeling cold and thinking that I must have a lot of vitamin D in my body. People wondered if I was African or American. Everyone was talking about me. I was the only Black person at that school and the only Black deaf person. That first night I could not sleep. So the next day in class, I couldn't pay attention. I went back to my dorm and slept and slept. My body finally became adjusted to the time difference. That first winter, my mouth would bleed because I wasn't used to the cold. The signing was also different. I would sign something, and everyone would laugh. For example, one sign I used for "pen" is a sexual sign in ASL. I was so embarrassed. After that, every time I signed "pen" they would laugh at me, even though I was signing it correctly.

(continued)

ESSAY 3.2   CONTINUED

Here in America, I noticed that many students were living on Vocational Rehabilitation money. They played around a lot and didn't study. I worked so hard because the government was paying my way, and I wanted to make sure that I got good grades. I took everything very seriously. Others did a lot of partying and drinking. I saw girls drinking, and I was surprised because in Africa, girls don't drink much or at all. It was a culture shock for me to see the differences between America and Africa. In Africa, when you go to a party, you dress very nicely. In America, girls would wear jeans, and I'd say, "Is this a party?" In my culture, if you're invited to a party, it means there is food and nice dancing. It was so different here. One time I was invited to a banquet. I thought I should wear jeans. Of course everyone else was dressed up. I couldn't believe it. I started asking my teachers what different things meant. I shared a dormitory room with an interpreter for a while before I was married, and she told me not to be like the deaf students who fool around, wasting the tax dollars being spent on their education. I remembered what she told me, and I always worked hard in school.

I was married shortly after coming to America. When my husband received his associate's degree, he transferred to Western Oregon State College. They didn't have a home economics education major, so I transferred to Oregon State University and graduated with a BS degree. The students at Western Oregon and Oregon State worked much harder than the students in Idaho. I studied the way the hearing students studied. If they did better, it made me want to do better. In Idaho, the deaf students played around a lot, and I didn't really like working with them.

During the years I was in school, I became pregnant three times. Sometimes, I brought the babies with me to class. When I was a sophomore, I was pregnant with my first child. I had to take my exams a week after I had my baby. When I was pregnant the second time, the same thing happened. I brought the baby to class, sometimes feeding the baby or sometimes leaving if the baby became fussy. My husband and I took turns taking care of the children. I was so worn out after finishing my bachelor's degree that when I started my master's program, I only took two classes each semester. Ultimately, I earned my master's degree.

All that hard work gave me strength and courage and made me realize that I could get through anything. I know that other deaf people can do the same.

Reprinted by permission of the author.

Transmission of Culture

With only 5 to 7 percent of deaf individuals having two deaf parents, Deaf culture must be transmitted in ways that are different from almost any other culture that is passed on from parents to their children. It is assumed that Deaf culture has traditionally been transmitted to succeeding generations through the home-away-from-home environment of residential schools for the deaf. Indeed, a great concern among Deaf adults has been the erosion of schools for the deaf subsequent to the passage of Public Law 94-142, the Individuals with Disabilities Education Act, in 1975, which mandated a least restrictive environment for children with disabilities. This mandate was interpreted as meaning the public schools by many local educational agencies.

At residential schools, Deaf children are with Deaf houseparents, older Deaf students, Deaf workers, and Deaf teachers. In addition, hearing teachers in residential schools appear to be more knowledgeable of Deaf culture than hearing teachers in public schools. Woodward and Allen (1993) found that a much larger number of Deaf teachers are employed by residential schools than public schools, and the hearing teachers in residential schools have "adapted themselves in striking ways to Deaf culture, by attempting to adopt sociolinguistic characteristics valued in the U.S. Deaf community" (p. 373).

Patterns in the Culture

Deaf culture is more than a shared language. The community shares a pattern of beliefs, values, behaviors, arts, customs, institutions, social forms, and knowledge. Study of the culture is relatively recent, so understanding of these patterns is still quite incomplete.

Political activity, such as the Deaf President Now movement, is part of the culture. Art forms are also part of the culture. Storytelling has a long tradition in the community. Poetry in the community is performed rather than read. Deaf artists often make their connection with the Deaf community clear in their work, and when they do, it is considered Deaf art (Gregory, 1992). Deaf theater has a long and rich history. The National Theatre of the Deaf is widely respected and performs throughout the world. Deaf individuals share a history that is increasingly documented by publishers such as Gallaudet University Press. Members of the community come together in community social groups, organizations, churches, synagogues, fraternal orders, and sororities. Stories, poetry, plays, and folklore are available in print and video formats. Poetry, for example, is a unique genre because unlike poetry written in English, Deaf poetry is based on handshape, location, movement, direction, and other nonmanual components. Rutherford (1988) noted that "the folkloristic tradition of Deaf America is over 175 years old and is replete with legends, naming practices, tall tales, folkspeech, jokes, sign play, games, folk poetry, customs, ritual, and celebrations" (p. 137).

The culture of Deaf individuals developed over time, and it endures because the Deaf community shares a history, a present, and a future. Schein (1989) titled his book about the Deaf experience *At Home Among Strangers*, because it expresses the feeling of comfort, relaxation, and sharing when Deaf people come together. In this book, he wrote, "Deaf people have demonstrated their talents for adaptation, for finding ways to work with and move around barriers. These adaptations and the accompanying folkways and values form Deaf culture" (p. 67).

Home Cultures and Ethnicities

Knowledge of other cultures and ethnicities is as critical as knowledge of Deaf culture. Deaf individuals have the same diverse racial, ethnic, and linguistic backgrounds as hearing individuals. These communities also share patterns of beliefs, values, behaviors, arts, customs, institutions, social forms, and knowledge. The research on home cultures and ethnicities has focused largely on the differential achievement levels of deaf children from diverse backgrounds. And almost all of the studies address race exclusively.

Educators of children who are deaf seem less likely to acknowledge the differential educational experiences of children from minority backgrounds than educators of hearing children. There appears to be an attitude that cultural differences are not significant in the lives of Deaf individuals. Yet studies have shown that African American and Hispanic students perform significantly lower on measures of achievement than white students who are deaf (Cohen, Fischgrund, & Redding, 1990; Kluwin, 1993, 1994a). As Kluwin noted, "Race is a pernicious factor in the school achievement of deaf students" (1993, p. 79).

Involvement of parents from diverse cultures, particularly parents who do not speak English, is important in educational programs for all children, whether deaf or hearing. It is also critical for teachers to understand cultural differences, family values, and child-rearing practices. Without this understanding, deaf children can be caught between conflicting expectations for thought and conduct (Yacobacci-Tam, 1987). In addition, parents who do not see themselves as respected by the school system are likely to be privately critical but publicly uninvolved with their child's education (Bennett, 1988).

Assessment presents a problem if professionals are not aware of the influence of culture on assessment tools and practices. In both school and counseling settings, individuals conducting assessments must be knowledgeable of assessment instruments and procedures that are culturally sensitive and aware of the potential for bias within the instrument and by the examiner (Eldredge, 1993; MacNeil, 1990). The examiner also needs to take into account the languages and possible language mixing of a child who may be using a home language that is not English and a sign language that is not ASL (Gerner de Garcia, 1995).

Deaf individuals from minority groups must deal with issues of stereotyping, prejudice, and discrimination. They must figure out the respective influences of their multiple cultures as well as the subcultural groups of which they may be a part. For example, it is believed that African American Deaf, Hispanic Deaf, Native American Deaf, and Asian Deaf are just a few cultures within cultures (Anderson & Grace, 1991; Martin & Prickett, 1992; Page, 1993; Stewart & Benson, 1988). Dual minority membership appears to place Deaf individuals in double jeopardy. According to research conducted by MacLeod-Gallinger (1993):

> Racial and cultural minority status are associated with lower socioeconomic status. And minority within minority status appears to act as an exponential factor in this regard.... In general, the deaf population endures depressed labor force, occupational and earnings conditions relative to the hearing population. The data have indicated that those who are also members of ethnic minorities face additional disadvantages. (pp. 26–27)

In the mid-1980s, Delgado wrote in the introduction to *The Hispanic Deaf* (1984) that the bicultural Deaf child "is in the batter's circle, but the pitchers are sitting in the bullpen and nobody in the stands seems to know what's going on" (p. 2). During the last quarter of the twentieth century, educators and researchers devoted considerable attention to issues of bilingualism and biculturalism. Bilingualism meant ASL and English. Biculturalism meant Deaf culture and hearing culture. However, many families of deaf children speak languages other than English, many deaf children are exposed to sign languages other than ASL such as Mexican Sign Language, increasingly greater numbers of Americans are described as having diverse ethnicities, and although there is a dominant culture in the United States, it really cannot be described as hearing culture. The challenge is to develop broader understanding of cultural identities, deeper knowledge of the cultures that are represented among deaf children and adults, and greater sensitivity to cultural differences.

SUMMARY AND CONCLUDING THOUGHTS

This chapter discussed the development of language in deaf children—face-to-face language, reading, and writing. It described the languages that deaf children and adults use including ASL, spoken English, manually coded English systems, and pidgin sign. It also discussed the multiple cultures of deaf individuals, but most particularly, Deaf culture. The relationship between language and culture is inextricable. It seems appropriate to conclude this chapter with the passage that closed the book *Deaf in America* by Padden and Humphries (1988).

> Deaf culture is a powerful testimony to both the profound needs and the profound possibilities of human beings. Out of a striving for human language, generations of Deaf signers have fashioned a signed language rich enough to mine for poetry and storytelling. Out of a striving to interpret, to make sense of their world, they have created systems of meaning that explain how they understand their place in the world. That the culture of Deaf people has endured, despite indirect and tenuous lines of transmission and despite generations of changing social conditions, attests to the tenacity of the basic human needs for language and symbol. (p. 121)

CHAPTER FOUR

COGNITIVE ABILITIES

FOCUS QUESTIONS

- Why is it important to consider the factors that influence the performance of deaf children and adults on measures of intelligence?
- What is the relationship between cognitive development and language development?
- How are the cognitive demands placed on deaf children in classrooms different from the cognitive demands within everyday conversations?
- Why should educators and parents be concerned about improving the thinking abilities of deaf children?
- Should the school curriculum for deaf students include instruction in cognitive skills?

Until the mid-1960s, the research indicated and the rhetoric presumed that deaf individuals had inferior cognitive development because of their linguistic deficiencies in English. When researchers such as Vernon (1967b, 1968), Furth (1966), and Myklebust (1964) examined the assumptions underlying this conclusion, they initiated a body of research that influenced the education of deaf children for the next several decades. Almost simultaneously, researchers and educators considered the relationship between language and cognition in deaf individuals, examined the linguistic features of ASL, and investigated the cognitive benefits for children who were immersed in a sign language environment early in life. Much of this research focused on the intelligence of deaf persons.

INTELLIGENCE

Subsequent to carrying out a series of investigations on intelligence among deaf individuals, Braden (1994) conducted a meta-analysis of the research literature on the effect of deafness on intelligence. He found a nearly identical IQ distribution between deaf and hearing individuals. His own studies and those that he reviewed confirmed the seemingly logical presumption that deaf individuals will score lower on verbal intelligence tests and with procedures that are oral only. But on tests of nonverbal intelligence, no significant differences are evident. "The most remarkable feature of this meta-analysis is the similarity between deaf and normal-hearing people. Deaf people have similar nonverbal IQs and their IQs mirror the trends found for demographic groups in the normal-hearing population" (p. 105).

The results of investigations indicating that deafness has no effect on IQ (for example, Braden, 1985a, 1985b) led researchers to examine other factors such as parental deafness, educational setting, gender, and race.

Factors Related to Intelligence

Deaf children of deaf parents have been found to score significantly higher on performance IQ tests than deaf children of hearing parents and hearing children (Conrad & Weiskrantz, 1981; Kusche, Greenberg, & Garfield, 1983; Sisco & Anderson, 1980; Sullivan & Schulte, 1992; Zwiebel, 1987). Braden (1987) found that these apparent differences in IQ actually represent differences in rates of encoding information. The deaf children of deaf parents seem to have superior speed of information processing, which shows up as higher scores on timed tests. He hypothesized that sign language use promotes response speed.

Deaf children attending residential schools for the deaf have lower verbal IQs than deaf children attending either day schools for the deaf or public school programs (Braden, 1994). Two reasons have been suggested. One reason is selection. It is possible that students who have greater ability to succeed academically tend to attend public schools or day school programs, whereas students at residential schools tend to have less ability to succeed academically and a higher percentage of these students have multiple disabilities. A second possible explanation is the effect of the residential school environment on IQ. According to this possibility, students at residential schools have lower IQs because the school program has a deleterious effect on cognitive development. The results of two studies by Braden and his associates indicate that the first reason explains these differential IQ scores between students at residential schools and students in other types of educational programs (Braden, Maller, & Paquin, 1993; Paquin & Braden, 1990). They found that the IQs of deaf students increased over time after enrollment in residential schools for the deaf. They found no changes for students attending day school programs. Though students with lower IQ scores typically attend schools for the deaf, the residential placement appears to foster increased IQ scores rather than depress them.

Gender differences in intelligence have also been investigated among deaf individuals. Given that verbal IQ tests are regarded as less valid measures of intelligence, the tests where gender differences typically favor females are not used with deaf individuals. It is, therefore, more crucial to know whether performance IQ differences are gender biased or reflect true differences in intelligence. Although small differences on a few subtests have been identified, no significant differences in IQ have been found between male and female deaf children or adults (Ensor & Phelps, 1989; Phelps & Ensor, 1987).

Race differences are a fourth area that researchers have examined. The differences in IQ between African American deaf children and Caucasian deaf children mirror the differences found between African American and Caucasian hearing children (Braden, 1984, 1989b, 1994; Jensen, 1985). Explanations have included environmental factors, test bias, sampling bias, language, culture, genetic effects, and the interaction of these (Braden, 1994; Isham & Kamin, 1993). Clearly, much is unknown that might explain these IQ differences.

Intelligence and Academic Achievement

Educators are considerably less interested in simply knowing the IQ of the deaf children they teach than in using this information to understand their academic achievement. What is the relationship between intelligence and academic achievement?

Although the performance IQ of deaf children has been found to correlate with academic achievement, the correlations have been quite variable, and relatively small correlations have been found in some studies (Brooks & Riggs, 1980; Hirshoren, Hurley, & Kavale, 1979; Paal, Skinner, & Reddig, 1988; Padmapriya & Mythili, 1988). Making predictions about potential achievement based on IQ measures, therefore, would seem to be a questionable practice unless greater consistency in correlations could be found. Phelps and Branyon (1990) suggested that these discrepancies could be accounted for by the differences in tests of nonverbal intelligence. They found that the Kaufman Assessment Battery for Children Nonverbal scale equaled the correlation with achievement that is commonly accepted for hearing populations. They recommended that educators use the Kaufman in preference to other tests of nonverbal ability. The Hiskey-Nebraska Test of Learning Aptitude has also been found to correlate well with tests of achievement, but the Wechsler scales have not (Watson, Goldgar, Kroese, & Lotz, 1986).

Naglieri, Welch, and Braden (1994) suggested that the PASS model is a better approach to measuring the intelligence of deaf individuals than any of the intelligence nonverbal scales. The PASS model conceptualizes intelligence as a relationship among cognitive processing tasks—planning, attention, simultaneous, and successive. Planning involves aptitude for asking questions, solving problems, and self-monitoring. Attention involves orienting to a task and selectively attending. Simultaneous and successive processing involve the acquisition, storage, and retrieval of knowledge. PASS cognitive processing tasks have been developed by Das and Naglieri (Das, Naglieri, & Kirby, 1994; Naglieri & Das, 1988, 1990) and used to measure the intelligence of deaf children.

Intelligence is one aspect of cognitive abilities. Memory is another. Both are strongly related to academic performance.

MEMORY

The information-processing model that cognitive psychologists use to represent cognition includes four steps—acquisition, storage, retrieval, and use of information (Reed, 1995). Memory involves the storage and recovery of information. If information is best stored and recovered with a verbal code or inner voice, then deaf individuals would be at a disadvantage in processing information. However, if alternative codes are just as effective, then no disadvantage would exist, but the implications for instruction might be significant. Several researchers have pursued questions about the importance of verbal code in memory storage and retrieval.

Verbal and Other Encoding Memory Processes

On memory tasks that involve verbal encoding or sequential processing, deaf children have been found to perform less well than hearing children, but as well or better than hearing children on tasks with visual, motor, or spatial aspects (Heinen, Cobb, & Pollard, 1976; Krakow & Hanson, 1985; O'Connor & Hermelin, 1976; Parasnis, Samar, Bettger, & Sathe, 1996; Siple, Fischer, & Bellugi, 1977; Tomlinson-Keasey & Smith-Winberry, 1990; Wallace & Corballis, 1973).

Bebko conducted a series of studies in which he and his colleagues examined the verbal memory performance of deaf children (Bebko, 1984; Bebko, Lacasse, Turk, & Oyen, 1992; Bebko & McKinnon, 1990). These researchers found that deaf children were less likely to spontaneously rehearse new information, and when they did, they used the strategies inefficiently and less effectively than hearing children. They also found that rehearsal strategies showed up later among deaf children.

Tsui and Rodda (1990) examined the memory performance of deaf children and adolescents. They attributed the limited memory capacity of the subjects in their study to less successful use of what they referred to as executive cognitive strategies, which included planning, monitoring, and evaluating information.

Memory Performance

Another difference in the memory performance of deaf individuals seems to involve memory monitoring. Krinsky (1990) examined the memory monitoring of deaf adolescents by asking them to judge their feelings of knowing words they were unable to define. Her purpose was to learn whether deaf learners can effectively apply this cognitive strategy because "without accurate memory monitoring, a person might persist in trying to remember what he or she had never learned or had forgotten, and not persist in trying to remember information that might be remembered with more effort" (p. 389). She found that the deaf adolescents were unable to assess their feelings of knowing, unlike hearing adolescents who were able to do this. The memory monitoring of these deaf adolescents was considerably weaker than the hearing adolescents.

Memory and Language

If memory and language are interrelated, then the earliest memories of children with delayed language development should show up later than the earliest memories of children who acquire language at representative ages. Given that deaf children with hearing parents typically acquire language later than both hearing children and deaf children with deaf parents, Williams and Bonvillian (1989) hypothesized that the initial recollections of deaf individuals with hearing parents would occur significantly later than the initial recollections of hearing individuals, and that the initial recollections of deaf individuals with deaf parents would parallel hearing individuals. They found, however, no significant differences between the three groups. All of the subjects reported their initial recollections between three and four years of age. It appears as if the onset of language does not relate to one's earliest memories.

Memory and Aging

It is generally assumed that memory loss will accompany old age. The research has been equivocal, with some studies finding memory decline as inevitable and some finding that memory loss is not a predestined part of the aging process (Holland & Rabbit, 1992; Johansson, Zarit, & Berg, 1992; Lachman, Weaver, Bandura, Elliott, & Lewkowics, 1992; Light &

Burke, 1988). If memory loss is not inevitable, what are the factors that contribute to maintaining memory function? Levy and Langer (1994) suggested that cultural beliefs about aging result in a self-fulfilling prophecy. They compared six groups—old and young Chinese hearing, American hearing, and American Deaf individuals. They found that the Chinese and Deaf individuals, who were held in high esteem within their cultures, performed significantly better on memory tasks than the American hearing individuals, who were held in much lower esteem within mainstream American culture.

In addition to intelligence and memory, educators are interested in the development of cognition in deaf children.

COGNITIVE DEVELOPMENT

The relationship of language and thought has lead researchers in deafness to place cognitive development as a focal point of research. From investigations designed to understand development to studies devised to assess interventions (discussed later in this chapter), researchers have been interested in how the deaf child acquires and uses knowledge in increasingly complex ways.

Piagetian Tasks

The cognitive development of deaf children has typically been studied by using Piaget's developmental tasks. Research since the mid-1960s has consistently shown that deaf children progress through the same stages of cognitive development and perform similarly as hearing children, but somewhat later on certain tasks (Cates & Shontz, 1990b; Chang & Gonzales, 1987; Furth, 1966; Murphy-Berman, Witters, & Harding, 1985, 1986; Witters-Churchill, Kelly, & Witters, 1983).

Dolman (1983) examined the relationship between deaf children's syntactic development and their performance on four Piagetian tasks designed to evaluate their attainment of concrete operations—conservation, classification, seriation, and numeration. He found that operational abilities were significantly related to English syntactic comprehension.

Unlike others who have viewed the deaf child's cognitive skills as similar to the hearing child's, Rittenhouse proposed that deaf children exhibit cognitive differences (Rittenhouse, 1981, 1987b; Rittenhouse & Kenyon, 1991; Rittenhouse, Kenyon, Leitner, & Baechle, 1989; Rittenhouse & Spiro, 1979). These differences, he and his colleagues postulated, are the result of language delay and experiential deficit and not cognitive capacity. The debate about cognitive differences would be strictly academic if the cognitive development of the deaf child was an unimportant consideration in planning instruction. But of course it is important. Rittenhouse and Kenyon advised teachers to "examine each child's individual pattern of task mastery instead of expecting every student to follow the same emerging pattern. This might enable the teacher to take advantage of already developed skills and to better accommodate the specific needs and capabilities of the individual child" (1991, p. 320).

Non-Piagetian Tasks

Several researchers have used non-Piagetian tasks to examine the cognitive development of deaf children. The results are more mixed than studies using Piagetian tasks. Bond (1987) used three subtests from the McCarthy Scales of Children's Abilities—Block-Building, Puzzle-Solving, and Draw-a-Design. She found that the 2½- to 5½-year-old deaf children in her study did not significantly differ from the hearing children on any of the tasks.

Jamieson (1994) examined the interactions between mothers and toddlers from the perspective of Vygotskian theory involving the relationship between adult–child communication and the cognitive development of the child. According to Vygotsky's zone of proximal development, cognitive development occurs within the context of a task that a child cannot carry out independently but can carry out with support from a more knowledgeable and skilled individual. As the child is supported, the child ultimately develops the ability to carry out the task independently. Jamieson found that hearing mothers of deaf children were less likely to use interactional strategies that were supportive of cognitive development compared to hearing mothers of hearing children and deaf mothers of deaf children.

Peterson and Siegal (1997) used a set of tasks that they described as "theory of mind" tasks (that is, designed to understand the individual's thoughts and wishes). In each task, the child was presented with a scenario that required taking multiple perspectives. For example, in one scenario, a girl doll hid a marble in a basket and left. A boy doll took the marble from the basket and put it in another place. Then the girl doll returned. The child was asked where the girl would look for the marble, where the marble really was, and where the girl put the marble in the beginning. The researchers found that the performance of deaf children with deaf parents was more like hearing children than that of deaf children with hearing parents.

The analogic reasoning of deaf adolescents was investigated by Sharpe (1985). In order to control for language bias, she used two types of analogies, figure analogies and word analogies, with vocabulary at the second-grade level or below. The deaf adolescents performed equally well on the figure analogies and word analogies, which indicated that the task was truly measuring their analogic reasoning rather than their linguistic abilities. When compared to hearing adolescents, the deaf adolescents demonstrated significantly poorer performance on all of the analogic reasoning tasks, which supported the conclusion that they were not developing this particular complex cognitive skill as well as their hearing peers.

Parasnis (1983) examined the cognitive skills of young deaf adults and found no differences on tests of cognitive skills between deaf and hearing subjects and between male and female subjects. She also found no differences between the students who had learned to sign from birth and the students who had learned to sign between ages 6 and 12.

Visual Tasks

The visual modality is a keystone for learning and communication among deaf individuals. The importance of vision has led researchers and educators to look at the role it plays in cognition and whether vision is a modality of enhanced abilities for deaf individuals.

Chovan, Waldron, and Rose (1988) observed that deaf middle- and high-school students found visual problem-solving tasks to be easier to solve than hearing students did. In order to distinguish the effects of deafness per se from use of sign language, Parasnis, Samar, Bettger, and Sathe (1996) analyzed the visual spatial skills of deaf nonsigners. They found no enhancement of visual spatial cognition in deaf children who did not sign.

In addition to research that has focused on how the deaf child acquires knowledge and uses information, the relationship between cognitive development and language development has been of particular interest to educators and researchers.

COGNITION AND LANGUAGE

The relationship between cognition and language acquisition is an interdependent one. Language acquisition occurs as a result of the interaction between the child's innate cognitive abilities, cognitive strategies, and conceptual knowledge. As noted in Chapter 3, Rice and Kemper (1984) described this interaction with the analogy of a growing plant. The seed of the plant is the child's innate cognitive abilities. The seed provides the child with the cognitive capacity to make sense of the language used with the child by individuals in the child's environment. The root system is the child's developing conceptual knowledge as he or she interacts with the environment. The stem, branches, and leaves are the child's developing language as he or she interacts with individuals. This root system supports the above-ground plant when it sends its roots in the direction of water, just as cognitive development supports language development. The above-ground plant supports the root system when it sends its leaves in the direction of light, just as language development supports cognitive development.

Deaf children begin life with a language seed that is full of cognitive potential. They need a fertile environment that will enable the language seed to grow into a mature language plant.

Although many articles and books discuss the issue of language and cognition, there is actually little research about the relationship between language development and cognitive development in deaf children. And there is even less that provides strategies for improving language through cognition and improving cognitive development through language. Two areas of study have offered this perspective.

Cognitive and Linguistic Demands

Classrooms place cognitive and linguistic demands on children that are quite different from the conversational demands of everyday communication. Researchers such as Cazden (1988), Heath (1983), and Wells (1986) have examined the differences between school discourse and home discourse. One common type of school discourse, for example, is "question–answer–evaluate," sometimes called *question–answer routines.* In a question–answer routine, the teacher asks question after question, as in the following scenario:

> **Teacher:** Lynn, what is the capital of Ohio?
>
> **Lynn:** Columbus.
>
> **Teacher:** That's right. Tina, where is the Olentangy River?
>
> **Tina:** In Cleveland?

The child who is called upon is supposed to give a brief answer. And the teacher's next question does not necessarily follow logically from the child's answer. If the same topic were being discussed conversationally, it might progress as in the following scenario:

> **Teacher:** Lynn, tell me about the capital of Ohio.
>
> **Lynn:** It's Columbus.
>
> **Teacher:** Columbus is …

Lynn: Well, Columbus is in the center of Ohio. Maybe that's why it's the capital.

Tina: I'm moving to Columbus. My mom is going to work at Ohio State University.

Teacher: I know that Columbus has a river running through it.

Tina: Yes, it has a funny name, like old and tangy.

Lynn: You mean Olentangy.

Another feature of school discourse is the amount of language produced by the adult when compared to the child. Classroom discourse is marked by a high proportion of teacher language and a relatively small proportion of individual child language.

Other features of school discourse involve the kinds of control over the interaction that is maintained by the teacher. Unlike conversations with parents and peers, the teacher controls the choice of topic, takes longer turns, monitors who takes turns and how long their turns are, and determines when the topic should be changed or terminated.

The patterns of discourse in classrooms with deaf children may be similar but not identical to patterns of discourse in classrooms with hearing and deaf children. Johnson and Griffith (1986) examined a spelling lesson in two fourth-grade classrooms. They found that the regular classroom was characterized by rapid conversational shifts, complex academic tasks, and complex language structures. In contrast, the deaf education classroom was characterized by routinized academic tasks and relatively simple language structures.

When children are not fluent in the language of instruction, cognitive and linguistic demands may make it difficult or even impossible for the child to be an engaged learner. Cummins (1984, 1987) conceptualized the cognitive and linguistic demands of classrooms as being on a continuum, with context-embedded and cognitively undemanding communication at one end and context-reduced and cognitively demanding communication at the other.

Figure 4.1 conceptualizes Cummins's continuum in a school environment with deaf students. At the level in which the communication is context-embedded and cognitively undemanding, such as a basketball game during recess, the deaf child would interact quite effectively both receptively and expressively. However, as context was reduced and cognitive demands were increased, the language proficiency needed by the deaf child would increase commensurately. Without the language skill to understand complex and abstract concepts within minimal communicative context, the deaf child would have extreme difficulty understanding

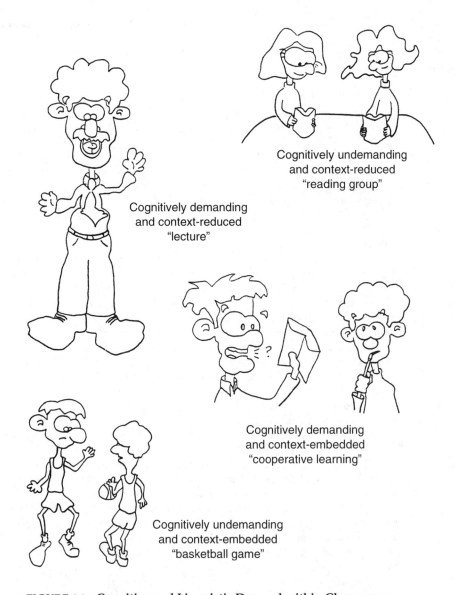

FIGURE 4.1 **Cognitive and Linguistic Demand within Classrooms**

the teacher and the content being taught. This context-reduced and cognitively demanding context is quite typical of much instruction, particularly at the high school level.

Two young deaf men are described in Essays 4.1 and 4.2. Their ability to handle classroom communication reflects contrastive needs.

ESSAY 4.1

Signs of Success

JOE HENDERSON

This story doesn't have anything to do with distance running—at least not directly. But it has everything to do with the values that runners hold dear—enduring and overcoming obstacles.

My son Eric dabbled in track during high school, and he'd gotten pretty good at sprinting (nearly qualifying for the state meet twice in the 100 meters) before leaving the sport. He found bigger "races" to run as he picked up speed academically and socially.

Eric was born with limited hearing. When this was discovered at age 3, he was fitted with hearing aids (which so annoyed him that he tried to flush one down the toilet and fed the other to the family dog).

He hadn't yet voiced his first word at that time, and without signing he had no access to language. The advice given us at the time was, "Put him in an oral program. This will give him a better chance of learning to speak than if he relied on sign as his first language." He wouldn't speak in sentences until his sixth year, and because of this his mainstream classes made little sense to him. He had to repeat an early school year.

Eric hit a bigger wall when he started middle school. He joined a new group of strangers at the worst of all ages. He was the only boy like himself at a time when the greatest sin is to be different. Each school day became a lonely, threatening ordeal.

He needed a change, and his younger sister, Leslie, pointed the way. She, too, is hearing-impaired, and that year she'd started attending the Oregon School for the Deaf (OSD). Eric visited there, saw kids like himself working in classrooms, and said, "I want to come here next year."

The move seemed like a mistake at first. "It was like I'd been sent away to prison," Eric said later. "I thought my life was over." He now felt lost between two worlds—at home with neither the deaf nor the hearing.

Staying at the school for the deaf depressed him, but going back to his old school terrified him. So that summer he decided to "stay at OSD, try to get along with everybody and improve my life." He later came to realize that "in regular school I would have always been 'that deaf kid.' Here, at OSD, I'm just another kid."

He did things there that he would never have tried at a regular school: ran track and played football, coedited the school's yearbook and literature magazine. He traveled to an academic competition against other schools for the deaf. He appeared before the state legislature on behalf of a bill to allow out-of-state students to attend his school—and shook hands with the governor at the law's signing.

At graduation he walked first to the stage among members of his class, and began speaking, "I am Eric Joseph Henderson," he said, "salutatorian of the class of 1997." He simultaneously signed and spoke his welcoming remarks. He now attends a regular university, not one for the deaf. He has held jobs among the hearing, and has some friends who hear and some who don't.

The boy who was caught between the worlds of speakers and signers is now a 21-year-old man equally at home in both. Eric, the nondistance runner, has taught his dad and many others some new meanings for enduring and winning.

Reprinted with permission of Joe Henderson. Originally published in *Runner's World*, December 1998.

ESSAY 4.2

David Brandel

I attend Amherst High School in New York. I am 20 years old and a senior. I have had the opportunity of experiencing both Deaf culture and hearing culture through my education.

I went to Windermere Elementary School in Amherst, which is a public school. Then I changed schools and went to St. Mary's School for the Deaf in Buffalo. This was in 1991. I had no idea what it was like to be in a deaf school. I had to learn how to adjust to both speaking and signing at the same time. My classmates seemed wild and crazy. That first year I failed most of my classes.

A year and a half went by. My mother, teachers, district officials, and the principal of the elementary department had a meeting to discuss moving me to the B.O.C.E.S. (Board of Cooperative Educational Services) program. They agreed that I should be placed in a special education class at Amherst Middle School, and I moved there in January of 1993. During my two years in middle school, my educational test scores improved a lot, and I received good marks on my report card.

It took a lot of time for me to change from Deaf culture to hearing culture because of the way deaf people used to communicate with other people. But I also felt comfortable going into hearing culture because I had dealt with a lot of hearing people, including my family. During this time, I changed my attitude. I started working very hard to succeed and to achieve better marks. Also, my behavior improved when I moved from the Deaf school to the hearing school. It was easier for me to communicate with other people during a conversation by using speech instead of signing. I was able to make more friends, and it was easier to deal with my family issues using speech. For example, my parents make sure I am looking at them when they are talking to me.

I graduated in the class of 2000. I felt wonderful to be part of my class. I worked hard through my high school years to keep up my grades. My teachers were very happy with the quality of my work. My plans for my future are to go to a two-year college and become a building maintenance worker in the construction field. I am also thinking about going into the automotive field.

Reprinted by permission of the author.

Wood (1991) noted that the deaf child is also confronted with the issue of divided attention during instruction.

> When a hearing child is struggling to put a jigsaw puzzle together, we can help by talking to the child about his or her actions. The child, meanwhile, is left free to look at what he or she is doing. We might go further in attempting to help or to teach by talking to the child while we point to or show a piece of the puzzle. We pace the timing of our talk to fit the child's actions. What we say can be brought to life by what the child sees. So much is obvious and mundane. The deaf child, however, faces additional cognitive demands in this situation. If we say or sign something to the child, he or she must look away from the object of communication to what is being communicated. At the least, it seems likely that these memory demands make learning through instruction more difficult for the child. (p. 250)

Wood postulated that the experiential deficits and cognitive delays that have been observed among deaf children might be the result, in part, of these patterns of classroom discourse. When Strassman (1997) examined the relationship between metacognition and reading in children who are deaf, she found that instructional practices used to teach reading seem to be hindering rather than strengthening the deaf child's ability to strategically reflect on his or her own thinking processes and learning. For example, she found that deaf children typically think that the purpose of reading is to complete worksheets, answer teacher questions, and memorize vocabulary words, and that these are the activities on which they spend most of their instructional reading time in school.

Symbolic Play and Language Development

The child's ability to symbolize is manifested in the emergence of language and imaginative play during the second year of life (Musatti, 1986; Vandenberg, 1981). As aspects of the child's semiotic function, both language and play require that the child be able to represent reality in thought (Piaget, 1962). This relationship between the early development of language and the beginnings of symbolic play have also been found in studies of children with developmental delays, mental retardation, and language delays (Casby & Ruder, 1983; Lombardino & Sproul, 1984; Terrell, Schwartz, Prelock, & Messick, 1984).

Investigations into the imaginative play of deaf children have shown a similar correspondence between language development and symbolic play, with delays in language corresponding to delays in imaginative play (Blum, Fields, Scharfman, & Silber, 1994; Casby & McCormick, 1985; Darbyshire, 1977). Schirmer (1989) found that the 3- to 6-year-old deaf children in her study engaged in imaginative play, and these imaginative play behaviors were related to their language development level but not to their chronological ages. The deaf children at later stages of language development demonstrated higher percentages of time engaged in imaginative play and greater use of higher level symbolic play behaviors such as telling about a scenario that they intended to carry out, which is called *planned play,* and developing a scenario for the play action, which is called *story line.*

The cognitive abilities of deaf individuals have been studied from both theoretical and applied perspectives. Much of the research on intelligence, memory, and cognitive development is theoretical in nature. The research on thinking skills is typically applied in nature, as researchers have tried to determine how to improve the critical and creative thinking and problem-solving skills of deaf students.

THINKING PROCESSES AND SKILLS

Deaf individuals have stereotypically been characterized as concrete thinkers. Indeed, Myklebust (1964) described deaf individuals as having a more concrete intelligence than hearing individuals. Zwiebel and Mertens (1985) found that the deaf children in their study, who were between ages 6 and 15, tended to rely on visual/perceptual skills, whereas the hearing children, who were 10 to 12 years of age, relied on abstract thinking skills. Tzuriel and Caspi (1992) obtained a similar finding with deaf and hearing children between ages 4 and 6. Although there is no evidence to indicate that deaf individuals are unable to think abstractly, it appears that deaf children need to be guided in developing their thinking at levels beyond the concrete.

Laughton (1988) used art lessons as a medium for encouraging creativity among elementary students at a day school for the deaf. The creativity curriculum was designed to develop four nonverbal components of creative thinking—fluency, flexibility, originality, and elaboration. Every lesson started with a brainstorming session, and during the lesson, the children were encouraged to engage in these four components of creative thinking. Results indicated that the children improved significantly in flexibility and originality but not in fluency and elaboration. Laughton concluded that deaf children "can be taught strategies for developing their creative abilities within a typical school setting. This type of information should encourage reexamination of the stereotypes regarding divergent thinking deficiencies of deaf students" (p. 262).

Several researchers have attempted to improve the reasoning skills of deaf children. Peterson and Peterson (1989, 1990) approached reasoning from a social cognitive perspective. They explored whether deaf children who were confronted with a situation that engaged them in cognitive conflict would make progress in their reasoning skills. In one study, they used a positive justice task to improve reasoning. The students were shown a video with a boy, a smaller girl, and an adult male. In the first sequence, the boy and girl load bricks into a wheelbarrow, wheel it to a spot where other bricks have been stacked, and unload the wheelbarrow. During the wheeling, the girl clearly struggles with the weight of the bricks. After doing this several times, the adult enters with chocolate candy bars in his hand. The video is stopped, and the children in the study were asked to give as much chocolate to the boy and girl as they deserve, and then asked to explain why they chose the number they did. The video is then resumed, and the father is shown giving more chocolate to the boy than the girl. The children were then asked if the father was right to do this and after replying, to reallocate their own chocolate again and explain why. The researchers found no delay in the justice reasoning of the deaf children when compared to the hearing children in the study, but being confronted by an adult-generated contradiction did not improve the deaf children's reasoning ability. In a second study, Peterson and Peterson used a peer debate procedure. They paired deaf children and asked them to solve a logical problem that neither child would have been able to solve independently. Results indicated that peer debate promoted reasoning among the deaf children.

Geisser (1990) addressed reasoning from the perspective of logical thinking. At the Rhode Island School for the Deaf, a curriculum was developed to teach logic to the students, which they called the "Philosophy for Children" program. The curriculum engaged the children in thinking and discussing syllogisms such as the following:

All _____ are _____ . No _____ are _____ . Some _____ are not _____ . Some _____ are _____ .

She found that the curriculum improved the students' ability to draw conclusions, make inferences, and develop thoughtful inquiry.

In addition to creative thinking and reasoning, educators have been interested in improving the problem-solving skills of deaf children. As Luckner and McNeill (1994) noted, bodies of knowledge become outdated, but problem solving transcends time, place, and kinds of knowledge. Their research indicated that deaf and hard of hearing students do not perform as well as hearing students on problem-solving tasks, but the gap narrows with age. The reason for the low performance in problem solving may be that it is not taught, which is what Luckner found in a 1992 study. According to Luckner and McNeill:

> If deaf students are to participate successfully in society, they must be provided with learning experiences in school that adequately prepare them for successful participation. In a society that is becoming technologically more

advanced and that requires increasingly diverse skills, deaf individuals may benefit from opportunities to develop problem-solving strategies and abilities that can be generalized to postschool employment and independent living situations. (1994, p. 376)

Schirmer and Woolsey (1997) used a thinking skills hierarchy to develop questions that encouraged deaf children to think abstractly and critically. These questions were then used as a template during reading instruction. The questions required the children to analyze, synthesize, and evaluate what they were reading. The set of questions in Figure 4.2 were found to be effective in encouraging higher level thinking and, indeed, did not need to be supported with questions that also required literal level thinking, such as questions related to story details. In the early 1980s, David Martin and other researchers began to study a cognitive skills program called Instrumental Enrichment.

Instrumental Enrichment

Instrumental Enrichment was originally developed by Feurstein, a cognitive psychologist who was a student of Piaget. The program was developed to provide what Feurstein called a mediated learning experience for culturally disadvantaged groups emigrating to Israel in the early 1950s (Martin, 1992). The program was a supplement to the curriculum, and it was designed to engage the children in a series of increasingly difficult tasks that were contrived to develop and enhance cognitive skills (Martin, Rohr, & Innes, 1982). The objectives of Instrumental Enrichment

FIGURE 4.2 **Questions That Encourage Higher Level Thinking**

Why did (the character) do (the action)?

What's the main idea of this story?

What kind of story is this?

What does (the author or the character) (believe or assume) ?

What would have happened if …?

What would be a better (action or ending)?

How would you have solved (the character's) problem?

What doesn't make sense? Is this (action or behavior) logical?

Do you see any (errors or inconsistencies or fallacies) in the story?

What are the (strengths or weaknesses) of this story?

are to improve spatial reasoning, ability to manipulate several sources of information simultaneously, and to understand cause-and-effect relationships (Martin, 1983). The program consists of fifteen instruments, which are curriculum guides and paper-and-pencil exercises. They are taught for approximately one hour per day, three to five days per week, for two to three years. The program, therefore, is intended to teach thinking skills separate from content area instruction.

The first study of the Instrumental Enrichment program was conducted after a two-year pilot project at the Model Secondary School for the Deaf at Gallaudet. Martin (1984) found that the students involved in the program showed improvement in problem solving, nonverbal logical thinking, abstract thinking, reading comprehension, and mathematical computation. Other researchers found equally positive results with deaf students in a variety of educational programs including residential and day schools (Haywood, Towery-Woolsey, Arbitman-Smith, & Aldridge, 1988; Huberty & Koller, 1984; Johnson, 1988; Keane & Kretschmer, 1987). Martin also conducted studies of the Instrumental Enrichment program with deaf college students and found similarly positive results in logical reasoning, reading comprehension, math concepts, and math computation (Martin & Jonas, 1989).

After more than a decade of using Instrumental Enrichment with deaf students, Martin noted that "progress is not made overnight and there is no 'quick fix' when one is serious about teaching higher order reasoning to learners at any level. Incorporating these strategies into the student's repertoire is an incremental process" (1993, p. 86).

Although Instrumental Enrichment is a supplementary curriculum, some approaches to thinking skills instruction are incorporated within content area instruction.

Promoting Thinking during Instruction

Marzano and his associates (1988) developed a framework for curriculum and instruction that they called *dimensions of thinking.* They did not intend this framework to be used as a taxonomy or a scope and sequence chart. Rather, they hoped it would be used in conjunction with learning regular classroom content and "as a means to comprehending a theory, solving a problem, or drafting an essay" (p. 5).

Figure 4.3 is a conceptualization of how the dimensions of thinking interrelate and can be used with other taxonomies and thinking skills frameworks. The four dimensions include metacognition, critical and creative thinking, thinking processes, and thinking skills. Metacognition involves monitoring one's own thinking. Metacognition is viewed as overarching in that deaf children should always be examining when they

know and when they do not, what they know and do not, what they
need to know, and what to do. At the next level, deaf children should be
continuously engaged in thinking critically and creatively. Critical thinking involves making evaluative judgments, and creative thinking involves generating new ideas. Again, regardless of the specific thinking
process or skill in which the child is engaged, he or she should be evaluating the idea and combining ideas in new ways. The next level involves
thinking processes. Marzano and associates identified eight processes—
concept formation, principle formation, research (called *inquiry* here),
comprehending, problem solving, decision making, composing, and oral
discourse (called *communicating* here). Each are defined in Figure 4.3.

Thinking skills should be placed at the center of the framework.
Marzano and associates identified eight core thinking skills:

- *Focusing.* Defining problems and setting goals
- *Information-gathering.* Observing and formulating questions
- *Remembering.* Encoding and recalling
- *Organizing.* Comparing, classifying, ordering, and representing
- *Analyzing.* Identifying attributes and characteristics, relationships
  and patterns, main ideas, and errors
- *Generating.* Inferring, predicting, and elaborating
- *Integrating.* Summarizing and restructuring
- *Evaluating.* Setting criteria or standards and verifying

This list is not exhaustive nor does it represent the core thinking
skills that other authors have developed, which is why these specific
ones were not included in Figure 4.3. Teachers, psychologists, speech/
language pathologists, tutors, parents, and others can use any of the taxonomies and frameworks that have been developed. The most frequently
used taxonomy is Bloom's classification. He and his associates (Bloom et
al., 1956) classified the intellectual objectives of education into six lower
to higher levels: knowledge → comprehension → application → analysis
→ synthesis → evaluation.

Another popular taxonomy is Barrett's (1976), which was specifically designed to distinguish among the cognitive and affective dimensions of reading comprehension through four major levels: literal →
inferential → evaluation → appreciation.

Pearson and Johnson (1978) proposed a taxonomy of questions that
was designed to distinguish between information from the child's prior
knowledge and information from a written source.

- Textually explicit questions have answers that are obvious in the
  written material.

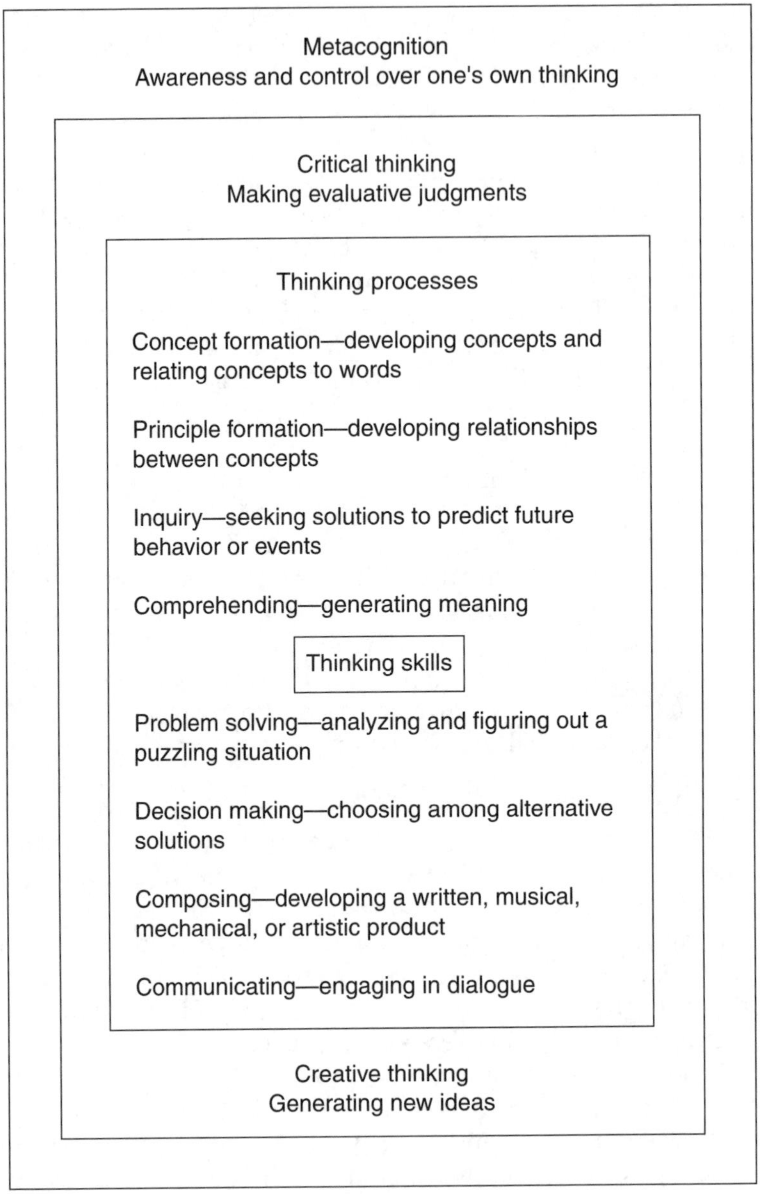

Metacognition
Awareness and control over one's own thinking

Critical thinking
Making evaluative judgments

Thinking processes

Concept formation—developing concepts and
relating concepts to words

Principle formation—developing relationships
between concepts

Inquiry—seeking solutions to predict future
behavior or events

Comprehending—generating meaning

Thinking skills

Problem solving—analyzing and figuring out a
puzzling situation

Decision making—choosing among alternative
solutions

Composing—developing a written, musical,
mechanical, or artistic product

Communicating—engaging in dialogue

Creative thinking
Generating new ideas

FIGURE 4.3   Framework for Developing Thinking

- Textually implicit questions have answers in the written material, but the answers are not obvious.
- Scriptally implicit questions have answers that come from the child's prior knowledge; the question is related to the written material, but the answer cannot be found there.

Raths and his associates (1986) suggested that teachers use the following list as a core group of thinking operations:

- *Comparing.* Observing similarities and differences
- *Summarizing.* Briefly stating the substance of information
- *Observing.* Watching, noting, and perceiving
- *Classifying.* Sorting things into groups according to some principle
- *Interpreting.* Putting meaning into an experience
- *Criticizing.* Analyzing and evaluating
- *Looking for assumptions.* Deciding what is being taken for granted
- *Imagining.* Perceiving beyond the idea that has actually been presented
- *Collecting and organizing data.* Independently seeking information and collating the findings
- *Hypothesizing.* Proposing a possible solution to a problem
- *Applying facts and principles in new situations.* Determining which facts and principles are relevant and using the relevant ones to predict what will happen in a new situation

The framework can be used by teachers and others who work with deaf students as a method for monitoring the continuous incorporation of thinking into instruction and interaction.

SUMMARY AND CONCLUDING THOUGHTS

This chapter discussed the cognitive abilities of deaf individuals from the perspective of several bodies of information—intelligence, memory, cognitive development, cognition and language, and thinking processes and skills. The relationship between cognition, language, and experience is complex. The deaf learner has the same cognitive capability as the hearing learner, but linguistic and experiential factors often impede the cognitive development of the deaf child. As Martin (1993) noted, "Cognitive potential is not equivalent to achievement. The purpose of systematic cognitive strategy instruction is to incorporate techniques found to be most effective with deaf learners, along with the strong and proven principles of cognitive strategy instruction for all learners, so that deaf learners indeed can reach their full cognitive potential" (p. 85).

CHAPTER FIVE

PERSONAL AND SOCIAL DEVELOPMENT

FOCUS QUESTIONS

- Why did early research indicate that deafness imposes a variety of personality problems and disorders whereas recent research does not attribute disordered personality constellations to deafness?

- Is there reason to believe that deaf children will have more difficulty than hearing children in social development?

- What is the role of language in the social interaction of deaf children, adolescents, and adults?

- What are the barriers to social integration between deaf and hearing individuals?

- How successful are programs designed to improve social skills?

Personal and social development often seem to take a backseat during the early and adolescent years of deaf children because of the focus on language development and academic progress. The importance of social interaction and personal growth is never, of course, underestimated by the deaf person and rarely overlooked by parents. It is, perhaps, only educators and other professionals who seem to forget at times that the personal and social dimensions are equally important as the academic ones, and that language ability is connected irrevocably to using language with others. This chapter begins with the personal dimensions of development.

IDENTITY AND PERSONALITY

This book views identity as the child's sense of self and personality as a set of characteristics that are shared, consistent, and observable.

Identity

How does the deaf child develop a sense of self? Finn (1995) asserted that self-concept and identity could only be developed successfully "through the ongoing process of social interactions with people surrounding the child, either hearing or deaf. The key to this interaction is communication. The most effective communication for hearing children is through their sense of hearing, but for deaf children through their sense of vision" (p. 2).

The deaf individual's identity is multifaceted, including a set of unique, as well as culturally shared, characteristics and attributes. One aspect involves degree of hearing loss. A profoundly deaf individual has an identity different from a hard of hearing individual. Lutes (1987) described hard of hearing individuals as "caught between the normal hearing and the deaf, in 'no man's land' without a clear identity" (p. 74). Mottez (1990) distinguished between the oral deaf identity, which views the world "as a continuum with no sharp divisions, ranging from the hearing all the way to the deaf," and the signing Deaf identity, for whom "the division of the world between deaf and hearing is cultural and clear cut" (pp. 214–215).

Weinberg and Sterritt (1986) examined the identity patterns in adolescents attending a state school for the deaf. They found that the students with a primary hearing identity were rated poorest in academic placement, social relationships, personal adjustment, and perceived family acceptance. Students with a primary deaf identity were rated higher on all measures than the students with a primary hearing identity. However, students with a dual identity (that is, they identified with both hearing and deaf populations) were rated highest on all measures. The authors recognized that it is not possible to determine whether a dual identity resulted in better adjustment or whether adolescents who were having better academic and social experiences were more likely to develop a dual identity. They did, however, suggest that the deaf child should be encouraged to identify with both hearing and deaf groups.

This difference between identity groups was not found by Cole and Edelmann (1991) when they investigated the self-perceptions of deaf adolescents. The adolescents with a hearing identity, deaf identity, and dual identity did not differ significantly in their responses and did not report having greater problems than their hearing peers. Interestingly, their teachers reported the students as having greater problems than the students self-reported, which the authors suggested may account for the relatively high incidence of behavior difficulties that have been found in studies based strictly on teacher ratings.

One of the issues discussed in Chapter 3 is multiculturalism. As the deaf child develops an individual identity, his or her multiple cultures will influence the shaping of this identity. For example, the Deaf child who is African American has two obvious cultural influences, but this view is undoubtedly narrow. Anderson and Grace (1991) noted that this child's "multicultural reality is presumed to include at least four distinct cultures: African-American, European-American, hearing and Deaf cultures" (p. 73). A fifth culture might be added if the child is also influenced by a separate Deaf/African American culture.

Personality

Much of the research on personality constellations of deaf individuals has suggested a variety of problems and disorders. Some of these issues are addressed in Chapter 6 on mental health. But it is important to note in this chapter that we have relatively little information on the development of personality in deaf children. Rather, the research has focused almost exclusively on how personality structures of deaf individuals deviate from normal and healthy structures. The critical question is whether these constellations are an accurate depiction.

Studies during the 1960s and 1970s profiled the deaf individual as typically egocentric, rigid, immature, lacking empathy, constricted, deficient in social adaptiveness, impulsive, suggestible, and lacking an inner locus of control (Altshuler, 1971, 1978; Freeman, Malkin, & Hastings, 1975; Vernon, 1967a; Williams, 1970). Later studies, however, contradicted these findings.

Feinstein conducted a series of studies with deaf adolescents utilizing a case study approach and found that they were more vulnerable to adjustment difficulties because of the stress associated with communication and not because deafness presented a particular deviant or deficient personality structure (Feinstein, 1983; Feinstein & Lytle, 1987). Chess and Fernandez (1980) viewed the difficulties of rubella children as directly related to neurologic damage rather than deafness or communication. Sinkkonen (1998) found no inherent deaf personality among Finnish deaf and hard of hearing children. The deaf and hard of hearing children in this study, who virtually represented the complete population in Finland, were not more impulsive than the hearing children in the sample, and when impulsivity was a characteristic, it was connected specifically to communication problems.

Another possible explanation for the deaf personality constellation is the language of the testing situation. Edmunds, Rodda, Cumming, and Fox (1992) proposed that difficulties with written English underlie the performance of deaf individuals on tests of personality. After examining the research describing the personality of deaf individuals as deviant, they concluded, "There is good reason to suggest that descriptions of the personality structures of deaf people parallel those that address the written language of deaf people" (p. 108).

One aspect of personality involves the individual's attribution for success and failure. Individuals with an internal locus of control believe that they can control life's events. Individuals with an external locus of control believe that life's events, such as rewards and punishments, are the result of factors such as chance, luck, or fate (Pervin, 1996). Research with deaf student populations has indicated that they hold patterns of locus of control beliefs similar to hearing populations, which tend to be internal more than external. In a series of studies, Wolk found no support for the commonly held belief that deaf children and young adults have a locus of control orientation that predisposes them to place blame on others and environmental factors (Wolk, 1985; Wolk & Beach, 1986). Instead, this research provides support for the conclusion that deaf students vary their attribution of causes and solutions of personal and academic problems, depending on the type of problem, and they tend to maintain a stronger internal than external locus of control.

Another aspect of personality involves an individual's tolerance for ambiguity. Brice (1985) hypothesized that deaf children would have a higher tolerance for ambiguity because they are so used to being in situations and in conversations that are not fully clear to them. He presented hearing and deaf children with a set of pictures that changed slowly from one animal to another. He found that the hearing children responded significantly more quickly to changes in the pictures than the deaf children, and the hearing children were more likely to demand an explanation from the experimenter.

One deaf child's personality is described eloquently by her father in Essay 5.1, Fast Finisher.

■ ■ ■ ■ ■ ■ ▬▬▬▬▬▬▬▬▬▬▬▬▬▬▬▬▬▬▬▬▬▬▬▬▬

ESSAY 5.1

Fast Finisher

JOE HENDERSON

My daughter, Leslie, was a slow starter in life. She arrived late, on Labor Day 1982, and was late leaving the hospital because of a blood disorder.

In her first six months, Leslie gained only 2 pounds, then nearly died during heart surgery. Her recovery was complicated by anemia so severe she required several transfusions.

Oh, yes, Leslie also has Down syndrome and is deaf. She didn't sit up until she was 2 years old and didn't walk until she was almost 4. She'll never talk.

If you picture Down syndrome kids as slow moving, forget it. If you think of deaf kids as wordless, forget that, too. Neither description fits Leslie.

From the day she stood up and took her first steps, she's been making up for lost time. And for what Leslie lacks in voice, she compensates with sign language.

She and her mother live next door to a dairy, and Leslie once took me there to make the appropriate introductions in signs. "Cows, this is Dad. Dad, these are cows." She lives in a world where animals know her language, where there are no bad people and where the future is never more than a day away.

Of my three children, Leslie is the most high-energy. She makes Sarah (who's on the fast track in her newspaper job) and Eric (who was a good 100-meter-dash man before his school dropped track) look sleepy by comparison.

Leslie is Ms. Sprinter. One of her favorite ways to spend a morning is playing at Hayward Field, the famous University of Oregon track. This has been true since I first took her there soon after she began walking.

Leslie doesn't know Hayward's name, but she has signs for it: "run" (as in around the track); "climb" (as in up and down the grandstands); "jump" (as in on top of the pole-vault pit); and "dig" (as in into the long-jump sand).

So, when the opportunity arose, it seemed only natural that Leslie would choose to enter the Special Olympics. We went to a meet this spring.

"What does Leslie want to do?" asked the woman in charge.

"She likes to run," I told her. "Which distances do you have?"

"We can start her with the 50 meters. If she likes that, she can also do the 100."

Leslie lined up, with two other runners, in the eighth heat of the 50. She knew about the starting line and about running in lines. Some other things she didn't comprehend so well.

She signed an "8" to me, indicating this was her favorite lane. Fine, but the other two runners were in lanes 1 and 2. This left her all alone on the outside of the track. I had to coax her over to lane 3.

Leslie didn't understand about starts, either. The other two runners took off when signaled. Leslie held her ground. She didn't start after them until they were about 10 meters down the track.

Even with the delayed start, Leslie caught one of the others. After finishing, she flopped dramatically onto her back, arms spread wide, eyes closed, tongue hanging out. (She and I like to watch televised track meets together; no doubt she was mimicking the runners she's seen on TV.)

The idea at a Special Olympics meet is to award lots of medals to everyone, if possible. Often this is achieved by limiting every heat to just three participants and by counting each heat as a separate event with its own gold, silver and bronze medal winners.

As a result, the awards ceremonies last almost as long as the competitions. The announcement for Leslie's race came as, "The winners in the eighth heat of the 50 meters are..."

She knew just what to do on the victory stand. After having the medal draped around her neck, she pumped both arms for 10 seconds of triumph.

For everything she has achieved in the last 14 years, Leslie deserved her moment on the victory platform. I quietly but emotionally celebrated *all* her triumphs.

Reprinted with permission of Joe Henderson. Originally published in *Runner's World*, October 1996.

In addition to the development of identity and personality, personal and social development involve morals, ethics, and values.

MORALS, ETHICS, AND VALUES

There is little information available on the development of morals, ethics, and values in deaf children. Investigators who have studied these issues have become somewhat mired in definitions, instruments, and bias.

Sam and Wright (1988) examined the structure of moral reasoning in deaf adolescents. The adolescents in this study exhibited a lag in their moral reasoning ability that appeared to be directly related to their language development level. The researchers observed that some of the adolescents were highly egocentric in their thinking and had little inclination to compromise or take another's perspective. Many of the adolescents demonstrated their knowledge of social rules but not any real understanding of the reasoning behind them.

Markoulis and Christoforou (1991, 1993) found no differences between the sociomoral reasoning of deaf and hearing children, but suggested that the deaf child may have difficulty acquiring more complex sociomoral reasoning structures because of the relationship between peer interactions, reciprocal role taking, cognitive development, and sociomoral reasoning. Arnold (1993) argued, however, that Markoulis and Christoforou's suggestion is ungrounded, given that the deaf children in their study exhibited no lag in sociomoral reasoning.

When teachers of deaf children were asked to prioritize the personal and social competencies needed by deaf students, White (1982) found that they identified three areas as most in need of improvement— accepting responsibility for one's actions; awareness of one's values, strengths, weaknesses, interests, and goals; and making sound decisions. The teachers also identified self-confidence, initiative, and dependability as important but not urgent.

Keenan (1993) explored the apologies of deaf adolescents. She found that their written apologies had a routinized feel and were seen by others as being a rather blunt response to the situation in large part because of their inability to express themselves adequately in written English.

Although personal development has received relatively little attention by researchers, the social development of deaf individuals has been a venue of great interest, particularly social integration and social skills.

SOCIAL INTEGRATION AND SOCIAL SKILLS

In the mid-1980s, a colleague and I examined the literature on the social development of deaf children and their integration within classrooms

(Hummel & Schirmer, 1984). In light of the attention being given to increased mainstreaming at that time, we were interested in understanding our state of knowledge about the social skills of deaf children and the impact of integrated education. We found research indicating that deaf individuals have adequate social development but poorer social adjustment and problems of social integration with hearing peers. The studies we read supported the development of social skills training programs for deaf students as part of their school curriculum. It is interesting to examine subsequent research to see whether our conclusions are still well founded, to evaluate the progress made in developing social skills programs, and to determine whether these programs have been effective.

Social Abilities and Adjustment

When compared to hearing children, some studies indicate that deaf children demonstrate lower levels of performance on measures that are designed to assess social abilities whereas the opposite finding has emerged in other studies. One explanation for the discrepancy may be language level in English or ASL. Weisel and Bar-Lev (1992) suggested that the deaf child's social ability is strongly related to language ability; when language ability is weak, social ability will suffer. Another group of researchers found that delayed language has no obvious effect on the social skills of young deaf children, but early language difficulty appears to impede long-term social development and adjustment (Musselman, MacKay, Trehub, & Eagle, 1996). This finding leads to age as a second possible explanation for the discrepancy. However, when Cole and Shade (1985) examined the social adjustment of deaf adolescents, they found similar patterns of well-being for deaf and hearing adolescents.

Comparisons between groups of deaf children have provided insight into the influence of factors such as sign language, degree of hearing loss, and educational setting (Furstenberg & Doyal, 1994; James, 1986; Macklin & Matson, 1985; Minnett, Clark, & Wilson, 1994; Weisel, 1988b). The following observations seem to be reasonable based on the available research:

- The social adjustment of deaf children with deaf parents is not better or worse than the social adjustment of deaf children with hearing parents.
- The social functioning of deaf children is not better or worse than the social functioning of hard of hearing children.
- Deaf students in residential school settings are less socially mature than deaf students in mainstream settings.

Social abilities are developed within multiple social contexts including sports and extracurricular activities. The importance of sports to the social development of deaf children and the social lives of deaf adults was investigated by Stewart and his associates (Stewart, 1993b; Stewart, McCarthy, & Robinson, 1988; Stewart, Robinson, & McCarthy, 1991). They were particularly interested in exploring what they referred to as *deaf sport,* which is a term that "encompasses both the activities that surround the organization and planning of games and the socialization aspects in which participants and spectators are involved. There are no differences in the rules and playing of games by the deaf, as no physical impairments are present that would require them; a deaf athlete is not a disabled athlete" (Stewart, 1986, pp. 196–197). Deaf sport involves the organization of sporting events by deaf individuals and for deaf participants. They found:

- The effect of equity among deaf participants and the ease of communicating in a common language serve to draw deaf individuals into deaf sport rather than hearing sports activities.
- Schools for the deaf and deaf friends are the typical conduit for bringing deaf individuals into deaf sport.
- Deaf sport is more preferred for recreation and socialization, whereas hearing sport is more preferred for competition among deaf athletes.
- As increasing numbers of deaf students are educated in inclusive settings, public school programs and hearing sport clubs will become important arenas for recruiting deaf individuals into deaf sport.
- Deaf sport is a milieu for socialization among spectators as well as the participants.

In addition to deaf sport, extracurricular activities can provide deaf students with socialization opportunities that positively influence their social development. Stewart and Stinson (1992) observed that extracurricular activities initially provide an entry to socializing with peers, which then naturally leads to unstructured, out-of-school social interactions. "In addition, extracurriculars provide deaf students with opportunities to enjoy themselves, to experience school in a more relaxed environment divorced from the threat of grades (although participation in some activities may require that students maintain at least a minimum grade in all subjects), and to interact with others on a common ground and in some instances in a more equitable fashion" (p. 140).

Social ability and social interaction are intertwined. The quality of social interaction in the deaf individual's life and the influences of social interaction on educational accomplishment have been studied from the vantage point of young childhood through adulthood.

Social Interaction

Social interaction is often equated with social integration in educational settings. During the mainstreaming movement of the 1970s, the regular education initiative of the 1980s, and the full inclusion movement of the 1990s, educators and parents were concerned about improving the educational opportunities of deaf children while simultaneously enhancing their ability to negotiate social relationships across and within minority and majority cultures.

Social Interaction during Preschool and Kindergarten

The social interaction of young deaf children has been examined from a number of perspectives. It should be no surprise that the research has been equivocal, given difference in characteristics of children, the variance in school settings, and the small numbers of children included within individual research studies. Much of the research has been conducted by Antia and Lederberg.

When social integration first became a focus of attention, researchers were interested in determining whether deaf children in public school classrooms were socially interacting with hearing children or whether they were simply sharing the same physical environment (Antia, 1982; Brackett & Henniges, 1976; Kennedy, Northcott, McCauley, & Williams, 1976; McCauley & Bruninks, 1976). As expected, deaf children tended to interact more often with teachers than with their peers. Also, as expected, the reason for greater or less interaction involved communication. Deaf children with better oral skills interacted more often with hearing children than deaf children with poorer oral skills. Antia (1982) concluded that "physical proximity is a necessary but not solely sufficient condition for promoting interaction" and, therefore, educators must structure the educational environment in ways that foster social interaction (p. 24).

The role of language in social development and social interaction is a pivotal issue that has been confounded by the possible differing effects of oral English and ASL. Cornelius and her associates examined the play behaviors of deaf preschool and kindergarten children and found that the children in signing classrooms demonstrated higher levels of social play behavior and lower levels of aggression than the children in oral classrooms (Cornelius & Hornett, 1990; Cornelius & Sanders, 1987). Williams (1993) observed deaf preschool children interacting with one another as they worked at the classroom writing table during free-choice time. She found that the deaf children in the oral classroom interacted with one another less frequently than the deaf children in the signing classroom. Minnett, Clark, and Wilson (1994) observed that deaf and hard of hearing children in an auditory preschool environment tended to engage in more solitary play, whereas deaf and hard of hearing children in a signing preschool environment tended to engage in more parallel social play.

Regardless of communication, most of the research indicates that language plays an important role in social interaction. In a series of studies conducted by Antia and associates, deaf preschool children were consistently shown to engage in nonlinguistic interaction more frequently than linguistic interaction (Antia & Kreimeyer, 1987; Antia, Kreimeyer, & Eldredge, 1994; Kreimeyer & Antia, 1988). Lederberg (1991) examined the social interaction among deaf preschoolers and found that language and social skills develop independently of one another. However, she also found that language ability affects social interaction and play in a few key ways. Compared to deaf children with low language ability, deaf children with high language ability were more likely to engage in play activities that required linguistic interaction, such as playing in a group of three or more; they were more likely to choose playmates who also had high language ability; and they tended to use more language and expect playmates to use more language. When Spencer, Koester, and Meadow-Orlans (1994) analyzed the communicative interactions of deaf and hearing 2- and 3-year-old children in a day-care center, they found that language ability, not hearing status, was associated with the frequency of communication that the deaf child experienced. In other words, language ability mattered considerably more than being deaf.

Lederberg and her associates (1985, 1986, 1987, 1991) studied the social interaction of young deaf children from the standpoint of playmate preference. They found many similarities and few differences in the types of peer relationships developed by deaf and hearing preschoolers:

- Deaf and hearing preschoolers have two types of relationships, maintained and nonmaintained friendships. Nonmaintained friendships are temporary and change frequently. Maintained friendships are enduring and typically involve just one or two other children. Deaf preschool children tend to have fewer long-term friendships than hearing children.
- Nonlinguistic communication between deaf and hearing preschoolers seems sufficient for engaging in temporary play activities as well as for developing long-term friendships.
- Deaf and hearing children prefer to play with others of the same ethnicity, gender, and age.
- Social interaction between hearing and deaf playmates is more dependent on their familiarity with one another than the hearing child's prior experience in playing with other deaf children.

Classroom configurations offer differing opportunities for peer interactions. A deaf child in a classroom with other deaf children may exhibit different patterns of interaction than a deaf child in a classroom with hearing children. And these interactions may be different from the deaf child in a classroom with some deaf and some hearing children. For example, Esposito and Koorland (1989) found that young deaf children are more likely to engage in nonsocial, parallel play when in an environment with all other deaf children and in social, associative play when in an environment with hearing children. In environments where deaf children have deaf peers, they appear to prefer playing with deaf children and in these settings, hearing children also prefer playing with hearing children (Minnett, Clark, & Wilson, 1994; Spencer, Koester, & Meadow-Orlans, 1994).

Programs designed to facilitate the interaction between young deaf and hearing children will be discussed later in this chapter. The research since the 1970s has confirmed the importance of doing more than simply placing deaf children in an integrated environment and hoping that effective interaction would take place. Antia and Dittillo (1998) examined the peer social behaviors of deaf and hearing preschool, kindergarten, and first-grade children. They found the behaviors of these deaf and hearing children to be remarkably similar in an environment that facilitated social interaction. However, the adults in the environment are an important factor in developing a facilitative environment. For example, in one case study of a deaf preschooler, the strategy taught to the child by the teacher was ineffective for accessing social interactions, and the child's perseverance in using the strategy hindered interaction with his peers (Messenheimer-Young & Kretschmer, 1994).

Social Interaction during Childhood and Young Adolescence

The social interaction of school-age children and adolescents has been studied from a variety of different positions and points of view. Researchers have used child self-ratings, peer ratings, and teacher ratings. And some researchers have scrutinized social interaction by observing deaf children and adolescents with peers and adults.

Hagborg explored the social acceptability of deaf adolescents at a residential school by using sociometric ratings (1987, 1989b). He found that the students rated highest by their peers had been enrolled in the school for the deaf for longer periods of time, were more likely to be female than male, exhibited better behavioral adjustment, and were more likely to be Caucasian than from a minority culture. Coyner (1993) used sociometric ratings with deaf and hard of hearing students who were mainstreamed in a public junior high school. They were assessed as having relatively poor self-concepts, and yet their hearing peers rated them high in social acceptance. As with the Hagborg studies, Coyner found that females were rated higher than males in social acceptance. She also found that academic success was strongly related to social acceptance by hearing peers. In a study of the social adjustment of oral deaf children integrated into first- through sixth-grade general education classrooms, the researchers found that the deaf and hard of hearing children were more likely to be rejected by peers than the hearing children, and they were quite aware of their low social status (Cappelli, Daniels, Durieux-Smith, McGrath, & Neuss, 1995).

The self-perception of socialization and social ability would seem to be a basis for social interaction. If the deaf child perceives his or her social-ization as inadequate and social ability as poor, effective social interaction is not likely to take place. Hurt and Gonzalez (1988) found that deaf chil-dren often feel apprehensive about communicating with hearing peers, and this apprehension both inhibits them and makes them feel that the in-teraction is less than satisfactory. This finding was echoed in a study by Maxon, Brackett, and van den Berg (1991). The deaf children in this study reported themselves as less able to express their emotions verbally and less verbally aggressive than their hearing peers, though their actual lan-guage abilities were almost on level with their hearing peers. When Cart-ledge, Cochran, and Paul (1996) asked deaf adolescents to self-evaluate their social skills, the ratings of the students in mainstreamed settings were significantly higher than the students in residental school settings. The authors suggested that students in a public school setting have greater opportunities to observe and try out a variety of social behaviors among a greater number of peers and situations than students in a resi-dential school and, therefore, feel more competent socially.

Beyond early childhood, language plays an increasingly larger role in social interaction. Linguistic competence in English or ASL can be offset by social communication strategies such as access rituals (Antia, 1985; Gaustad & Kluwin, 1992). These seem to play a particularly impor-tant role in the social acceptance of deaf adolescents. According to Stin-son and Whitmire (1992), deaf students using oral communication report that they interact more frequently with hearing peers, and students using ASL or simultaneous communication report that they interact more fre-quently with deaf students. In addition, deaf students who participate in class, school, and social activities are more likely to see themselves as so-cially competent and emotionally secure in their peer relationships.

Within the classroom, while language differences and difficulties can deter social interaction, communication strategies can enhance inter-action. Shaw and Jamieson (1995) observed one 8-year-old deaf child in a school setting with no other deaf children. This child preferred to com-municate with individuals who signed, and so he interacted most fre-quently with his interpreter. He consistently chose to interact with individuals who could sign over his peers who could not sign. He also preferred to interact with girls more than boys, which seemed a result of their greater facility in communication. When Antia and Kreimeyer (1994–1995) conducted a case study of a deaf child who was fully included in a regular classroom, they found that the teachers, aides, and hearing children started learning sign language so they could communicate directly with the deaf child. Their efforts were encouraged by the interpreter, who assisted them in learning new signs.

Intuitively, it has been believed by some educators that the best environment for the development of social skills is the school for the deaf because this is the milieu for comfortable and culturally appropriate social exchange. Others believe that the public school setting offers the best opportunity for deaf children to develop appropriate social skills because it provides a multicultural context. In one study of teachers' perceptions of the social skills of deaf adolescents, no differences in the social–emotional behaviors between deaf adolescents in a residential school for the deaf, a high school program using oral communication, and a high school program using simultaneous communication were found (Cartledge, Paul, Jackson, & Cochran, 1991). Stinson and Whitmire (1992) reported that deaf students who are mainstreamed in public school programs differ in how connected they feel toward their peers. Students who spend the highest amount of time in the self-contained class with other deaf students show a high need for closer relationships with peers in general. Students who spend the highest amount of time in regular classes show a high need for closer relationships with deaf peers. Musselman, Mootilal, and MacKay (1996) found that deaf adolescents in segregated educational settings had lower perceived social competence than deaf students in partially integrated and mainstream educational settings. The results of this study "suggest that deaf students can benefit from placement with both deaf and hearing peers. They show that partially integrated students were able to be actively bilingual/bicultural, studying and interacting in both deaf and hearing settings, an experience that was associated with a strong sense of personal competency.... The findings also support the contention that relationships with deaf peers are essential to the social and emotional health of deaf persons" (p. 61).

Social Interaction during Late Adolescence and Young Adulthood

Studies of social interaction beyond young adolescence have largely focused on the interaction between deaf and hearing students within integrated high schools and colleges. Much of this research has relied on the population of students at the National Technical Institute for the Deaf (NTID). NTID is housed at the Rochester Institute of Technology (RIT), and this educational environment affords the opportunity for a substantial degree of social as well as academic interaction between hearing and deaf students. In essence, Rochester Institute of Technology provides a real-life laboratory for researchers interested in understanding the factors that improve and interfere with social interaction.

One way that researchers have explored the social interaction of deaf individuals during high school is by asking college-age students and college graduates to reflect back on their experiences. Deaf individuals who attended public high schools typically described their high school experience as less positive socially and more positive academically than deaf individuals who attended residential schools for the deaf (Foster, 1987b, 1988, 1989a; Mertens, 1989). Foster noted that deaf students find themselves in a trade-off situation, trading superficial peer interaction for enhanced academic opportunities or trading opportunity for social interaction with peers for lower quality education. In her 1987 study, the deaf subjects reported feeling "like outsiders in school. They were rarely included in parties or other kinds of social events. Conversations and friendships were often limited or superficial. While they used a variety of strategies to make friends or learn to live with the loneliness, the isolation described by these respondents was a critical part of their experience" (Foster, 1987b, p. 22). The results of Foster's 1988 study were not so clear-cut. Several subjects recollected having a very good social life in high school, where they had many hearing friends and attended parties and other social events. Others reported feeling isolated and lonely.

Magen (1990) examined the nature and intensity of positive experiences among deaf adolescents from the perspective of their own memories. The deaf adolescents reported positive experiences that were similar in intensity to those reported by hearing adolescents, and these experiences revolved around interpersonal experiences rather than solitary experiences. Charlson, Strong, and Gold (1992) analyzed the experiences of deaf high school students who had been nominated by their respective public school and residential school programs as outstandingly successful. The researchers observed that regardless of school setting, most of the students experienced some level of social isolation. The mainstreamed students often felt isolated from their peers and the residential students often felt isolated from their families. However, most of the students also possessed positive coping strategies.

Stinson and Kluwin (1996) observed that healthy social development can take place along the spectrum of segregated to integrated educational programs. But the program has to take into account the child's social orientation. They noted that deaf adolescents arrive in high school oriented to deaf peers, hearing peers, neither, or both.

> Both features in the school program and in individual characteristics contribute to peer orientation. In regard to school programs, deaf and hard-of-hearing students are unlikely to form good relationships with hearing peers unless

some efforts are made to bridge the communication barrier and to structure situations where positive interaction can occur. Also, deaf students will not form relationships with other deaf peers unless they have regular opportunities for interaction with each other and unless there is a group big enough to provide some choice in relationships. (p. 130)

Is social interaction in college different from social interaction in high school? Foster and DeCaro (1991) examined the interactions between deaf and hearing students living in the same residence hall at Rochester Institute of Technology. They found that interactions were influenced by a number of individual and environmental characteristics. For example, deaf students chose a particular dormitory because it afforded them an opportunity to learn how to interact with hearing people, whereas hearing students typically chose the same dormitory because it was one of the nicest on campus. Both hearing and deaf students described their communication as good enough to complete routine tasks or accomplish a personal goal, but as not fluent or easy. Some behaviors, such as drinking illegally, mitigated against interaction because students kept their doors closed so as to avoid notice by the school authorities. The segregation of many classes was also a barrier to social interaction. Although the students observed that interaction improved over time, the transience of dormitory life made it less likely that deaf and hearing students would share a common living space for extended periods of time.

Brown and Foster (1991) interviewed thirty hearing students at the Rochester Institute of Technology and found that they believed the deaf students at RIT were as competent and successful academically as hearing students but less competent socially. The classroom was not a strong catalyst for the formation of friendships and did not serve to dispel stereotypes about differences between deaf and hearing people. The authors concluded that "to meet the challenge of integrating deaf and hearing students in social contexts, it may be necessary to focus intervention efforts on providing the students with information and strategies that they can implement themselves and that will enable them to accept one another as individuals, rather than as typical or exceptional members of a group" (p. 27).

When Coryell, Holcomb, and Scherer (1992) probed the social interaction of deaf and hearing students at RIT, they found that personal contact, communication strategies, and understanding of cultural diversity contributed to positive attitudes. They observed little meaningful interaction, however, between the deaf and hearing students. Murphy and Newlon (1987) examined the experiences of deaf students attending eight universities in the United States. They found that deaf students were   lonely than hearing students. Alternately, first-year students, male students, and hard of hearing students were not more lonely than sophomore through senior students, female students, and deaf students. They also found that satisfaction with parental and peer relationships, adjustment to disability, and comfort with speech for hard of hearing students and comfort with sign language for deaf students were inversely related to loneliness.

Social Interaction during Adulthood

Beyond school, there are few environmental structures that serve to encourage social interaction among deaf and hearing individuals. Indeed, most structures such as Deaf churches, clubs, and sports promote social interaction within the Deaf community. Deaf adults often report feeling socially rejected by hearing individuals and socially alienated from the hearing community.

Foster (1989b) suggested that the development of the Deaf community is the consequence of social rejection by the hearing community and social acceptance by deaf peers. From interviews with deaf adults, she found recurring themes of social alienation among hearing individuals and rewarding social experiences among deaf individuals. The deaf adults in her study reported turning to other deaf individuals for real conversation, information, close friendships, and intimacy.

Not all deaf individuals find social satisfaction within the Deaf community. In one study, 95 percent of the deaf individuals who were interviewed reported having deaf friends, but only 81 percent noted that they meet with friends for leisure time activities (Backenroth, 1993). This group of deaf individuals also reported being lonely 5 to 10 percent of the time.

In Essay 5.2, Ruth Maddox discusses her issues with social interaction, the ways that she has coped, and the individuals in her life who have provided support, love, and friendship.

■ ■ ■ ■ ■ ▬▬▬▬▬▬▬▬▬▬▬▬▬▬▬▬▬▬▬▬▬▬▬▬▬▬▬▬▬▬

ESSAY 5.2

Ruth Maddox

My mom was a writer. Once she tried to write about me. She was on chapter three when she died. I lost her notebook that she used for writing about me. I decided to try to write a book about me, but now I will wait until my daughter, Cassie, is older. I have two daughters. Cassie will be two next month, and Alex is four. My husband, Mike, is hearing, but he knows sign language. He learned sign before he met me. I met him in Virginia. I had transferred from the Philadelphia College of Performing Arts to Shenandoah University in Winchester, Virginia. He was once a student, but he was visiting Shenandoah because he grew up in Winchester. I was the only deaf student. He didn't know that. I was walking down the hallway, and he was walking with his friend. Mike tried to say hello to me, but I did not hear him. My friend told him, "Excuse me, she is deaf." He started to say "Oooohhhh." (Once he told me that he thought to call me a bad word because it wasn't nice that I didn't say hello. I laughed and told him that it wasn't a nice word. It's funny. But I hate bad words.) A few days later, he tried to find me. He learned where I lived in the dorm. So he brought a sign language card with him. When I opened the door, he and I both looked at the card. I told him that I could talk. He said, "Oh." We were just friends for a while, and then we started dating. We were engaged for a year and were married on April 30, 1989. I know we were married very fast.

I lost my hearing when I was eight years old. It is so hard for me to remember myself as a hearing child. I traveled around the world with my family and remember everything, but I do not remember about my hearing. I stopped talking when I was a small child after my father left. I was a very silent small child. I had spoken four languages and spoke very pretty. I remember my mother saying that my voice was beautiful. But after my father left I did not talk. I was only a smile without talking. I forgot my name and many many words. It was so hard for me to understand any words. I still forget what some words mean.

Before I went to the Beebe Clinic in Easton, Pennsylvania, my mom hired a private speech teacher after school. The A. G. Bell Clinic in Washington, DC, told my mom about the Beebe Clinic. Mrs. Beebe urged my mom to work hard with me. I know that Mrs. Beebe and my mom cared about me and always thought about what's the best for Ruthie. She was a wonderful mother. She fought for me for a long time. My father did not agree with my mom about me. But it was not their choice. It was my choice what I wanted to be. I wanted talking and not sign language. Mom listened to me. She wanted what was best for me. My father did not listen or believe in me. He wanted me to learn sign language. I refused. I loved talking too much. Mom supported me a lot. She and I were so close. I had no relationship with my father. I knew he was my father and I loved him, but I was fighting with him. I tried to be a good daughter, I loved him, and I know he loved me. It's a long story. He lived in Africa for many years. I am a funny girl and stubborn and spoiled and I talk too much (smile).

I was the only deaf family member, so I felt uncomfortable. I would just smile all the time when I did not hear or understand when family members talked. My mom was my interpreter, only without sign language. I understood her perfectly. My brother, Elihu, was my interpreter, too, but he was so busy playing with his friends or doing schoolwork. So I often felt sad because he did not help. But I was a young girl. My family would talk to me, and they understood me, but I did not understand or hear anything. At Passover, I did not want my mom to help me because I knew the service. But at other times it bothered me. At family dinners, my brothers, Elihu and Dani, and my mom talked a lot but I did not hear or understand. I was mad. I told them, "What are you talking about all the time?" I was so tired of it. It's not their fault. It's just a deaf thing. I understand that's how I feel being a deaf person. Of course my mom knew how I felt. She interpreted for me when they talked, but some of them did not tell me what they talked about until I became frustrated. I yelled and asked them to please tell me what they talked about. They were so surprised. They'd say, "Oops."

(continued)

ESSAY 5.2   CONTINUED

After my mom died, Paige, my sister-in-law, learned to help me, and sometimes Elihu did too. I have known him for almost thirty-four years. He sometimes did not help me, but it's ok. He started learning to help me after my mom died. He did well. My husband, Mike, is great to me. He helps me lots. His family supports me very much. They love me and my mom and Elihu and other family members. Since my mom died, I try to stay strong and be happy. I am ok that I am deaf, and I am fine. I have family and friends who support me. It makes me so proud, and I know my mom is proud of me.

I miss her so much. After she died, many family members and friends called to check up on me because they knew that she was my best friend. She died just after my oldest daughter, Alex, was born. Mom died at age sixty-five on April 2, 1995. It was so hard. It was a terrible year for me. My grandfather died before I became pregnant. Then my father died when I was about five months pregnant. Then my grandmother died when I was about seven months pregnant. Then after Alex was born, my mom died. It was terrible. But I am very grateful to God for waiting until my mom held Alex before she died. Mom told Elihu at the hospital (Elihu told me that) she could not believe that she stayed alive so long until she saw Alex because she had a bad heart after I was born. She worked hard to stay strong until Alex arrived. I thank God for that.

Elihu and I used to be close. I smile now because we were not always close, like when we were mad at each other, you know, a brother and sister thing. I don't see him often now, but sometimes we talk on the phone. Elihu is working hard at his job and playing with his boys, so he has no time to see me. Dani, my oldest brother, lives in India. He is so far away from me and Elihu. Every year he comes to America to see us for a while. He sounds like my father.

Mike's parents are very supportive to me. They help me a lot. They loved my mom. They became best friends to her. Mike's mother and she were close like sisters. She misses my mom a lot. My aunt is very close to me. And other aunts are great. So I have friends, and they support me. None of them are my best friend, but they are wonderful friends. Now I am a full-time mother. I have no time to visit my friends, but we talk on the phone and sometimes we see each other. So I am lucky to have family and friends who support me.

Cassie's birthday is next month, and she will turn two. I think she is a beautiful gift from God and Mom and my family in heaven. Alex started to learn sign language and spoke very well at about seven months of age. Cassie is almost two but does not talk yet. She's too lazy. But she is a sweet little girl. I tried to teach her to speak and learn sign language. Alex helps me a lot. Sometimes she interprets for me when I need her. I taught her about manners that my mom taught me. Alex is very well mannered. I teach Alex in home schooling before she goes to kindergarten.

I was a ballet teacher and actress. It was so easy for me to dance without music. I had a good memory when the teacher taught me to dance. I could feel something next to the piano. When I was the teacher, my students helped me with the music. I enjoyed teaching, and I miss it. But I enjoy being with my children.

Reprinted by permission of the author.

Backenroth (1995) probed the social interactions of deaf individuals in their work situation. He was interested in the particular experiences of deaf individuals who were connected to both the hearing and Deaf cultures. He chose individuals who also had both hearing and deaf coworkers. Most of the deaf individuals noted that they socialize with hearing and deaf coworkers during breaks, wished that their hearing coworkers would learn sign language, and were relatively satisfied with their social contacts at work. They defined the most important factors for well-being in their working life as cooperation, social relations, positive attitudes, openness, and equality.

Clearly, most research has centered on the socialization of deaf individuals. Very little information has been gathered on the similarities, differences, and unique experiences of hard of hearing individuals. The same is true of the curricular and intervention programs that have been created to help children develop social skills and to enhance their social abilities.

Social Skills Improvement

Although some deaf children will learn the intricacies, subtleties, and nuances of social behaviors by observing others and noticing reactions, many deaf children need more obvious, direct, and systematic instruction about social skills. The interventions and curricula that have been developed tend to concentrate at the points of early childhood, childhood, and adolescence.

Social Skills Improvement during Early Childhood

Early childhood is a critical time for children to learn appropriate social skills and to use these skills in effective interaction with peers, both deaf and hearing. During the preschool years, socialization is a primary educational goal for all children. Given the research discussed previously about the social abilities of deaf children and their social interaction patterns, social skills training has been a high priority among preschool educators.

One group of researchers directed social skills training toward hearing children in an attempt to improve their interactions with deaf peers. Vandell, Anderson, Ehrhardt, and Wilson (1982) provided a three-week training program to a group of hearing children who were attending a preschool that was described as low-key mainstreaming. The hearing and deaf children were together for part of most days in cross-class activities, lunch, recess, and gym. During the training program, the hearing children were read stories about deafness and stories with deaf characters, learned some sign language, played games that simulated hearing loss, learned about hearing loss, and were paired with a deaf child for activities. The results were disappointing. Instead of increased interaction as a consequence of the intervention, they interacted less with their deaf peers. The researchers concluded that "in the current study the burden of change was on the hearing children who were doing the rejecting. Ultimately, a difficult but critical task may be having the hearing children see a value to interacting with deaf peers" (p. 1363).

Kluwin and Gonsher (1994) used a team teaching approach within a kindergarten class of hearing and deaf children. Each deaf child was assigned a communication buddy and the class was taught by two teachers; one was a certified early childhood teacher and the other was a certified teacher of the deaf. The hearing children made significant progress in learning to sign, and with the improvement in sign skills, social relationships developed and positive acceptance increased. Kluwin and Gonsher concluded that "facilitating communication and presenting opportunities for mutual interest, as in the communication buddies, is a necessary part of socially integrating the children with hearing losses into regular education settings" (p. 86).

Antia and Kreimeyer conducted a series of studies that were designed to assess the effectiveness of social skills training programs with preschool deaf children. In one study, five deaf preschoolers using oral communication and four using simultaneous communication were engaged in activities that provided them opportunities to practice greeting peers, sharing materials, assisting others, complimenting and praising, playing cooperatively, and inviting other children to join an activity. The teacher modeled these social skills and prompted the children both verbally and physically. They found an increase in positive peer interaction, though it decreased at the conclusion of the intervention. They also found that the intervention was more effective in increasing sharing than conversation (Antia & Kreimeyer, 1987).

They conducted a similar study with a different group of preschool deaf children in which the activities were designed to provide practice in greeting, sharing, assisting, refusing appropriately, conversing, complimenting and praising, cooperating, and dealing appropriately with others' emotions. Teacher modeling and prompting were used while the children were engaged in three types of activities. In shared product routines, the children worked together to create a single product. In cooperative game routines, they played simple, noncompetitive games. In role-play routines, they took turns acting out various roles of familiar experiences. As with the prior study, Kreimeyer and Antia (1988) found an increase in positive interaction, sharing, and conversation. They also found that the children generalized these social skills to play situations outside of the intervention activities, but only when the toys were the same ones as those used during intervention.

With a third group of preschool deaf children, Antia and Kreimeyer (1988) used arts and crafts activities as the backdrop for social skills training. The teachers again modeled and prompted the children to share, cooperate, and compliment while the children made a product that no child could make alone because the children had to share supplies or it was a product that was best made by more than one child. They found that the intervention resulted in high levels of positive peer interaction that were maintained when the intervention was gradually withdrawn, but not when the intervention stopped abruptly. They also found that the children's linguistic interactions increased, which they had not found in the previous two studies.

Subsequent to the studies of deaf children in segregated preschool settings, Antia, Kreimeyer, and Eldredge (1994) conducted a study in integrated settings. In addition to the social skills intervention that they had used previously, they implemented an integrated-activities intervention during which small groups of deaf and hearing children worked together on various activities. They found that total positive interaction increased, the integrated-activities intervention was more effective than the social skills intervention, deaf children interacted more frequently with deaf peers and hearing children interacted more frequently with hearing peers, and deaf children interacted with deaf peers as frequently as hearing children interacted with hearing peers. In a second study, Antia and Kreimeyer (1997) examined the play behaviors of this group of children during the intervention. They found that the frequency of the children's solitary and parallel play decreased and associative play increased, and these changes were maintained over time.

In a third study, Antia and Kreimeyer (1998) compared a social skills intervention with a familiarity-based intervention in preschool, kindergarten, and first-grade classrooms with deaf, hard of hearing, and hearing children. In the social skills intervention, the teachers designed activities to promote interactions, modeled social skills, and prompted the children to use specific social skills. In the familiarity-based intervention, the children worked together regularly, which allowed them to become familiar with each other. The social skills intervention increased interaction among the deaf and hard of hearing children but not interaction with the hearing children. The familiarity-based intervention increased recognition among all of the children but did not result in increased acceptance of the deaf and hard of hearing children by the hearing children.

Based on their research, Antia and Kreimeyer (1991) suggested that interventions must provide more than information. They need to teach social interaction and communication skills to both hearing and deaf children over a lengthy time period so that the children are very familiar with one another. Antia (1994) noted that several strategies can be used successfully in promoting positive interaction. The teacher should provide children with social toys, set up role plays and interactive games, keep adult interaction to a minimum during play, make sure that deaf and hearing children have long-standing and frequent contact with one another, and use social skills training approaches with deaf children who need help in effectively interacting with their peers.

Social Skills Improvement during Childhood

Several social skills training programs have been developed and used successfully with school-age deaf children. Some are sets of materials, some are teaching techniques, and some are curricula.

Murphy-Berman and Whobrey (1982) developed four types of materials that were designed to facilitate deaf children's social and affective skills. The first type required the children to identify the emotions experienced by characters at different points in a television program by using a series of five faces depicting degrees of feeling—happy, sad, proud, mad, afraid, and worried. The second type elicited the children's opinions regarding the personality traits of the major characters from the television program by choosing the picture that best represented which character was more tall, old, fat, mean, brave, smart, nice, or likeable. The third type asked the children to predict how the characters would behave in new situations by requiring them to choose from several pictures depicting various situations. The fourth type asked the children to express their opinion of the television program and particular scenes by showing them a picture of a scene with a five-face rating guide of "like very much" to "do not like," with the faces representing these emotions. These materials were used with 80 deaf children from five schools for the deaf. The researchers reported that the materials seemed to help the children focus on their affective responses and suggested that these types of materials could be used for improving empathy.

Greenberg and Kusche (1993) developed a curriculum to promote self-control, emotional awareness, and interpersonal problem-solving skills in deaf children, which they named PATHS (Promoting Alternative Thinking Strategies). In the curriculum, teachers were provided detailed lesson plans, scripts, guidelines, and objectives. The curriculum was designed to help deaf children do the following:

1. Develop specific strategies that promote reflective responses and mature thinking skills;
2. Become self-motivated and enthusiastic about learning;
3. Obtain information necessary for social understanding and prosocial behavior;

4. Generate creative alternative solutions to problems; and
5. Learn to anticipate and evaluate situations, behaviors, and consequences. (p. 68)

Their research on the effectiveness of the curriculum indicated that it was successful in improving social problem solving, social behavior, and emotional understanding.

Circle of Friends (Perske, 1988) was developed for hearing children, but has been used successfully with deaf children. In one school, a group of one deaf and eight hearing children were brought together with two teachers and an interpreter for one hour, once each week, for eight weeks (Luckner, Schauermann, & Allen, 1994). They carried out activities designed to help them clarify what a friend is, find common interests, learn to trust one another, celebrate diversity, and interact with each other. At the end of the eight weeks, the students reported the following:

- They felt more confident about making friends.
- They were better able to deal with problems by talking about them rather than resorting to physical outbursts.
- They had learned new ways to communicate with friends; using the relay service, for example.
- They felt they had a better understanding of what a friend really is, and really does. (p. 4)

Several researchers have targeted social skills programs to deaf children with language delays or difficulties. Curl, Rowbury, and Baer (1985) gave the 4- to 6-year-old language-delayed children in their study picture cues to indicate their choice of a play partner and a play activity as a technique for facilitating social interaction and minimizing teacher intrusion into their play behavior. The researchers found a dramatic increase in appropriate social interaction and a decrease in teacher involvement through the use of this relatively simple technique. Rasing and Duker conducted a series of studies designed to assess the effectiveness of a social behavior training program (Rasing, 1993; Rasing & Duker, 1992, 1993). The language-disabled deaf children in these studies ranged from ages 7 to 13. The program involved role-play situations, reinforcement of appropriate behaviors, and a correction procedure for inappropriate behaviors. They found increases in greeting, turn waiting, initiating interaction, interacting with others, and giving help.

Social Skills Improvement during Adolescence

As communication becomes more elaborate and complex, and peer relationships become more consequential, social skills become at once more important and more intricate. Schloss and his associates proposed that the classroom program can have a positive effect on the deaf child's social competence when the teacher consciously employs strategies that promote social development (Schloss, Selinger, Goldsmith, & Morrow, 1983). They classified these strategies as environmental management (including interpersonal interactions between student and teacher, creating a classroom schedule that maximizes social learning, systematic instruction that promotes a positive view of self and socially appropriate behavior, and motivational approaches) and student competency development (including counseling activities within natural settings, self-control training, and social skills training that involves identifying the needed skills, reinforcing appropriate behavior, modeling, practicing, and providing effective feedback). One of the techniques that Schloss and his associates used to promote social competence was a card game (Schloss, Smith, & Schloss, 1984). The game followed the rules of rummy, described fourteen consumer-related situations, and required the deaf students to ask questions, criticize, respond to small talk, and respond to suggestive selling. The students' skills improved during the game and generalized to situations outside of the classroom. A number of other strategies are described in Schloss and Smith's book, *Teaching Social Skills to Hearing-Impaired Students* (1990).

Role-play scenes were used by Lemanek and Gresham (1984) to improve the social skills of one deaf adolescent. The combination of modeling, rehearsal, feedback, and social reinforcement served to increase her ability to give and accept praise and to give and accept help. She also became more appropriately and effectively assertive. Role play was also used in a study by Barrett (1986). A group of deaf high school students at a residential school for the deaf, who participated in a sociodrama class, were found to experience increased social adjustment and positive feelings about themselves.

Structured learning approaches have been used with both hearing and deaf adolescents to teach social skills. Structured learning consists of four basic steps—modeling, role playing, performance feedback, and transfer of training. Each skill is taught as a sequence of parts or steps, the students are shown examples through role play conducted by skilled individuals, the students rehearse or practice the steps by role-playing their own situations, other students act as observers and provide feedback, and the students practice the new skill in real-life situations (Goldstein, Sprafkin, Gershaw, & Klein, 1980). In one study using structured learning with deaf students, Lemanek and her associates found improved social behavior during role play and generalization to new situations (Lemanek, Williamson, Gresham, & Jensen, 1986).

Lytle (1987) used a two-pronged approach to social skills training. The goals were to improve social behaviors and the thinking skills involved in social problem solving. During a period of eight weeks, a group of deaf adolescent boys were engaged in activities that encouraged participation, discussion, cooperation, and support for others. Lytle found that the curriculum was successful in helping the students to develop more effective patterns of social behavior and to understand social problem solving. At the end of the study, the students expressed feelings of greater self-confidence, ability to make new friends, and skill in communication.

Tripp (1993) focused specifically on values and decision making with a group of adolescent deaf students within the context of a one-semester curriculum. She found that the students who completed the course:

- Were aware of the importance of taking the time to think through decisions
- Recognized that actions have consequences and they must make choices that are, therefore, not always the most obvious or easiest
- Realized the value in making decisions that reflect personal standards rather than peer pressure
- Understood the importance of choosing actions based on one's own internal logic
- Maintained an internal locus of control and did not get stuck in helplessness or blaming

Social integration and social skills ultimately lead to social status and roles in adulthood. A principal reason that deafness has been traditionally referred to as invisible is because during nonlinguistic interactions, deafness is not physically apparent. And even during linguistic interaction, deaf individuals have been known to be highly skilled at masking their hearing loss. My own grandmother made her way through Ellis Island during the early twentieth century without any customs agent being aware that she was deaf. In contrast, some deaf individuals mask their ability to use oral communication in their interaction with both hearing and deaf individuals. These decisions can lead to different levels of status within cultures, both hearing and Deaf.

SOCIAL STATUS AND ROLES

In the 1980s, the research was largely concerned with the differences in social status and roles between hearing and deaf youngsters. For example, Klansek-Kyllo and Rose (1985) examined independent social behavior and found that deaf youth who were mainstreamed for some of their educational programming demonstrated equivalent behaviors in the areas of motor development, personal living, and community living. In contrast, these deaf students demonstrated significant problems in the areas that related language to social development. In another study, Rachford and Furth (1986) compared the understanding of friendship and social rules among deaf adolescents. For friendship, the deaf and hearing adolescents were asked the following questions:

- How do people become friends?
- What do friends do together?
- What do close friends talk about?
- What is the most important thing friends do for one another?
- How are conflicts between friends resolved? (p. 393)

For the social rules, the deaf and hearing adolescents were asked to respond to the following questions about the rules involved in the game of kickball, the school rule about no running in the halls, and the law specifying 16 years as the minimum age for obtaining a driving license:

- Could the rule be changed?
- Has this rule always existed?
- How did the rule originate?
- What is the purpose of the rule?
- Must the rule be obeyed in all cases?
- If the rule is modified, which rule, the old or the new one, is the right rule? (p. 393)

Rachford and Furth found that the deaf adolescents exhibited similar understanding to hearing adolescents about friendship, but quite different understanding of game rules, which is one aspect of social rules.

In a similar theme, Haley and Hood (1986) investigated perceptions based on hearing aid usage and found that hearing junior high school students tended to rate deaf peers with hearing aids as less intelligent and less intelligible, but also rated them as more likely to be hard workers. Cox, Cooper, and McDade (1989) observed that college-age hearing students rated individuals with hearing aids as lower on achievement but higher on other aspects such as appearance, personality, and assertiveness. Silverman and Largin (1993) obtained a different result with a group of students at a parochial school with hearing and deaf students. They found that the pictures of students with an obvious hearing aid were rated more positively on scales that included good, happy, friendly, kind, beautiful, healthy, strong, pretty, smart, popular, friendly, likeable, intelligent, outgoing, and nice. The researchers suggested that by the early 1990s, there was greater sensitivity and acceptance of individuals with a hearing loss than previously.

When Rittenhouse (1987a) examined the attitudes of high school students toward school and each other, he found that both hearing and deaf students expressed similar kinds of fears about their adult future. Furthermore, the deaf students in self-contained settings felt significantly more negative about their school situation than deaf students who were mainstreamed for some of their educational programming. Weisel (1988a) investigated the attitudes of hearing students and found that those with moderate contact with deaf students expressed the most negativity and attributed the greatest degree of functional limitation to deaf individuals when compared to hearing students with virtually no contact and hearing students with a high level of contact. No differences in attitudes were found among the students with no contact and high contact. Another way to approach the issue of attitudes was used by Rienzi, Levinson, and Scrams (1992). They asked hearing university students to rate the suitability of unmarried individuals to adopt a child. The subjects in this study were most biased against hearing men and deaf women.

One of the issues that became apparent in the mid-1980s was the discrepancy between attitude and behavior. Hearing individuals who were given information about deafness might change their attitude toward deaf individuals, but they were considerably less likely to change their behavior. In one study, first-year college students were provided with information about deaf persons and subsequently asked questions designed to measure their attitudes. Kottke, Mellor, and Schmidt (1987) found that the information affected attitudes but not interpersonal acceptance.

The negative attitudes that emerge when individuals from separate cultures develop stereotyped beliefs have been found to be an issue when hearing and deaf individuals are brought together, such as in an educational setting, with little information about each other. Dampier, Dancer, and Keiser (1985) asked first-year college students to listen to an informative tape about deafness and a tape designed to elicit empathy. They found that the empathy tape was significantly more effective in changing attitudes toward elderly deaf individuals. Martin (1987) recommended the following strategies for reducing ethnocentrism:

- Provide multiple opportunities for deaf and hearing students to interact on a regular basis, preferably on joint projects or activities.
- Give opportunities to discuss openly why they react positively or negatively to one another.
- Encourage expression of ways that their own culture might appear strange to a person from the other group.
- Discuss the fundamental ways in which all human groups are similar (kinship, division of tasks, language, prolonged childhood dependency, belief system, use of symbols, tool systems, etc.). Deaf and hearing people are equally "human" because each group has established its own specific responses to those same needs.
- Teach about the processes by which humans develop stereotypes.
- Teach about the wide variation of behavior within any culture.

- Point out nonstereotypic behaviors of both groups.
- Teach about the positive contributions to human life by both groups.
- Help students create and analyze a model culture as a thinking tool for understanding both cultures. (p. 7)

Educational settings can orchestrate the kinds and accuracy of information provided about deafness and deaf individuals, but most hearing individuals gain most of their information about deafness via the media. Haller (1992) examined how two well-regarded newspapers covered issues of deafness during a four-year period that included the Deaf President Now movement at Gallaudet University. Her purpose was to determine whether deaf individuals were being covered by the media along traditional or progressive disability models. She found that during that period of time, the issues of deaf persons were not prominent news unless they were involved in a civil rights movement, such as Deaf President Now. At these times, the two newspapers showed deaf persons as a legitimate minority group within a culturally pluralistic society. In contrast, when deaf individuals were covered within general news or feature articles, they tended to be portrayed as medically or economically deficient. During the four-year period, presentations within these two newspapers tended to become more evenhanded, with traditional forms of presentation falling and progressive forms increasing.

When Poon (1996) examined the literature on attitudes toward deaf and hard of hearing individuals, she noted that stereotypical attitudes and negativity were largely related to lack of knowledge about deafness. She also determined that when hearing and deaf individuals were engaged in cooperative activities and one-to-one activities, positive attitudes and understanding were fostered.

The personal and social development of deaf individuals certainly does not stop when they complete high school or college. At the point in time when educators typically disengage professionally from the life of deaf individuals, but not on personal levels, other professionals continue to be as interested and concerned about their development.

PERSONAL AND SOCIAL DEVELOPMENT THROUGH THE LIFE SPAN

Much of the research on the personal and social development of deaf individuals through the life span has concentrated on the adventitiously deaf, elderly deaf, and oral deaf.

As individuals age, they generally lose hearing. Though acquired deafness is not only caused by aging, it is the most common cause of adventitious deafness. Individuals with acquired hearing loss typically experience increased feelings of isolation. Stevens (1982) found that social isolation was the principal handicap associated with adventitious deafness. Nordeng, Martinsen, and von Tezchner (1985) observed that adults who became deaf experienced a breakdown of social life. In a study of loneliness among very old adults living in rural settings, Dugan and Kivett (1994) found that while loss of a spouse accounted for emotional isolation, diminished hearing acuity accounted for social isolation.

Deafness beyond childhood but before late adulthood imposes a variety of life changes and challenges. As Rutman (1989) contended, "Acquired deafness must be considered, first and foremost, a social and psychological loss which affects all communication and interpersonal interactions, and which deprives individuals of the type of social relationships, occupational goals and overall quality of life to which he or she was accustomed and which gave life meaning" (p. 305). Whereas prelingual deafness is viewed as a difference, acquired deafness is viewed as a loss. Individuals who are late-deafened are typically found to experience loneliness, and their sense of identity is disrupted and often confused (Meadow-Orlans, 1985). Adventitious deafness will be discussed in more depth in the next chapter on mental health.

As individuals age, hearing takes on greater importance because of decreased mobility and activity. Hearing provides access to entertainment, information, and, of course, others. It is estimated that more than 11 million elderly individuals in the United States have a significant hearing loss, and approximately 3 percent of these individuals became deaf prelingually, a percentage that has changed relatively little during the last half of the twentieth century (Northern, 1996; Walsh & Eldredge, 1989). For elderly adults who have never learned to communicate without hearing, meaningful contact with the world can diminish tremendously. However, even among individuals who are deaf prelingually or postlingually during childhood, adjustment to the aging process includes changes in social life. Tidball (1990) found that long-lasting friendships, many of which were established during their school years, were a principal source of social and emotional support for older deaf adults. She also found that ties with nuclear families tended to be strong, though these ties often did not extend to grandchildren who had not learned how to communicate with their deaf grandparents.

One study specifically focused on the factors that contribute to life satisfaction among oral deaf adults. McCartney (1987) surveyed members of the Oral Deaf Adults Section of the Alexander Graham Bell Association for the Deaf. Among the issues related specifically to social satisfaction, these oral deaf adults felt that the key to their social life was involvement in social groups, such as exercise clubs, volunteer organizations, and civic groups. They also believed that their success was in part attributable to their ability to get along with others and taking an active role in social situations.

SUMMARY AND CONCLUDING THOUGHTS

This chapter discussed personal and social development from the point of identity formation in early childhood through the development of social skills in childhood and adolescence and to the social issues encountered by deaf individuals in adulthood. In his autobiography, David Wright (1993) related his feelings about social situations as a teenager aboard a ship bound for Africa:

> My deafness did, and still does, often make me feel at a disadvantage; but that is quite a different thing from feeling inferior. What made me suddenly conscious of deafness, rather than sensitive about it, was the awful incertitude in which I found myself—not knowing what was going on. How can you break into a group of people, join them, introduce yourself, if you have no notion what they may be talking about? Specifically there was the realization that I had no idea how to strike up an acquaintance. How does one break the ice—what does one actually say to a complete stranger? Having started, what then? I was at a loss because I had no way of finding out except by trial and ignominious error. Deafness prevented me from overhearing how it was done. (p. 98)

Deaf individuals "overhearing" the social milieu of hearing individuals, and deaf individuals with limited sign language proficiency "overseeing" the social milieu of signing individuals, confront similar challenges in learning the social rules of the respective cultures and finding satisfaction in their social lives.

CHAPTER SIX

MENTAL HEALTH

FOCUS QUESTIONS

- In what ways can self-esteem affect overall mental health of deaf children, adolescents, and adults?
- What factors are most important to the psychological adjustment of deaf individuals?
- How does the Deaf community view sexuality issues and sexuality information?
- Are certain emotional and behavioral problems more prevalent among deaf persons?
- What are the major hurdles facing a deaf individual seeking counseling or therapy?

Mental health is the emotional and intellectual response of a person to his or her environment. In a book that details the history of deaf education, *The Conquest of Deafness*, Bender wrote, "The child today who is born with a hearing loss can look forward to a warm, happy acceptance in his family and his community, to a rich and complete education, and to full citizenship in society" (p. 181). She wrote this book in 1970. The deaf child born in 1970 is an adult today. If Ruth Bender was correct, then the deaf adult's response to the environment is presently both positive and healthy. Yet the literature on mental health rarely includes research on "health" but, rather, focuses on disorders and difficulties. Indeed, John Denmark's book, *Deafness and Mental Health* (1994), does not contain the term *mental health* anywhere except within the title and when discussing mental health legislation.

Chapter 5 discussed the development of identity and personality in deaf children. This chapter will extend that discussion to issues of psychological adjustment, relationships, behavioral problems, mental disorders, and counseling.

SELF-ESTEEM

Self-esteem is a principal component of mental health. It is important to understand both the factors that contribute to the self-esteem of deaf individuals and ways to improve self-esteem. Bat-Chava (1993) found four factors to be the major contributors to the self-esteem of deaf persons—hearing status, family environment, school environment, and group identification.

Hearing Status and Self-Esteem

When Bat-Chava reviewed twenty-two studies comparing the self-esteem of deaf people with hearing people, he found overall findings of lower self-esteem among deaf people. However, the ways that test instructions were communicated appeared to affect the results in some of the studies. For example, in a study by Cates (1991b), the self-concept of hearing and deaf students were comparable when the instrument measuring self-concept was administered to the deaf students by an individual fluent in ASL.

Brooks and Ellis (1982) suggested that the reason for lower self-esteem can be found in society's negative labeling of deaf individuals. They hypothesized, "If individuals have a stigma, and are in a social setting that allows the internalization of the standards of the wider society, and they perceive that others adhere to the standards which negatively differentiate them, and they perceive that others negatively differentiate them, then they will have negative self-esteem" (p. 63). They also postulated, "If individuals have a stigma, and are in a social setting that allows the internalization of the standards of the wider society, but others mediate the standards with regard to the stigma, and they perceive that others do not negatively differentiate them, then they will have positive self-esteem" (p. 63). Their study comparing the self-esteem of deaf and hard of hearing individuals appeared to support their hypothesis. The hard of hearing adolescents in their study demonstrated higher self-esteem than the deaf adolescents because, according to Brooks and Ellis, deaf individuals tend to be more stigmatized than hard of hearing individuals.

Beck (1988) obtained a similar finding when he compared the self-esteem of deaf, hard of hearing, and hearing adolescents. The highest self-esteem was found among the hearing adolescents, followed by the hard of hearing adolescents. The lowest self-esteem was found among the deaf adolescents. He observed that language was the principal contributory factor to self-esteem, which was also the observation of Kusche, Garfield, and Greenberg (1983) in their study of the affective understanding of deaf adolescents. Loeb and Sarigiani (1986) found that the hard of hearing 8- to 15-year-old children in their study reported similar self-satisfaction as hearing children, and when asked what they would like to change, mentioned many things, such as their rooms and homes, but did not cite themselves.

Hilburn, Marini, and Slate (1997) examined the self-esteem of deaf and hearing adolescents. The deaf adolescents with hearing parents exhibited significantly lower self-esteem than the hearing adolescents with hearing parents. However, no statistically significant difference was found between the deaf adolescents with hearing parents and the deaf adolescents with deaf parents, or the deaf adolescents with deaf parents and the hearing adolescents.

Adventitiously deaf individuals have unique issues with self-esteem. It is believed that acquired deafness is an emotionally traumatic event that dramatically impacts the individual's self-esteem. Luey (1980) viewed the event to be catastrophic, similar to events such as serious illness or the death of a loved one, due to the loss of a sense on which the person has depended for communication and enjoyment of life. David and Trehub (1989) interviewed deafened adults who expressed their need for "help in restructuring their world and affirming their role or identity within that new structure" (p. 203). In Orlans's (1988) study of hard of hearing adults, he found that those who lost their hearing as adults felt great difficulty in adjusting to their hearing loss and often described themselves as reclusive because of their difficulty in interacting with even close family members.

Family and Self-Esteem

Self-image has its origins in the connection between the deaf child and his or her parents. Love, caring, and support can be expressed in multiple ways. Although the hearing parent can be just as effective as the deaf parent, it appears as if deaf children with deaf parents are more likely to have higher self-esteem than deaf children of hearing parents, and deaf children whose hearing parents use sign language are more likely to have higher self-esteem than deaf children whose parents use oral only communication (Bat-Chava, 1993; Desselle, 1994).

Yachnik (1986) found that among deaf college students, those with deaf parents had higher self-esteem than those with hearing parents. He suggested one reason might be that the deaf individual with deaf parents has greater access to social relationships within the Deaf community outside of the school setting, and this ease of social activity may positively affect self-perception. He cautioned educators and others not to assume, however, that lower self-esteem meant low self-esteem, because the studies on self-esteem do not incorporate any absolute value of adequate self-esteem against which the scores can be compared.

Searls (1993) investigated self-esteem among the children of deaf parents. He found that hearing college students with deaf parents demonstrated comparable self-esteem to deaf college students with deaf parents. When Warren and Hasenstab (1986) attempted to determine which variables would be the best predictor of self-concept, they found a strong relationship between child-rearing attitudes and self-concept among deaf children. Parental indulgence, protection, and rejection correlated negatively with self-concept. Parental acceptance and discipline correlated positively with self-concept.

In Essay 6.1, Ashli-Marie Grant tells about her feelings for her hearing family in an essay that she wrote for school.

ESSAY 6.1

Ashli-Marie Grant

My name is Ashli-Marie Grant. I am nine years old. When I was two years old, my family found out that I was deaf. The people I think have courage, a big heart, and a smart brain are my family! I love them very very much. When they found out I was deaf, my grandparents, my parents, my aunts, uncles, and cousins all learned sign language so we could communicate. They did this because they love me. My mom and dad were very courageous and went to court with the state to get summer school for me and won! I am happy because I want to learn more education for school! I love my brother and sister because we play together and can communicate and have fun.

Reprinted by permission of the author.

School and Self-Esteem

When researchers have examined the influence of schooling on self-esteem, they have typically taken into account two factors—type of school and communication. No significant effects have typically been found for either factor. Although changes in school environment, such as residential to public or vice versa, can adversely affect self-esteem for a period of time, one setting has not been found to be superior to another in enhancing self-esteem (Bat-Chava, 1993; Lytle, Feinstein, & Jonas, 1987).

The type of school may not affect self-esteem in a direct way but self-esteem assuredly affects school achievement. Koelle and Convey (1982) found that self-concept was a significant predictor of academic achievement among deaf adolescents attending residential schools for the deaf. Chovan and Roberts (1993) assessed the relationship between achievement and self-concept among 9- to 19-year-old deaf students attending a school for the deaf. They found that the deaf students' concept of self was particularly associated with reading success.

Group Identification and Self-Esteem

Group identification involves having friends who share an identity, being involved in a community with shared values and identity, and feeling a sense of shared characteristics with members of a group. Bat-Chava (1994) investigated the relationship of group identification and self-esteem in 267 deaf adults and found that having primarily deaf friends and being highly involved in the Deaf community had a positive effect on self-esteem. He also found that deaf individuals who are members of the Deaf community but do not identify with it are more likely to have low self-esteem.

Bat-Chava noted that membership in a minority group results in low self-esteem if that group is perceived by the majority culture to be inferior. However, this effect can be mitigated by identification with a minority group that prides itself on its unique qualities and characteristics. His research with adult Deaf individuals appears to support this hypothesis. If true, deafened and hard of hearing individuals reap the benefits of identifying with groups of deafened or hard of hearing individuals such as through the organization Self-Help for the Hard of Hearing (SHHH).

Glickman (1996a) proposed that deaf and hard of hearing persons are either culturally hearing, culturally marginal, culturally Deaf, or bicultural. The culturally hearing are primarily deafened individuals who see their condition as a medical pathology and strive to be as hearinglike as possible. The culturally marginal are deaf or hard of hearing individuals who do not feel a part of either the Deaf or hearing communities. The culturally Deaf are primarily individuals who grew up within Deaf families or residential schools for the deaf and identify strictly with the Deaf community. The bicultural are deaf or hard of hearing individuals who feel comfortable in both hearing and Deaf communities. According to Glickman's analysis, the culturally hearing and culturally marginal are the most likely to suffer poor self-esteem.

As Bat-Chava (1993) noted, "Having a community of people who share one's minority group membership, both in childhood and in adulthood, protects deaf individuals from the majority's negative attitudes" (p. 229).

In Essay 6.2 Cara Frank discusses her experiences with friends, family members, and teachers.

■ ■ ■ ■ ■ ▬▬▬▬▬▬▬▬▬▬▬▬▬▬▬▬▬▬▬▬▬▬▬▬▬▬▬▬▬

ESSAY 6.2

Cara Frank

I'm fifteen years old, and I'm a ninth grader. I'm taking all the required courses right now, plus ASL and calligraphy. Calligraphy is only one semester; the other semester I'm going to take Driver's Ed. I'm looking forward to that. My parents haven't taken me out driving because I'm not really old enough yet. I won't get my permit until this summer.

I was six years old when I got my cochlear implant. I remember because it was pretty scary. All I remember is going down the hall on the stretcher, having the mask put on my face, waking up with a headache, and having a bad hair day because half of my hair was shaved off. I don't remember the very first time I put on my headphone, but I do remember noticing different changes in the sounds I heard. Before the implant, I couldn't hear the phone ringing, but now it's just the most annoying thing sometimes. I guess that was the first thing I remember hearing, the phone and also the doorbell.

I don't remember this, but my mom told me stories about how I acted after I got my implant. We were down in the park walking together, and I told her to stop walking. She stopped walking, there was silence, then I told her to walk again, and she walked again, tap tap tap, back and forth. I was trying to figure out what I was hearing. Then I realized I was hearing her footsteps. I could hear all the things that I couldn't hear before.

Before I got my cochlear implant, a lot of times I couldn't understand my brother really well, and I always had to depend on reading his lips. Now I can just rely on my hearing and not lipreading. But his voice is changing, so I kind of have to take a step back right now and get used to his voice. With males, who have really low voices, I have a lot of trouble understanding their voices. Also, people who have braces, I can't read their lips at all. So I depend on both hearing and lipreading. If it's a loud, clear voice, then I don't even have to lipread a person.

A funny thing happened to me about four weeks ago. I met this guy, and he had no idea that I have a hearing loss. He had a pretty low voice, so I had to read his lips. We were just getting to know each other, and, after a while, he asked me, "Do you want to kiss me or something, because you've been staring at my lips." I felt my face turn red! I said, "Um, no, not really. I've been looking at your lips because I've been lipreading you." I explained the whole thing to him, and he still said, "Oh, are you sure you don't want to kiss me?"

Some people are easier to understand than others. One of my teachers had a mustache and a beard, and I was always begging him to shave it off. My PE teacher had a mustache, but he had a loud, booming voice in a gym where it echoes. A loud booming voice is okay, but the echoing part is kind of confusing. When people do presentations and they put their paper in front of their mouth, I would like to say, "Could you pull the paper down, please?" But I can't do that. When I was younger, my speech teacher would cover her mouth so that I would concentrate on hearing her. I'm glad she did that because I don't want to be so reliant on lipreading.

I use the regular telephone with certain people, but boys, no, I ask them to call another way because they have that deep voice. Although I can hear them, I can't understand the words. I have to use the relay service and listen to what the relay operator says. One guy thought I was the relay operator. I said, "No, you got it wrong." I explained it to him, and then he said, "I heard a lot of typing noises, is it the computer?" I don't know how stupid they can be sometimes. I told him about it the day before I called, and he forgot or something. But this happens a lot.

I went to Tucker-Maxon Oral School until second grade, and then I transferred to an elementary school. We lived in Beaverton, Oregon, at the time. I was in mainstreamed classes all day long, but I got pulled out for speech. I don't remember how often. I had an itinerant teacher who worked with me for a couple of years, but I didn't like it. I thought it was kind of annoying. The other kids see this woman pull me out of class and none of them are being pulled out, at least by the teacher, so that was kind of awkward. They still do it now, and I still don't like it. People don't understand. They say, "You sound like you have a normal voice, why do you need speech?" And, I don't know, it's just a part of having an implant. I explain the whole thing to them, that I have to correctly learn how to pronounce words because the way words look is not always the way they're pronounced. The English language is messed up. I still get pulled out for speech every Tuesday or Thursday. Otherwise I take all of the regular classes with real-time captioning. In sign language class it's easy to get the information because they're signing. But in math, our teacher didn't even have a classroom at first, so we had to sit out in the hall. There was a lot of background noise, and I was missing a lot of stuff.

It's really annoying that every class has a class clown, and they're always interrupting the teacher or pulling some kind of prank that's distracting, and then I just miss what the teacher's saying. So, the captioning is good for that. You know, if the class clown's caught my attention and I'm not paying attention to the teacher, then I can just look back on the laptop and see what I've missed.

I've had the same captioner since the sixth grade, so we have a really nice relationship. It's funny because if there was somebody I liked, she'd caption something about him on to the screen to me. I would type back to her on the laptop, "Don't do that!" or make a joke out of it. Because, you know, other people can see that. She has a new computer now, so I can't do it anymore and I miss that because it was really fun.

A long time ago when my mom first told me that the school agreed to provide captioning, I didn't want it because I just wanted to blend in. I didn't want to stand out. It was also my very first year in Washington, and I didn't know anybody yet. I wanted people to see me, not the computer, because when I come to school with a computer, people pay more attention to that, usually, than me. They want to know about the captioning before knowing me. Then, once they've got the hang of it, which takes a long time, then they start to get to know me. At the end of a presentation I gave to the school about my hearing loss, in which I was reading from the laptop screen right in front of me, one kid asked, "Can you read?"

My science teacher last year was terrible. I thought that he would be understanding because he actually had a hearing loss, too. So it's kind of weird that he didn't understand. He would just talk to my captioner, Christy. He would tell her about the assignment or whatever. He did that all year long and never stopped. I would go up to him and tell him, "You can talk to me." When I would go up to him and ask questions, he would talk to me, but other times he

(continued)

would just talk to Christy, expecting her to relay the information. I didn't understand that. It was very annoying.

What Christy sends me on the screen isn't permanent, it's fleeting. But she also sends me notes later through e-mail, though I don't really need notes yet. She does it just in case. That just started this year. The district pays her to send notes for a couple of classes, because it's hard to be watching the teacher, paying attention, and taking notes at the same time. Sometimes the teacher has something on the overhead and also is talking, so if I'm watching the overhead, then I'm missing what the teacher is saying. I usually get some of the information. I miss more of it when I'm so focused on reading the words because I can't both read and listen at once. I'm not using the notes much yet because the teachers mostly give assignments and not lectures. I'm only a freshman. I might need those notes as the year goes on, but not right now.

I know there are some kids in my high school with hearing impairments, but I have not seen one single person. I think today I just saw a girl pass me with a hearing aid in her ear, but that's all I've ever seen. I've seen people use sign language, but they have no hearing problem, they just know it from ASL class. I thought this year would be so interesting meeting all of those people because I want to learn sign language. I feel like I should because it's kind of, sort of what I am. So, it'd be fun to sign back and forth. I only have actually one person who I can share with, she just got a cochlear implant two months ago. That's nice but I also want to meet other people. All the schools that I've been at, except Tucker-Maxon, I've been the only hearing impaired student. I don't really have any other deaf or hearing impaired friends at my school so sometimes I feel left out.

In elementary school, I was really shy, and I think nobody really wants to talk to a person who never talks. It's really hard to start up a conversation. In high school it's really different. People accept you more. I remember that in sixth grade I had to change to a different class for the captioning schedule to work. So, I had to switch classes, and I didn't like that because I was new, and I had already met new people. Now I was going to meet even more new people, and I already had enough of people pointing my implant out. So I didn't want to go through that again. Now I kind of know how to handle it.

I wear my cochlear implant all the time except when I go to sleep. So when I spend the night with friends, and they turn off the light, if we're still talking, I'll keep it on. I have to take it off to swim and things like that. Even if I could wear it while I swim I'm not sure if I would want to because you could see the entire implant on me and it would be distracting. I don't have problems with people seeing that, but it would probably bother some people and that would really annoy me because I'm a really active person. I used to put my hair in a ponytail a lot, or french braid it, but it can be annoying. Sometimes I do try to hide it because once they see that, they label me. So sometimes I avoid it for a little while and then tell them. Then they give me a chance. But sometimes they don't. So, during the first week of school I was wearing my hair down, but now I'm pulling it up in ponytails and stuff. On Monday I had my hair french braided and that's really obvious because you can see the whole thing. There was this girl sitting next to me in math, and we just had a new seating chart done, so I was sitting near nobody I knew. The girl kept looking, and I didn't know what to do. I turned to her and said, "Do you want to know what that is on my ear?" And she said, "Um, no." Sometimes people will just say, "What is that?" but not very often. Maybe they get a little nervous. Sometimes my friends tell other people. I think that when I was little, people pointed it out more.

Sometimes I have to go to Tucker-Maxon, to get the mapping changed in my implant (the computer inside my processor that changes the sounds into better ways for me to hear). It's good to get a change because I get used to the sounds and start falling asleep, and then once I get new sounds again I wake up.

I've thought about what I want to do in the future a lot, but I still have no idea. I think that I'll go to college. Most of the jobs that I'm interested in require a college degree. I don't want to work in a fast food restaurant. I mean, as a teenager that's okay, but not for the rest of my life. I want to do something that's going to help other people. I actually wanted to be a doctor for a while, but blood and stuff really grosses me out, so I couldn't handle that. And, I'm not that great with science, so I'm not meant to be a doctor. We had to do dissection, and I couldn't handle it. I felt really sick. I maybe want to become an artist or a writer. I do know that I want to become a role model for younger kids with hearing losses.

I know that my family pushed me a lot when I was younger to keep working hard with my speech. I remember one of my mom's friends talking about how hard my mom worked. Once they decided to go camping together, her family and mine, and my mom asked all these questions like, "Is this camp loud? Is it noisy? What kind of activities do they have there?" She was really asking if this would be a good camping place for me. It's really interesting hearing that because I never actually got to see my mom doing that. I've never seen my mom teach, and I don't really want to. My mom has probably told people stories about me, and I don't want them to know that's me.

My friend Andrea has a really high voice. She just got her cochlear implant, and so far she's doing really good. We went to the beach with this teen group. We were lying on the ground, and she could hear something. She asked me what it was, and I looked at her to make sure I understood what she was talking about. I asked, "What do you hear?" She said, "I hear somebody blowing or some kind of roaring." I said, "That's the ocean." I thought it was really nice to experience that. She had never experienced that before. It made me feel like a mother seeing her child experience something new. Another time there were trees with pine cones on them, and you know how they crackle when they open up. She could never hear that before. We were camping, being really quiet, and after a while she asked, "What's that?" We figured out that it was the pine cones. She's becoming aware of all the other sounds like crickets and sounds of spring, and she's really enjoying it. She's glad she got it.

In my ASL class, sometimes I get the impression that everyone thinks all deaf people are the same. It's kind of awkward because I want to raise my hand and tell them that's not true, but I'll take up the teacher's time and turn it into a lecture. Every once in a while I'll raise my hand and say something. I don't want everybody to think that all people who are born deaf or have a hearing loss use sign language. Most of them in my first period class only know about it because they know me. But people in other classes might not know somebody like me, and they might think that all deaf people use sign language and can't use speech.

(continued)

ESSAY 6.2   CONTINUED

> I don't really know if I'm happy with the choices my parents made for me because I never got to try out the other side by using sign language. But I think they made the right decision. It's really great what technology can do now. I probably would not enjoy using sign language all the time because you can't communicate with everyone. With the implant, I have the chance to try out both worlds, the deaf world and the hearing world. With sign language you stick to one world, the deaf world. I couldn't live with that. I would probably want to try out the other one. I also wonder what it's like in the actual hearing world, like what my voice really sounds like because it probably sounds different to me. Does my voice sound higher or lower? When I was younger, I started noticing that there were differences in people's voices, and so I asked my brother, "Jerry, do I have a female voice?" He said, "Yeah." I asked him, "Is it really high or is it low, or what?" He said, "If it were any lower it would be a male voice." It was good hearing the part about how my voice does sound like a female voice; however, I'm not sure if I like it being that low. A lot of people tell me that my voice is really outstanding.

Reprinted by permission of the author.

Programs for Building Self-Esteem

Chapter 7 will present some of the instructional programs that have been developed for Deaf awareness and Deaf studies in elementary, middle, and high school. Several programs have been developed specifically to build the self-esteem of deaf children and youth.

The Rotterdam Deaf Awareness Program was started in 1981 at the Rudolf Mees Institute to help deaf students to develop a Deaf identity and understand Deaf culture. According to de Klerk (1998), key aspects of the program have been interactive learning, active participation of Deaf adults, continuous self-reflection, and the direct involvement of the students in program development.

Outdoor education programs are often used as a milieu for teaching self-reliance and self-esteem. One outdoor adventure education program involved college students from Gallaudet University. The students traveled through the Rocky Mountains for ten days with three instructors. Luckner (1989) found a significantly positive effect on the students' self-concept. Another outdoor adventure program engaged deaf students in 14- to 16-day canoe trips in northern Minnesota, and Luckner (1988) also found significant gains in self-esteem among these students. He concluded:

> Outdoor adventure education provides students with an opportunity to learn from a natural environment. It allows individuals to experience real sit-

uations that do not require generalization. Through active involvement, one's attention is compelled to the problems at hand. Mastery of challenging tasks conveys salient evidence of enhanced competence. When combined with the provision of an interpersonal, social context through group interaction, outdoor adventure education offers a supportive and highly structured framework for promoting self-concept change. (1989, p. 48)

Classroom experiences can affect self-esteem both positively and negatively. Luckner (1987) recommended that when planning instruction, teachers should consider each lesson as an opportunity to promote the deaf child's sense of uniqueness, feeling of connection to others, feelings of accomplishment, and sense of control. As Clymer (1995) recognized, "Positive self-concept is a jewel of many facets—pride, acceptance, identity, achievement, success, responsibility, and independence" (p. 119). In addition to self-esteem, psychological adjustment includes the development of empathy.

EMPATHY

Empathy involves vicariously experiencing the feelings, thoughts, and experiences of another person. Empathy is often thought of as the ability to take someone else's perspective. Early research with deaf children indicated deficits in their empathy development (Bachara, Raphael, & Phelan, 1980).

One method for assessing empathy is through role-taking tasks. Kusche and Greenberg (1983) asked 4- to 10-year-old deaf and hearing children to guess which hand a penny was in and to hide a penny for the investigator. They found the younger deaf children in the study to be delayed in role-taking ability when compared to hearing children, but this difference disappeared by age 6. They concluded that deaf children are not more egocentric than hearing children, but on some tasks they have difficulty expressing their knowledge or feelings because of their English or ASL language abilities. "Role-taking tasks often confound the basic skill of differentiating perspectives with linguistic knowledge and social understanding" (p. 147).

Cates and Shontz (1990a) used a different role-taking task than Kusche and Greenberg. They asked 7- to 14-year-old deaf children to describe a four-cartoon picture sequence from their own perspective and then from the perspective of a character who was introduced halfway through the story line and who did not know what had transpired previously. They found that role taking was not correlated with social behavior but was correlated with emotional adjustment, self-image, and communicative effectiveness.

Another method for assessing empathy is picture interpretation. Sanders (1985) asked deaf and hearing children between the ages of 4 and a half and 15 and a half to identify the emotions expressed in drawings and photographs. She found that the deaf children were as able as the hearing children to identify emotions from facial expression and body language. However, in pictures that presented additional contextual elements, some of the deaf children had difficulty interpreting the emotions being expressed. It would appear that the deaf children were more reliant on the emotions expressed by the individual being depicted than on situations in which the individual was involved. In other words, they had no difficulty identifying emotions but some difficulty identifying emotional situations.

Weisel (1985) suggested that some of the difficulty deaf individuals demonstrate with empathy might be related to how emotions are expressed with and without sign language, and he hypothesized that they may actually be more able to interpret and understand others' emotions. He showed deaf college students films that included emotional expressions in sign language. The deaf actors signed two sentences that stated, in essence, they were going out, wouldn't be back, and to tell others they weren't here. As they signed these sentences, they nonverbally expressed one of six emotions—anger, disgust, fear, happiness, sadness, and surprise. Weisel did not find the deaf subjects to be more sensitive to the nonverbal messages than the hearing subjects. He concluded that studies using emotional expressions in English as well as sign language "do not suggest that deaf people naturally compensate and develop a superior sensitivity" (p. 521).

A final aspect of psychological adjustment is self-efficacy. Chapter 5 discussed locus of control as it related to social development. In this chapter, locus of control is part of self-efficacy.

SELF-EFFICACY

Self-efficacy is the individual's knowledge of his or her own power to produce an effect. One aspect of self-efficacy, according to Delgado (1982), is maturity or self-dependence. He postulated that deaf individuals are frequently characterized as immature because in the context of school and home, they are often encouraged to be dependent on others, particularly hearing teachers and parents. Therefore, they might reach the benchmarks of emotional development somewhat later than hearing individuals. Meadow and Dyssegaard (1983) noted that although many deaf individuals could be characterized as immature and dependent, many deaf children and adults could also be characterized quite differently. The variance can be found in the different ways that deaf students are encouraged to be self-motivated and to develop their abilities for leadership and independence.

Another aspect of self-efficacy is locus of control. Research with hearing college students has found a positive correlation between internal locus of control and academic motivation. Research with deaf college students has indicated that they tend to attribute their academic success to external factors and, therefore, demonstrate less motivation to work on improving specific academic areas (Dowaliby, Burke, & McKee, 1983; Hayes-Scott, 1987; Schultz & Pomerantz, 1976).

A third aspect of self-efficacy is impulsivity. Deaf children have been found to be more impulsive than hearing children regardless of communication used by the children, though deaf children with deaf parents appear to be less impulsive than deaf children with hearing parents (Altshuler, Deming, Vollenweider, Rainer, & Tendler, 1976; Harris, 1978; O'Brien, 1987). Deaf children become less impulsive with age, but so do hearing children, and the differences between them seem to remain.

Psychological adjustment occurs in the context of the deaf individual's interactions with others and the world. How well the individual has adjusted can be seen in his or her relationships, particularly the ones that require intimacy.

INTIMACY AND SEXUALITY

The ability to be intimate with others is a reflection of one's psychological adjustment, and intimacy enhances one's psychological well-being. With this in mind, it would be valuable to understand the issues involved in intimacy for deaf individuals. However, there appears to be little information available about intimacy among friends, partners, and spouses.

Historically, deaf individuals tended to marry deaf individuals, though the pattern appears to be changing as increasing numbers of deaf children are educated in programs with hearing children and larger numbers of hearing individuals are skilled in sign language (Rice, 1984; Updegraff, 1992). Hard of hearing individuals appear to choose hearing individuals as spouses and many deafened individuals have lost their hearing during their marriages. The stresses and adjustments seem to be similar to those within any marriage. As Rice (1984) noted, when deaf individuals marry,

> they proceed to establish a family relationship of reciprocal obligations and restrictions. They share, create, and maintain a common culture within the family structure. If they communicate easily with each other, and if they come from a similar family pattern of development and parenting, then their

adjustment problems will be minor and positive family relationships can be established easily.... When immaturity, indifference, lack of responsibility, or lack of emotional control come to the fore, a couple faces pain and frustration. (p. 19)

As in the broader society, domestic abuse exists in families with a deaf member. It does not appear that researchers, social agencies, or state agencies routinely isolate the statistics regarding domestic abuse in this population. In a 1982 study, Egley found no published documentation but inferential data to support the belief that substantial domestic abuse exists among and toward deaf people.

The aspect of intimacy that has received the most attention has been sexuality. Within the topic of sexuality, most of the research has been directed at how deaf individuals obtain sexuality information. There has also been some interest in understanding homosexuality among deaf individuals, sexually transmitted diseases within the Deaf community, and sexual abuse of deaf children.

Sexuality Information

It appears as if the sources and completeness of sexuality information has not changed over the decades. In the 1980s, Fitz-Gerald and Fitz-Gerald (1980, 1984, 1985, 1987) noted that deaf young people tended to obtain most of their information about sex from peers, observation, experience, and media such as television and movies. When Fitz-Gerald and Fitz-Gerald interviewed deaf adolescents, they found that more than half reported discussing menstruation, dating, marriage, body changes, and teenage pregnancy with their parents. However, the adolescents also reported rarely discussing sexual behavior, decisions for having or delaying sex, birth control, adolescent parenting, and personal relationships. In the 1990s, Joseph, Sawyer, and Desmond found that deaf and hard of hearing college students obtained most of their information about sex from friends, magazines, and television (1995). However, unlike the young people in the Fitz-Gerald and Fitz-Gerald studies, they also obtained information from their doctors.

In the mid-1980s, Tripp and Kahn asked deaf and hearing adults, who ranged in age from 20s to 80s, about their sexual knowledge. The hearing adults demonstrated significantly greater knowledge of sex, physiology, slang, pregnancy and fetal development, contraceptives, and male and female anatomy than the deaf adults.

Fitz-Gerald and Fitz-Gerald (1987) asked parents why they find it difficult to discuss sex with their deaf children. The parents reported the following reasons:

- Embarrassment and discomfort
- Lack of knowledge for answering all of the child's questions
- Uncertainty about personal values and feelings regarding sexuality issues
- Fear that discussion will encourage sexual experimentation
- Reticence by the child to ask questions
- Communication problems
- Uncertainty with how and when to open the discussion
- Belief that the information is being provided in school
- Belief that the child already knows the information

When Love (1983) asked parents at a school for the deaf what would be the most desirable place for instruction in human sexuality, about three-quarters felt it was the home and one-quarter felt it was the school. Almost all of the parents wanted their children to participate in school instruction.

What is the sexual knowledge and behavior of deaf young people? Joseph, Sawyer, and Desmond (1995) surveyed deaf college students and found the following:

- More than 80 percent reported being sexually active, and of these, 11 percent reported having 10 or more sexual partners. About one-third reported becoming sexually active at 19 years or older and about one-tenth at 14 years or younger.
- Alcohol or other drugs were used by 13 percent during their last sexual encounter.
- Approximately one-third used a condom during their most recent sexual encounter, most believing that having a regular partner negated the need.
- Just over half reported being worried about contracting HIV/AIDS or other sexually transmitted diseases, and just under half reported being worried about pregnancy. One-third had been tested for HIV.
- The most common method of contraception was withdrawal, followed by condoms and oral contraceptives.
- More than 80 percent of the females reported having had a pelvic exam and Pap test, and half stated that they performed monthly breast self-examinations.
- Just over half of the males reported having had a testicular exam, and 17 percent stated that they performed monthly testicular self-examinations.
- When given an exam testing their knowledge of human sexuality, the students answered just under half of the questions correctly, with the females outscoring the males. The knowledge test consisted of items

about ovulation, HIV, reproduction, and the effectiveness of various forms of birth control.

Knowledge of sexually transmitted diseases is one particularly critical aspect of sexuality knowledge, and so it is no surprise that educators and counselors have been very concerned with how well young deaf people are being educated in this area. Luckner and Gonzales (1993) surveyed more than 200 deaf adolescents and found that they had a general idea about what HIV and AIDS are, and also a general idea of the impact. However, these adolescents demonstrated gaps in their knowledge about transmission and prevention of HIV, as well as poor awareness of personal risk factors. For example, almost half of the adolescents did not realize that heterosexuals could contract HIV, and more than 40 percent thought that all homosexuals are HIV positive or have AIDS.

A survey of the policies at schools for the deaf indicated that by the mid-1990s, most schools serving deaf and hard of hearing students were aware of the importance of establishing policies regarding students with HIV and AIDS, though the policies varied from highly comprehensive to very brief. Almost all of the policies dealt with issues of the student's right to attend school, the student's right to privacy, the protection of other students, and how placement decisions are made. Almost none of the policies dealt with HIV testing. Approximately half of the policies included an HIV/AIDS education provision but without specifically describing how and what kinds of information would be provided. Three-fourths of the schools reported providing HIV/AIDS education to employees, 90 percent to students, and less than 10 percent to parents. The survey's author, Deyo (1994), concluded that although administrators at most of the schools considered it important to establish and refine policies and procedures, "in many cases the policies are insufficient as clear guidance for handling the complexities of placing and providing services for students in a residential school setting" (p. 91).

Homosexuality

Attitudes toward homosexuality changed dramatically during the last half of the twentieth century, yet in the arena of sexuality, no issue has provoked as much passionate debate with the possible exception of abortion. Phaneuf (1987) commented, "In the context of an environment that espouses traditional attitudes towards homosexuality, a disability that impacts negatively upon communication and a lack of factual sexual information, the deaf young person who feels homosexual desires is unlikely to be prepared to deal with the situation" (p. 53). Parents are often concerned about the dual risk for discrimination that their child might face. And the gay deaf man or lesbian deaf woman feels the same degree of concern about letting others know about his or her sexual preferences as hearing homosexual individuals do.

Langholtz and Rendon (1991–1992) noted that deaf individuals have a smaller community with which to share their feelings about their homosexuality.

> If the parents are hearing, very often they will go through a grief that is reminiscent of when they discovered their child was deaf. For deaf parents of a deaf gay/lesbian child, there may also be a sense of loss. The loss could be in terms of closeness in their relationship with their child or with their standing in the Deaf community. There can be a sense of fear of ridicule by the fellow Deaf community members. (p. 33)

As there are pejorative words for homosexuals, there are pejorative signs. Many deaf gays and lesbians find their community in organizations specifically designed for them.

Sexual Abuse

In research studies reported by Sullivan, Vernon, and Scanlan (1987), a significantly greater percentage of deaf children than hearing children were victims of sexual abuse; they found 10 percent of hearing boys compared to 54 percent of deaf boys and 25 percent of hearing girls compared to 50 percent of deaf girls. Furthermore, whereas hearing girls tend to be abused more often than hearing boys, deaf boys are abused at a slightly higher rate than deaf girls. Although the numbers of children in these studies tended to be small, it appears that vans and buses bringing the children to and from school presented high-risk situations for the children because of the limited supervision and oversight. The researchers also found that deaf children will typically not discuss sexual abuse unless they are specifically asked, which means that their teachers and parents need to be knowledgeable of the physical, behavioral, and emotional indicators of abuse. If they do want to report it, the parent may not know the sexual signs that the child is using.

A serious issue at schools for the deaf has been a tendency to keep incidents of sexual abuse, as well as rape, in house. According to Sullivan, Vernon, and Scanlan, these actions result in inappropriate solutions, violations of legal statutes, and allowance of perpetrators to molest other children. "The key issue is that it must be reported, investigated, prosecuted and psychological help provided for the child victim" (1987, p. 258).

A related issue to sexual abuse is rape. In the study by Joseph, Sawyer, and Desmond (1995), approximately one-fourth of the deaf college students reported having been forced to have sex against their wishes on at least one occasion.

Mental health involves issues of psychological adjustment, intimacy, and sexuality, which were just discussed. Mental health also involves religion and spirituality, recreation and leisure. For Deaf individuals, the church and other religious organizations have traditionally been a central part of the Deaf community. Deaf clubs, deaf sport (as discussed earlier), and other deaf organizations have typically enriched the personal and social lives, and consequently the mental health, of deaf individuals. However, there is little documentation in the published literature about the role and function of these activities within the lives of deaf persons. There is, however, a substantial amount of information about the opposite end of the mental health spectrum—emotional and behavioral problems, counseling, and therapy.

EMOTIONAL AND BEHAVIORAL PROBLEMS

The literature during the past 100 years or more has indicated that emotional and behavioral problems are more prevalent among deaf individuals than other populations. Harry and Dietz (1985) examined the legal status of deaf individuals as a way of looking at emotional and behavioral problems. During the decade of the 1970s, the prevalence of prelingual deafness in defendants who were remanded to the maximum-security unit of a state mental hospital was five times greater than the prevalence of prelingual deafness in the general population. They postulated that either there is an association between hearing loss and criminality or the judicial system considers deaf individuals as incompetent and lacking criminal responsibility.

Given the conjecture about the prevalence of emotional and behavioral problems among deaf individuals, and the ramifications to the quality of life for deaf individuals and society, it seems vital to separate opinion from fact regarding prevalence and to determine the causes of emotional and behavioral problems as well as the types that are most common in the deaf population.

Prevalence

Much of the research indicates a substantially higher percentage of emotional and behavioral problems of deaf children when compared to hearing children. Aplin (1987) found prevalence figures between 4.8 percent and 19.7 percent for deaf students in mainstream settings and between 19.7 percent and 36.1 percent for students in schools for the deaf. When van Eldik (1994) investigated the behavioral problems of deaf boys between ages 6 and 11, he found that the deaf boys exhibited a significantly greater percentage of behavioral problems, with 28.4 percent of the deaf boys and 23.2 percent of hearing boys assessed as having behavioral problems. Hindley (1997) found a prevalence range of 43 to 50.3 percent among deaf and hard of hearing students.

Prevalence figures among adult deaf individuals are equally mixed. Harry (1986) reported that adult deaf individuals are diagnosed with mental disorders at a rate between 22 percent and 39 percent. Schizophrenia was diagnosed in 14 to 21 percent, personality disorders were diagnosed in about 15 percent, and other categories (such as situational reactions, bipolar disorder, and unspecified psychoses) accounted for the remaining 64 to 71 percent. Thomas (1984) found that the proportion of psychological disturbance in deafened individuals was 45 percent within the 16- to 19-year-old age range, 18 percent within the 39- to 59-year-old age range, and 14 percent within the 60- to 64-year-old age range. Among deaf individuals identified as intellectually gifted, Vernon and LaFalce-Landers (1993) found that 39 percent required treatment for mental illness.

Causes

It is unlikely that one or a set of factors within the early or later life experience of a deaf individual actually causes emotional or behavioral problems. However, it does appear that particular factors make it more likely that a deaf person will experience emotional or behavioral problems.

Greenberg, Kusche, and Speltz (1991) found that early parent–child attachment was a critical factor in the deaf child's later emotional stability. They also noted that language is central to the deaf child's ability to deal with internal motivation and external control. In other words, the deaf child who is able to use language for problem solving, either English or ASL, is also the child who reflects greater emotional adjustment.

Kluwin (1985) examined the discipline referral forms at five schools for the deaf in an effort to understand the factors that relate to behavioral problems. He found reading ability to be the factor that was most predictive of disruptive behavior in the classroom. Cohen (1991) suggested that student alienation and estrangement are at-risk factors for behavioral problems during this age because although these factors are common among virtually all adolescents, they are exacerbated when the adolescent is deaf, as a result of communication issues.

It is possible that deaf children and youth do not experience greater behavioral or emotional problems, but are misperceived to do so by teachers and parents who either do not understand the cultural factors underlying the child's behavior or expect certain traits in all deaf people. This view was not supported in a study conducted by Murphy-Berman, Stoefen-Fisher, and Mathias (1987). They found that neither deaf nor hearing teachers demonstrated bias toward the behavior exhibited by deaf children. It also might be expected that language difficulties between teachers and deaf students, such as teachers who are not fluent in ASL, would result in communication breakdowns, and miscommunication would lead to behavioral problems. However, there appears to be no research specifically examining communication as a factor in the behavioral or emotional problems of deaf children and adolescents.

Among deafened individuals, it does not appear that acquired hearing loss causes personality disorders; however, Thomas (1984) found that these individuals do experience higher levels of psychological disturbance characterized by anxiety, depression, sleep disturbance, listlessness, and panic attacks. Knutson and Lansing (1990) assessed deafened individuals between ages 22 and 71 who were seeking a cochlear implant and found that depression, social introversion, loneliness, and social anxiety were related to communicative functioning.

Altshuler (1986) studied the incidence of schizophrenia and found that while deaf patients tended to reside in state hospitals for longer periods of time than hearing patients, deafness itself was not associated with schizophrenia. He noted that "variation in environment and experience may alter the manifestations of genetic potential" (p. 127) and so explain the prevalence of affective disorders, such as depression, though not personality or other mental disorders.

Types

The same problems and disorders have been found in deaf and hearing children, youth, and adults. Types of problems that have been studied in deaf individuals include depression, eating disorders, and substance abuse.

Watt and Davis (1991) found a higher incidence of depression among deaf adolescents attending both public and residential school programs. Leigh and her associates conducted a series of studies on depression in deaf college students (Leigh, Robins, & Welkowitz, 1990; Leigh, Robins, Welkowitz, & Bond, 1989). They found a significantly higher level of mild depression in the deaf than the hearing college students but no differences in more severe depression. For both the hearing and deaf students, perception of low maternal care and high maternal overprotection were related to depression. They also found that when the deaf students felt a good match between their preferred mode of communication and their mother's communication, the deaf students were less likely to experience depression.

Eating disorders appear to be as much of a problem among deaf individuals as in the hearing population, though the research is quite limited. Hills, Rappold, and Rendon (1991) investigated eating disorders in deaf college students and found that 21 percent of the women and 12 percent of the men reported bingeing currently, 7 percent reported controlling their weight by vomiting and 14 percent by strict dieting and fasting, 39 percent reported a strong fear of gaining weight, and 46 percent perceived themselves as heavier than their actual weight.

Deaf individuals face the same risk of substance abuse as other populations. According to Lane (1989), a number of precipitating factors have been identified among deaf adolescents and adults:

- Lack of trust in oneself and others
- Dependence on the opinion of others
- Poor impulse control
- Poor communication skills
- Depression
- Immaturity
- Feelings of isolation
- Feelings of inferiority

It has been frequently reported that the Deaf community views substance abuse, and alcoholism specifically, as unacceptable and morally wrong. Sylvester (1987) stated, "Deaf communities tend to view alcoholism in moralistic and judgmental terms and, thus, perceive the deaf alcoholics among them as sinful" (p. 1). When Sabin (1988) assessed the attitudes of deaf high school students toward alcohol, she found that they distinguished between alcoholism and drinking. These deaf adolescents viewed drunkenness as unacceptable, but they did not view too much drinking as a character weakness.

When one or both parents are substance abusers, the children are directly and dramatically affected. Stevens (1987) noted that deaf children and adolescents are likely to have great difficulty dealing with this family situation, which may include domestic abuse in addition to the substance abuse. The typical silence about sharing family issues with others, along with the weak communication that sometimes exists between hearing parents and their deaf children, make it more probable that the deaf child will feel quite alone and helpless when a parent is abusing alcohol, drugs, or both.

The deaf substance abuser faces a number of barriers to recovery including the following (Guthmann & Sandberg, 1995; Lane, 1989; Rendon, 1992):

- There are relatively few treatment centers capable of treating deaf individuals, and few personnel are knowledgeable about deafness.

- Deaf substance abusers are widely distributed geographically.
- There appears to be limited awareness of substance abuse problems within the Deaf community.
- Deaf individuals are often mistrustful of hearing professionals.
- Concerns about confidentiality within the Deaf community serve to make Deaf individuals reluctant to seek treatment.
- Many deaf individuals lack information about resources.
- Communication with counselors and in self-help groups, such as Alcoholics Anonymous, can be complex and arduous.
- There is fear of losing the support of friends during recovery.

COUNSELING AND THERAPY

When deaf children, youth, and adults experience emotional or behavioral problems, they seek counseling and therapy from mental health professionals. The range of approaches to counseling and therapy that have been used with deaf individuals probably encompasses the range of approaches used with hearing individuals. And the problems for which they seek help also encompass the same range as those of hearing individuals. The results of Backenroth's (1992) study of deaf adults who are in counseling "suggest that deaf people do not constitute a single group and that, as in the hearing population, there is great variation in deaf people's problems, needs, and potentials" (p. 358). However, access to counseling and therapy by deaf individuals has been limited by communication issues as well as counselors' and psychologists' knowledge of deafness.

Access to Counseling and Therapy

Mental health services specifically designed for deaf individuals did not begin until the mid-1950s in the United States and later in some other countries such as England, and decades later researchers have continued to find that services are lacking. Pyke and Littmann wrote:

> Psychiatric services are not generally available to this group in the same sense that they are to the hearing population since most psychiatrists are not only unfamiliar with the chief mode of deaf communication, namely manual communication, but in addition have often had little opportunity to gain a good understanding of the psychosocial implications of deafness. Given such unfamiliarity, psychiatric assessment and treatment, be it through an interpreter or by means of writing, is both time consuming and difficult, with considerable risk for misunderstanding and mistakes on the part of examiner and patient. (1982, p. 384)

On a similar note, Gerber (1983) wrote, "As a unique minority group, deaf people have been virtually excluded from our mental health care system due to bias, lack of knowledge and skills by professionals, and significant language/communication barriers" (p. 50). As of the late 1980s, only 11 private psychiatric centers indicated that they provided inpatient care to deaf individuals (Gerstein, 1988). In state mental hospitals with specialized inpatient programs for deaf individuals, Dickert (1988) found more positive attitudes to deaf patients than in mental health programs serving deaf individuals within a general population, but he also found that regardless of the program, the deaf patients tended to be evaluated as having more severe mental illness and greater need for supervision and medication. Vernon and Daigle-King (1999) examined the inpatient and outpatient care of deaf mental patients and found that relevant research on mental illness had lagged even more dramatically than mental health services in the United States and Europe during the last half of the twentieth century. According to Steinberg, "Despite federal statutes mandating accessible mental health care for disabled persons, the mental health service needs of deaf Americans remain profoundly underserved" (1991, p. 387).

Not only have researchers observed a historical lack of mental health services for adults, but educators have also found the same barriers to counseling services for deaf children. When Briccetti (1987) compared the availability of mental health services of the mid-1980s to the mid-1970s, she found that although services had increased, the levels were still not adequate to meet the needs of deaf students. She concluded that "there is a limited availability of counseling services within the schools and there is not yet a sufficient number of community mental health services to which students can be referred" (p. 281). She also found that students with more severe problems were inappropriately served and underserved (Briccetti, 1988).

Accessibility goes beyond the availability of services to include the ability of deaf individuals to utilize the services. The difference lies in whether the deaf person has the same array of programs, counselors, and therapists from which to select and also whether the language used in these settings is shared by the deaf person. As Myers and Danek commented, "Too often, the deaf person has little choice of services, or little assurance that programs are staffed by professionals with expertise in deafness as well as other appropriate skills" (1989, p. 72). They conducted a survey of mental health providers in one large metropolitan community in the United States, and these providers expressed the following concerns:

- The deaf community was unaware of existing services.
- Outreach agencies were unable to work beyond their present capacities.

- Mental health services were perceived by the respondents as largely inaccessible to deaf people; often there was no place to refer a deaf client for mental health services.
- Front-line staff at generic social service agencies were unable to identify those deaf persons in need of mental health services and thus could not make appropriate referrals.
- When referrals were made, a gap existed between the referral agency and the receiving agency; the agency to which the client was referred frequently never received the client. (1989, p. 75)

Myers (1993) suggested that a basic level of accessibility includes interpreters and equipment such as TT, telephone amplifier, and television decoder. Beyond this level, mental health programs should also include staff members skilled in sign language who possess cultural knowledge and sensitivity. In a 1993 survey of services available in the state of Rhode Island, McEntee found that more than 70 percent of the service providers indicated that they had served deaf individuals during the past year; just 39 percent had TTs, 61 percent provided interpreters, and only 25 percent provided certified interpreters.

The section on mental health professionals will discuss the competencies of the counselors and therapists who work with deaf individuals. However, one point about mental health professionals seems important to make here; are the professionals who are being trained actually available to the deaf population? Wyatt and White (1993) surveyed counselor training programs that were specifically preparing counselors to work with deaf individuals, and they found that most of the graduates worked within rehabilitation settings rather than community mental health settings.

Therapies and Counseling Techniques

This section will present many of the therapies and counseling techniques that have been used with deaf children, youth, and adults. The purpose is to provide an overview of approaches, discuss why they have been successful or unsuccessful, and explain the underlying issues involved in implementing any type of therapy or counseling with individuals who are deaf. The purpose is not, however, to teach mental health professionals how to carry out these approaches.

Family Therapy

When family therapy is discussed, the predominant issue is communication. This literature typically addresses the family constellation in which the child is deaf and the parents are hearing. The flashpoint of differing viewpoints lies in the use of an interpreter within the therapy situation, particularly within families in which the members do not communicate fluently with one another. Sloman and Springer (1987) observed:

> The cultural clash in these families is often played out in the communication issue. When a lack of communication serves a systemic function, for example, by enabling parents to maintain their denial of their feelings about their child's deafness, the family may resist any attempt to explore how well they communicate. This, however, may run counter to a common therapeutic goal, which is to facilitate communication between family members. (p. 562)

Harvey (1982, 1984) suggested the following reasons for using an interpreter in family therapy:

- Therapists who are not fluent in sign language cannot communicate effectively with the deaf family member.
- Therapists who are fluent in sign language cannot interpret for all family members and provide treatment simultaneously.
- The interpreter's presence affects the interaction of family members and changes the power relationships, which influence the therapeutic process.

Harvey (1985) also noted that if an interpreter is used, the therapist should not assume that this person's presence provides all of the knowledge that is needed to work effectively with the deaf family member. The therapist must not only be knowledgeable about deafness, but he or she must also be informed about interpreter issues such as the code of ethics. Harvey further noted that the relationship between the therapist and interpreter must be mutually supportive and respectful.

Scott (1984) presented a viewpoint about the use of interpreters in family therapy that is in direct contrast to Harvey's view. In his work with families with a deaf member, he found that the issues within these families were not ones that were best addressed in a family therapy setting with an interpreter. His own experience led him to believe that in the therapeutic setting, it was best to maintain the communication already established within the family.

Therapy with Young Deaf Children

Two of the approaches discussed in the literature for conducting therapy with young deaf children are one-to-one therapy with the child and three-to-one therapy with the child and parents.

Zalewska (1989) suggested nonverbal therapy as a method for working with very young deaf children who appear to be experiencing disorders in the development of their personality. She described the principle of non-verbal therapy as a matching of therapist and child behavior in which the therapist is nondirective and follows the stages of play that the child experiences bodily, cognitively, and emotionally.

Fields, Blum, and Scharfman (1993) used a preschool setting as a therapeutic nursery for families with newly diagnosed children. They describe this method as a tripartite model of intervention in which the nursery setting is used to address the developmental needs of the deaf child and the emotional needs of the child's parents. The intervention "has the interrelated aims of alleviating parental distress, supporting the parent–child relationship, and facilitating the deaf infant's emerging ego capacities, as reflected in affective and cognitive functioning" (p. 41).

Sexual Abuse Therapy

As discussed previously, sexual abuse is one of the few mental health issues among deaf individuals that has received attention by the psychological and psychiatric communities. Boys Town National Research Hospital has been particularly active in addressing the needs of sexually abused deaf children.

In 1984, the Boys Town National Research Hospital established the Center for Abused Handicapped Children. According to Sullivan and Scanlan (1990), the goals of the program were as follows:

- To alleviate guilt engendered by the sexual abuse and to assist the child in regaining the ability to trust peers and adults
- To help treat the depression that is often manifested by children who have been sexually abused
- To help the child learn to express anger relating to the sexual abuse in appropriate and productive ways
- To teach basic information about normal human sexuality and interpersonal relationships
- To teach the child sexual preference and homosexual issues, when appropriate
- To teach sexual abuse issues, when appropriate
- To teach the child self-protection techniques
- The development of an affective vocabulary to label emotions and feelings
- The attainment of emotional independence
- Assistance in the establishment of a meaningful and stable identity
- Development of a personal value system
- The development of a capacity for lasting relationships and for both tender and genital love
- Treatment of secondary behavioral characteristics (pp. 25–29)

In a study of sexually abused deaf children, it was found that those who were treated at the Center for Abused Handicapped Children had significantly fewer behavior problems one year after therapy had begun than the children who had not been treated (Sullivan, Scanlan, Brookhauser, Schulte, & Knutson, 1992). For the boys, therapy was particularly effective in reducing aggression, hyperactivity, delinquency, immaturity, hostile withdrawal, and uncommunicativeness. For the girls, therapy was particularly effective in alleviating symptoms of depression, aggression, and cruelty.

Art Therapy

Art therapy has been used in individual and family therapy with deaf children. In individual therapy, Cohene and Cohene (1989) considered art therapy to be especially beneficial to deaf children because they are often unable or unwilling to discuss personally painful issues; expressing oneself through art can be less threatening than direct discussion, and art therapy is a relatively nonlinguistic approach.

Horovitz-Darby (1991) used art therapy within a family therapy setting. In her experience, the deaf child's expression of self through art symbols helped to mediate between family members and assisted parents in understanding their child's feelings. She observed that "the art materials help foster change both in communication and family systems functioning. The graphic components of the art mirror the visual aspects of sign language and pictorially aid the deaf child's ability to bridge the gap between the deaf culture and the hearing world" (p. 254).

Peer Counseling

Peer counseling capitalizes on the deaf adolescent's likelihood to seek advice about personal problems from a friend. In peer counseling, teachers nominate students who are representative of the school's population. The students who are chosen to be peer counselors receive training in basic counseling skills, which typically include active listening, avoidance of advice giving, paraphrasing, empathizing, and using body language that matches the sign or spoken message. The students then use these skills when interacting with peers who come to them for help or advice.

MacDonald and McLaughlin (1987) reported that at one school for the deaf, the peer support team developed their own code of ethics, which stated that peer counselors:

- Have a commitment to help people in solving problems
- Act confidentially and in a mature manner

- Are responsible for listening when people need to discuss personal problems
- Will not judge other people but rather will show acceptance of people
- Make sure that the environment respects their peers' privacy need
- Show understanding through actively listening to peers
- Only give ideas on options to solving problems and leave decisions to the person (p. 124)

Adult Therapies

Numerous therapies that are specifically meant for adult individuals have been discussed in the literature, and each presents both opportunities and challenges to the therapist, deaf individual, and sometimes others in the therapeutic environment.

One type of therapy used with adult deaf individuals is group therapy. Card and Schmider (1995) noted that when planning a group that includes at least one deaf or hard of hearing member, the therapist needs to consider the following factors:

- *Purpose of the group.* The purpose should determine membership, so the purpose should relate to the needs of all members being considered, including the deaf individual.
- *Selection criteria.* Selection should be based on ability to interact, ability to benefit from a group experience, and consonance between the person's needs and the group's purpose.
- *Size of the group.* Groups with a deaf member should probably be smaller in size than groups in which all members are hearing.
- *Communication.* The members of the groups should sit in a circle to facilitate communication, a hard of hearing member may need to use an assistive listening device, and a deaf member may need an interpreter.
- *Activities.* Group therapy tends to rely largely on verbal conversation, but with a deaf member, it is helpful to incorporate visual and action exercises.

Hittner and Bornstein (1990) pointed out that as the population of older individuals increases, the number of individuals with late-onset hearing loss who are seeking therapy will also increase. For example, in a group of eight adults over age 65, the therapist is likely to have two individuals with a hearing loss. The therapist's knowledge of deafness, including the implications of age of onset, and ability to use communication strategies that are inclusive for late-deafened and hard of hearing patients as well as Deaf patients, will be critical for the successful outcome of the group therapy.

Group therapy has also been used with deaf adolescents. Vernon and Hicks (1983) developed a group counseling program for adolescents with Usher's syndrome that helped the students develop bonds with other students going through the same experiences and assisted them in the first steps toward adjustment. Sarti (1993) used group therapy with deaf students entering their first year of high school who had demonstrated serious behavior problems during middle school. She found that the students developed improved self-concept, better impulse control, and enhanced reality testing.

Brief treatment was used by Harvey and Green (1990) to treat a hearing mother who had obsessional thoughts about her deaf child's future. In four sessions over a three-month period, the mother was helped to change negative internal images about her child and replace them with positive images supported through building external relationships with deaf adults.

Peterson and Gough (1995) suggested that the application of Gestalt therapy to working with deaf individuals is particularly appropriate within a rehabilitation counseling setting because of its focus on the whole person. Central to this therapy is building the deaf person's self-awareness, autonomy, and personal responsibility. Another therapy that has been suggested is provocative therapy. In provocative therapy, the therapist provokes the deaf individual's maladaptive behaviors, assumptions, and feelings and then uses the person's resistance and defenses to elicit more appropriate behaviors (Quedenfeld & Farrelly, 1983).

Rational–emotive therapy presents a special challenge because unlike many other therapies, a warm relationship between therapist and patient is not central to rational–emotive therapy. Because deaf individuals may enter the therapist–patient relationship with more suspicion toward a hearing therapist than hearing patients typically feel, Gough (1987) suggested that the therapist using rational–emotive therapy needs to pay more attention to establishing a trusting and accepting environment, given that the therapy itself is somewhat confrontative. Gough viewed this approach as well suited to helping the deaf patient "to think rationally, alter behavior to better satisfy needs, and experience less frustration and more pleasure in life" (p. 180). Unlike rational–emotive therapy, reality therapy is quite dependent on an empathetic, genuine relationship between therapist and patient. Indeed, the therapist is a friend who exhibits unconditional regard to the patient in this approach. As a therapy that focuses directly on the patient's present behavior, McCrone (1983) considered it very valuable for deaf individuals, especially within the rehabilitation counseling milieu.

Hypnosis is not a therapy itself but an adjunct to some therapies. As a vocal–auditory process, it presents singular challenges to both the therapist and deaf patient. Deaf patients must keep their eyes open and rely on sight for nuances that are communicated to hearing patients by voice. For the hard of hearing patient, the nuances of spoken language may be missed. Isenberg and Matthews (1991; Matthews & Isenberg, 1992) compared the hypnotic inductions of deaf and hearing college women and found that the deaf subjects were as hypnotizable as the hearing subjects. They also observed that the deaf subjects presented traditional trance indicators including flattened affect, change in breathing, glazed stare, autonomic head nods and finger twitches, and communication that was slower and sometimes produced with difficulty. Although hearing subjects often speak slower and use softer tones, several deaf subjects signed more slowly and one subject dramatically increased her signing space. Whereas Isenberg and Matthews used sign language via an interpreter to induce hypnosis, others have reported using fingerspelling and writing (Bowman & Coons, 1990; Wall, 1991).

Psychodrama is another adjunct to therapeutic approaches. Its use with deaf patients was first described by Clayton and Robinson (1971). Swink (1983, 1985) considered the "living out" nature of psychodrama to be well suited to deaf patients because instead of relying on verbalization, information is communicated "via signs, vocalizations, words, gestures, spatial boundaries, interactions, body movement and facial expression.... Emotional expression also becomes easier with less restriction on means of communication" (1985, p. 272). He found that signing deaf people tend to adapt to psychodrama more readily than hearing people, and it can be used effectively within individual, family, and group therapy.

Bibliotherapy, which uses literature to promote understanding, insight, and positive change, has also been used as an adjunct technique. Bryant and Roberts (1992) found that the use of bibliotherapy with deaf patients often reduces the amount of time spent in counseling because it allows individuals to assimilate information at their own pace outside of the counseling sessions.

Audiological counseling is typically thought of as informational in nature and more related to the issues of amplification, hearing aids, assistive listening devices, and audiograms that were discussed in Chapter 1. It has been suggested that audiological counseling can also provide an opportunity for deaf children, adolescents, and adults to discuss and deal with issues of adjustment, relationships, attitudes, and feelings (Grunblatt & Daar, 1994; Roberts & Wharton, 1991).

As awareness of the mental health needs of deaf individuals has grown and interest in working with this population has increased among counselors and therapists, approaches have been advocated but not yet implemented by mental health professionals. Sports psychology is one of these. As discussed in Chapter 5, deaf sports is an important part of the Deaf community, and deaf athletes participate in both hearing and deaf sports at all levels, from recreation to professional, and school varsity to Olympic competition. In 1991, Clark and Sachs found virtually no literature on sports psychology and deaf athletes. They noted that deaf athletes deal with the same issues about athletic performance and competition as hearing athletes such as anxiety, concentration, confidence, mental preparation, motivation, and teamwork.

Another approach that has been discussed is psychosocial rehabilitation, which is a mental health and rehabilitation model for individuals with persistent mental illness. The goal of psychosocial rehabilitation is to enable the individual to live successfully in the community. Cook, Graham, and Razzano (1993) recommended that for deaf individuals, the goal should be integration within the Deaf community rather than the larger hearing community. The "model's reliance on empowerment, client choice, service coordination, continuity of care, and situational assessment make it a firm foundation for program development" with individuals with mental illness who are deaf (p. 272). The importance of making therapy culturally relevant to deaf individuals has been echoed by many psychologists and researchers.

Culturally Affirming Therapy

Understanding the culture of the child or adult is essential for providing therapy that is appropriate, respectful, and helpful. In the absence of this understanding, the counselor or therapist can misinterpret the deaf individual's communication and behavior. For example, Harris, VanZandt, and Rees (1997) noted that deaf children tend to ask more personal questions than hearing children, and they use touch more freely to gain attention. Misiaszek and his associates (1985) cautioned mental health professionals about the potential errors in diagnosis that can be made when the clinician is unfamiliar with the psychosocial manifestations of deafness. The counselor who lacks cultural sensitivity is also at risk for imposing his or her own values because they are assumed to be shared.

A culturally affirmative program for deaf individuals often means quite specifically including information about Deaf culture and using ASL in sessions (Burnes, Seabolt, & Vreeland, 1992). It also means that deaf individuals should be involved in providing mental health services as counselors, role models, or liaisons between the deaf patient and the mental health community (Wax, 1990). More broadly, it means that the therapist recognizes the impact of minority culture membership on the Deaf individual's sense of self and ability to function in all aspects of life. And culturally affirmative therapy assumes that the goal of intervention is empowerment for the Deaf individual (Glickman, 1996b; Glickman & Zitter, 1989). Sue, Arredondo, and McDavis (1992) described the culturally skilled counselor as one who:

- Is aware of his or her own assumptions about human behavior, values, biases, preconceived notions, and personal limitations
- Attempts to understand the worldview of his or her culturally different client without negative judgments
- Develops and practices appropriate, relevant, and sensitive intervention strategies and skills in working with his or her culturally different clients (p. 481)

Therapists and counselors have also been advised to remember that deafness is only one aspect of an individual's cultural identity. Eldredge (1993; Eldredge & Carrigan, 1992) worked with Native Americans who are deaf and found that many of the issues with which they were struggling were more connected to their Native American culture than Deaf culture.

Henwood and Pope-Davis (1994) recognized the role of culture within the therapeutic environment with deaf individuals when they wrote, "It is not enough for psychologists to merely be skilled clinicians who can provide interventions and strategies to assist others. What is required is a comprehensive understanding of the cultural contexts in which these interventions and strategies are to be applied" (p. 500).

MENTAL HEALTH PROFESSIONALS

A recurrent theme among mental health professionals is that deaf individuals can be provided with effective therapy and counseling if the professional understands deafness, is sensitive to the deaf person's cultural identity, and is able to communicate effectively. This level of knowledge and skill has been slow to develop among the professionals who work with deaf children, adolescents, and adults.

Much of the literature about the competencies of mental health professionals has focused on two themes. The first theme is a discussion of the problem, which is that too few psychologists, psychiatrists, counselors, and therapists have sufficient background knowledge and skill. Much of this literature is an attempt to provide basic information about deafness (for example, Leigh, Corbett, Gutman, & Morere, 1996). The second theme is a discussion of the implications for deaf individuals who need, seek, and receive counseling or therapy. Much of this literature deals with the accuracy and completeness of assessments conducted when the professional doing the assessment has limited knowledge of deafness and skill in communicating (for example, Guthmann & Sandberg, 1998).

Outside of these two themes, a few studies have focused specifically on the communication between counselor and deaf person. It has been found that deaf individuals are much more willing to see a counselor or therapist who is able to communicate in sign language and much less willing to see one who is not and must use an interpreter (Freeman & Conoley, 1986; Haley & Dowd, 1988). Among school counselors, Zieziula and Harris (1998) found that the ability of school counselors to communicate with deaf students had improved greatly from the early 1970s so that by the late 1990s, they "appear to be better trained, feel more skilled, and feel that they can adequately communicate with the deaf students they serve" (p. 44).

SUMMARY AND CONCLUDING THOUGHTS

This chapter discussed issues pertaining to the mental health of deaf individuals. As stated at the outset, considerably more is known and has been written about mental health problems than any other aspect of mental health. For many years, the emotional response of deaf individuals to their environment has been defined as relatively disordered, which seems to account for a fairly large body of information about emotional and behavioral problems and substantial discussion about the issue of access to mental health services. More recently, there has been some conjecture that this characterization of deaf individuals has been based on a lack of cultural sensitivity and understanding. As researchers pay increasing attention to the "health" part of mental health, and consider mental health within a cultural context, all professionals will have a greater understanding of the mental health of individuals who are deaf and hard of hearing.

Livneh and Antonak (1997) summarized well the current state of knowledge about mental health among deaf individuals when they wrote the following:

1. Children and adolescents with prelingual deafness are somewhat more likely than are children without hearing impairments to display a range of social behaviors and emotional reactions, especially in school settings, that could impede psychosocial adaptation (e.g., withdrawal, loneliness, restlessness, acting out, impulsiveness, aggressiveness);
2. The prevalence of depression, anger, and anxiety among persons with adventitious postlingual deafness is somewhat higher than expected in the general population;
3. Increased risk of psychosocial maladaptation is not a necessary concomitant of severe, early onset, and long-lasting hearing impairment, but it may

be associated with poor communication abilities, the presence of additional disabilities, and poor educational experiences in segregated school settings;

4. Children with deafness raised by parents with deafness appear to be better adapted than children with deafness raised by parents without deafness;

5. Regardless of the presence or absence of deafness in the parents, a supportive family environment is conducive to psychosocial adaptation of persons with hearing impairments. (p. 282)

EDUCATION

FOCUS QUESTIONS

- Why is it important to have a continuum of educational placement options for deaf students?

- In what ways are oral/aural, bilingual, and total communication programs similar to and different from each other?

- Are English-as-a-second-language (ESL) methods and models developed for children learning a second spoken language applicable to bilingual programs for deaf children learning English and ASL?

- What are the essential differences between curriculum for deaf students and curriculum for hearing students?

- Given that a teacher of the deaf is certified to teach hard of hearing and deaf children from preschool through high school, which skills are most important?

Educators, parents, adult deaf individuals, and public policymakers are greatly concerned about the educational achievement of students who are deaf. In 1988, the Commission on Education of the Deaf issued a report to the Congress and the President of the United States that included fifty-two recommendations designed to improve the education of deaf students from the point of identification through postsecondary levels. In 1994, the Deaf Education Initiative Project of the National Association of State Directors of Special Education issued guidelines for enhancing educational programs. Since the 1960s, studies assessing the academic achievement of deaf students have consistently found that they lag far behind their hearing peers; even students with a unilateral hearing loss have been found to exhibit academic delays (Allen, 1986; Gentile & DiFrancesca, 1969; Holt, 1993; Oyler, Oyler, & Matkin, 1988; Trybus & Karchmer, 1977).

This chapter will discuss the educational program options for deaf students, curriculum and teaching strategies that are particularly valuable for deaf students regardless of the educational setting, the special needs of diverse deaf students, and the roles of professionals in the educational lives of deaf children and adolescents. Postsecondary education will be discussed in Chapter 8.

EDUCATIONAL PLACEMENT OPTIONS

The U.S. Department of Education (1996) defines six educational placements for students with disabilities—regular class, resource room, separate class, separate school, residential facility, and homebound/hospital environment. This range of options, often referred to as a continuum of services, is needed because individual children require different levels of support. The decision about placement is supposed to be made only after the child's needs are assessed. The Individuals with Disabilities Education Act mandates that students with disabilities be educated to the maximum extent possible with nondisabled students, which is the principle of least restrictive environment. Heward (2000) compared the right and wrong ways to determine whether a placement meets the federally mandated standard of least restrictive environment as the following:

> For many years special education operated like this: (1) a student found eligible for special education was labeled with a disability category; (2) the student was placed into a program for students with that particular disability; and (3) a not-so-individualized version of the already-in-place program was written down and presented as the student's individualized education plan, even though the program continued as usual whether the "new" student was in it or not. This is the wrong way, and has been the wrong way since IDEA first went into effect in 1977. The legally mandated and educationally sound process goes like this: (1) the school must determine whether the child has a disability and is therefore eligible for special education; (2) the child's needs must be determined and an IEP developed that specifies the special education and related services that will be provided to meet those needs; and (3) the child is then placed in the least restrictive environment in which an appropriate program can be provided and the child can make satisfactory educational progress. (p. 67)

The placements that most school districts provide for deaf students are regular classrooms at one end of the continuum and day or residential schools for the deaf at the other end of the continuum.

■ *Regular classroom.* The student with a hearing loss in the regular classroom receives all instruction from the classroom teacher or teachers. It is relatively unusual for deaf students to be placed in the regular classroom with no support services whatsoever. However, many hard of hearing students receive their full educational program under the direction of the regular teacher.

■ *Regular classroom with consultation from a teacher of the deaf or speech/ language specialist.* The deaf student in this placement option receives all instruction from the regular classroom teacher, but the teacher is supported by a teacher of the deaf or speech/language specialist who visits on a consultant basis. The consultant teacher monitors the student's attainment of goals and provides the classroom teacher with suggestions for including the deaf child in instructional activities.

■ *Regular classroom with supplementary instruction from a teacher of the deaf or speech/language specialist.* The deaf student in this placement option receives most instruction from the classroom teacher but is pulled out of the classroom for individualized or small-group instruction with an itinerant teacher of the deaf or speech/language specialist. The difference between a consultant teacher and an itinerant teacher is that the consultant teacher works directly with the classroom teacher, thus influencing the deaf child's educational program only indirectly. An itinerant teacher, however, works directly with the deaf child. The degree of contact varies significantly, depending on the child's needs. Contact time can range from being relatively small, such as once a week for half an hour, to relatively significant, such as several times a week for an hour or more. Because the U.S. Department of Education does not distinguish between types of regular education placements in the federal definition, only one statistic is reported for the regular class placement. According to the National Center for Educational Statistics (1999), 35.4 percent of students identified in the federal category of "hearing impairment" as the primary disability received education services in the regular class during 1995–1996.

■ *Resource room.* The deaf student in a resource room placement receives most instruction from the classroom teacher but spends part of each schoolday in a resource room, in which a teacher of the deaf provides instruction in specific subject areas or on specific skills. Sometimes the deaf child is grouped with other deaf children from the same school. Often the deaf child receives individualized instruction because the other children are likely to have different learning needs, given the relatively small number of deaf children who are likely to be attending any given school, even a school that acts as a kind of magnet school for students who are deaf. According to the National Center for Educational Statistics (1999), 19.1 percent of students with "hearing impairment" received services in a resource room during 1995–1996.

- *Separate class.* The deaf student in a separate class receives most or all instruction from a teacher of the deaf. The other students in the class are also deaf, though their ages and ability levels may vary quite widely. A deaf student in this setting is likely to interact with other students in the school for relatively small amounts of time. These interactions typically take place during lunch and recess, though the deaf student might also be integrated with hearing students in classes such as art and physical education. According to the National Center for Educational Statistics (1999), 28.5 percent of students with "hearing impairment" received services in a separate class during 1995–1996.

- *Special school.* The deaf student in a special school receives all instruction from teachers of the deaf within a segregated educational setting serving only children and adolescents who are deaf. These schools are typically referred to as day schools and residential schools. In day schools, the students commute back and forth from home to school each day. In residential schools, students are able to live at the school during the week and commute home on weekends and/or holidays. Special schools can be private or public. At one time, state-supported residential schools for the deaf were the primary educational setting for deaf students. According to a 1998 survey of educational programs for deaf students, 45 states still have residential schools for the deaf (*American Annals of the Deaf,* 1999). According to the National Center for Educational Statistics (1999), 16.8 percent of students identified in the federal category of "hearing impairment" as the primary disability received education services in the special school during 1995–1996.

- *Homebound/hospital environment.* Deaf students who receive all of their instruction in a homebound or hospital environment account for only 0.2 percent of the school-age population. Most of the children who are served in home or hospital settings are identified as health impaired or traumatic brain injury. It is likely that when children need to be served at home or in a hospital, hearing loss is rarely considered to be their primary disability. Therefore, it is possible that the percentage may actually be higher, particularly among children who are hard of hearing. ("Homebound" does not mean "home schooled," which is the education of children at home by a parent.)

The demographic data provided by the U.S. federal government does not distinguish between deaf and hard of hearing students. When Allen (1992) examined subgroup differences, he found patterns of educational placement that differed by degree of hearing loss, race, and age. Based on a 1990–1991 survey that tracked the educational and demographic characteristics of deaf and hard of hearing children who were receiving special education services in the United States, Allen found the following patterns in educational placements.

- Only 10 percent of students with profound hearing losses attend local schools and are integrated with hearing students for more than three hours a day.
- Less than 5 percent of the students with profound hearing losses attend schools having only one or two deaf or hard of hearing students. Two-thirds of the profoundly deaf students attend schools with more than 30 deaf and hard of hearing students.
- Placement in residential nonintegrated settings increases steadily from age 8 (13 percent) to age 18 (35 percent). As students get older, the proportion attending residential schools increases relative to the number attending other settings, the proportion attending local nonintegrated schools decreases, and the proportion who are integrated for three or more hours a day remains constant.
- White, non-Hispanic students are more likely than students from other racial and ethnic groups to attend local schools where they are integrated more than three hours a day with hearing students.
- The likelihood of attending a residential school with no integration is fairly equal for all disability groups, ranging from 21 percent for those with no additional disabilities to 28 percent for those with both physical and cognitive disabilities. (pp. 387–388)

A major concern among educators, parents, and deaf adults has been the reasons underlying educational placement decisions for deaf children.

Placement Decisions

Since the passage of Public Law 94-142 in 1975, deaf education has stood somewhat apart from other areas of special education in terms of how integration was viewed. Whereas other disability areas typically embraced the integration of all children in educational settings, professionals in deafness and parents of deaf children held to the belief that the integration of deaf children in classrooms of hearing children could not be assumed to be the best educational model. Whether integration was called mainstreaming or inclusion, it has been a source of contention and controversy because it seemed clear to most stakeholders that this type of placement could not meet the needs of all deaf children educationally, socially, emotionally, or culturally. Advocates for other disability groups viewed integration as a civil right, but advocates for deaf children viewed forced integration as a violation of their civil rights.

Each time that IDEA has faced reauthorization by Congress, fears were renewed that the continuum of educational placement options would be eliminated and all children with disabilities would be placed in regular education classrooms (Fields, 1994; Liu, 1995; Moores, 1993; Stoefen-Fisher & Balk, 1992). Stewart (1984) noted that "schools for the deaf were poorly served in the seventies during the mainstreaming crusade. They were positioned at the bottom of the cascade system of special education services and, in general, students were placed here only as a last resort.... The literature never refers to schools for the deaf as regular schools and teachers in these schools as regular teachers" (p. 102). Stewart could have written these words in 2000 and been as accurate as in the 1980s. Although the continuum of placement options has never been eliminated by law, the special school placement has certainly been seen by public policymakers as the most restrictive of educational settings and, therefore, the furthest from the core value of least restrictive environment (Dubow, 1989).

Rottenberg (1992) compared the integration programs in the United States, England, Italy, France, Switzerland, and Sweden. Based on her analysis of exemplary programs for deaf children, she recommended that integration policies must include the following attributes:

1. Integration is the normal pattern.
2. Support is provided to families in order to ensure parent involvement in their children's education.
3. Class size is limited in classes with deaf children.
4. Children are provided with a continuum of services based on their educational needs rather than provided a disability label that is used to identify their services.
5. Programs are locally designed to match the cultures and communities within which the children live.

When Wilson (1997) asked deaf adolescents to reflect on their experiences in public schools and schools for the deaf, these students offered several suggestions for making decisions about placement. First, they emphasized the importance of making sure that deaf students receive a social and cultural education as well as an academic education in whatever setting they are educated. Second, they considered IEP meetings the best place to provide parents with information about school placement options. Third, they urged their peers to be involved in their own placement decisions once they reach adolescence. Fourth, they encouraged deaf students to be exposed to different school placements through visitations, summer camps, and after-school activities. Fifth, they viewed socialization as an increasingly important factor in placement decisions during adolescence. And sixth, they pointed out that school choice must be a decision that is respected by others.

Components of Effective Placement
in Integrated Settings

Identifying the components of placements that promote learning for deaf students has been a difficult and less-than-satisfying enterprise. The complex nature of classrooms and students has confounded the ability of researchers to attain unequivocal evidence for the superiority of any setting or set of instructional practices (Kluwin, 1989). Factors that contribute to effective placement have been found in several studies of integrated classrooms with deaf and hearing students from preschool through high school (Kluwin, Gonsher, Silver, & Samuels, 1996; Luckner, 1991b; Lundeen & Lundeen, 1993; Weber, 1997; Winter & Van Reusen, 1997).

■ *Time to learn and plan.* The classroom teacher of deaf children needs time to learn about the child and deafness. The team of professionals working with the child needs time to share information and to plan instruction for the child. This team often includes the classroom teacher, consultant/itinerant/resource room teacher of the deaf, the interpreter, and others such as the speech–language specialist.

■ *Commitment to the model of education.* The professionals and the child's parents must feel committed to making the placement successful and confident about the child's ability to be successful.

■ *Support services.* The school principal and school district director of special education play key roles in providing the kinds of support that promote positive outcomes for deaf students. Examples of support include teacher of the deaf full-time, speech and language specialist, interpreters, paraprofessionals, volunteers, computers, and budget for purchasing materials and equipment.

■ *Clarity of program design.* Instead of simply an orientation to inclusion and the needs of the deaf child, the team of professionals should be engaged in activities that enable them to develop a common understanding of the program design, clarification of their individual roles and responsibilities, and identification of instructional strategies that are recommended in the research literature and reflect sound instructional principles.

■ *Parent participation.* Parents should be involved in their children's education on a daily basis and not be isolated to the process of planning IEPs and making placement decisions.

■ *Direct instruction by teachers of the deaf within the regular classroom.* From team teaching to occasional opportunities for teaching the whole class, contact with the teacher of the deaf within the regular classroom is very helpful for deaf students. When a teacher of the deaf is teamed with the classroom teacher and they deliver instruction together some of the time, both the hearing and deaf students benefit.

When Kluwin and Stinson (1993) conducted a study of deaf adolescents in local public schools, they found that some programs were working well and some were not. They concluded their book with the following remarks:

> Local public school education for deaf children is here and will no doubt continue in some form into the future. Sometimes it works miracles and sometimes it doesn't work at all. When the issue of the very existence of these kinds of programs is put aside, the problems of this system and the solutions to those problems become apparent. First, we saw children and teachers do better in programs where the political and governance integration of adult professionals was formalized. Second, regardless of the traits of the children, when goals were clearly defined and standards upheld, the children achieved higher than the average. Third, programs with "happy" individuals were programs where the students had more positive attitudes toward hearing peers and achieved at higher levels. Fourth, programs with more structured and supportive extracurricular opportunities produced graduates who were more interested in other people, regardless of their hearing status. (p. 152)

Academic Achievement

Relatively little research has been conducted to determine the factors that influence student achievement. Research exists on the effects of student placement and student background, but almost none exists on school-level variables (such as facilities, organization, and administrative support and attitudes), teacher characteristics, or students' attitudes toward one another (Mertens, 1990).

The influence of student placement on academic achievement has received some attention, particularly the effects of inclusive educational settings versus segregated ones. Much of this research on placement has shown that deaf students in general education classrooms demonstrate higher academic achievement than students in self-contained classrooms (Allen & Osborn, 1984; Holt, 1993; Kluwin, 1993; Kluwin & Moores, 1985, 1989). However, no one has satisfactorily taken into account the confounding effect of how students are chosen for inclusion. Are integrated students more successful than their peers in self-contained public school classrooms or schools for the deaf because the general education setting incorporates qualities that the other settings do not? Or are students placed in inclusive settings because they embody the qualities that will enable them to be successful?

Although the research has not provided firm answers to these questions, quality of instruction appears to be the primary determinant of achievement. The following features of quality instruction can certainly be found in both types of placement, but when researchers have examined the educational experience of deaf students, they have found these features to be considerably more characteristic of integrated classrooms.

- Teacher is trained in the academic content area being taught. In other words, science teachers are trained in science, math teachers are trained in math, and so forth.
- High expectations for student performance are maintained.
- Large amounts of content are presented.
- Time is devoted to direct instruction of content.
- Material is reviewed regularly.
- Students receive individual attention.
- Students are given effective and positive feedback.
- Relevant homework is assigned and monitored.

Academic achievement is supposed to be ensured through the IEP process. For school-age deaf children, once an evaluation team has determined that the child's hearing loss is adversely affecting his or her educational performance, an Individualized Education Plan (IEP) must be developed. IDEA requires that an IEP be developed and implemented for every student with a disability between ages 3 and 21. The members of the IEP team include the parents, at least one regular education teacher if the child is or will be in a regular education setting, at least one special education teacher, a representative of the local education agency, an individual who can interpret the instructional implications of the evaluation results, and the child if 14 years of age or older. All IEPs include the child's present levels of educational performance, annual goals, short-term objectives, special education services and related services, program modifications, extent to which the child will participate with nondisabled children and children with disabilities, how the child's progress will be measured, and how the child's parents will be regularly informed. IEPs must be reviewed on a yearly basis. In Essay 7.1, parents discuss their struggle to ensure that their deaf daughter received all of the services stated on her IEP.

■ ■ ■ ■ ■ ▬▬▬▬▬▬▬▬▬▬▬▬▬▬▬▬▬▬▬▬▬▬▬▬▬▬▬▬▬▬▬▬▬▬▬

ESSAY 7.1

Tami, Keven, and Ashli-Marie Grant

Ashli started school in Edmonds, Washington, when she was two years old. She was five years old when she started at Washington School for the Deaf, but she was in first grade because she has that late birthday and had actually started

(continued)

ESSAY 7.1   CONTINUED

kindergarten when she was four. We were so fortunate. She had wonderful teachers during the first three years. The first day there I just cried all the way home. Ashli had sat in the car and watched some older kids walking by us on their way to the nurse. And she looked at me and said, "Mom, they're signing! And what they're saying is..." and she parroted it back. And she came home that day and said, "Mom, the secretary can sign!" And the next day it was, "Mom, the janitor signs!" Well, we came from Edmonds where the teacher and the interpreter signed. Nobody else did. So she was just thrilled. That year the secretary left, and I came in as a parent volunteer. Then they hired me temporarily from April till June. During the summer, they made Lynn Woolsey the supervising teacher, and they appointed me permanently. Ashli was learning, she was happy, she was excited. I just loved the school. I felt, where else could she get this kind of self-esteem and pride?

Then everything changed. We got all new administrators. Lynn had left three sets of plans for the next supervising teacher in the elementary school because she was moving to Ohio to attend graduate school at Ohio State. We called these the brown files. All of the teachers and Lynn had sat down and developed groupings for the kids based on what would be best for them academically, socially, and emotionally. They poured hours into developing these. I was really impressed by that.

During the summer after Ashli had completed third grade, I had a sense that things were changing but thought I'd wait and watch. Then I got a call from a teacher about a week before I was due to report back to work for the fall. She told me that the teachers had finally gotten their class lists, and Ashli was placed in the second-/third-grade class. There was one other girl who was a fourth grader and was placed in this class. I talked with the teacher, and she told me that she'd make sure that Ashli got what she needed. But I told the teacher that I would insist that she get one-on-one or two-on-one time with Ashli and the other fourth grader to get them ready for the state fourth-grade proficiency test.

We called a meeting with the new supervising teacher, and she brought in the new director of education. It became apparent that they had never opened the brown files before changing all of the placements. I know the birth dates of these kids, not because I worked there but because the kids had gone to each other's birthday parties, and the placements had obviously been made strictly on birth dates. They hadn't looked at the brown files to see where the kids were academically, who was a good match, who wasn't. They had split the fifth graders and put half in the elementary school and half in the middle school. Again, they didn't split them up by needs but by birth date. So there were some kids who really didn't belong in middle school. When they saw Ashli's birth date, they put her in third. I pointed this out at the meeting, and the director said that he would be the kind of parent who would be concerned about my child being with older kids. I looked at him and said, "You know nothing about my child or me and my husband. Ashli has been here for three years with these kids and now I should suddenly be concerned about her being with them? You might have a deaf brother, you might have a deaf spouse, and you might be hard of hearing. But you don't know what it's like to raise a deaf child so don't try to tell me you know what's best for my child without asking me what my child needs." By the end of that meeting, it was decided that Ashli would stay in the second-/third-grade class, and they would get an assistant so that the teacher could get the two girls ready for the fourth-grade proficiency test. The very next day the decision was changed.

They put Ashli with a group of kids that she had been with when she first came to WSD. A lot of those kids had blow-ups and were silly. I went home and said to Ashli, "I'm sorry but they've changed your placement again. You're going to be with this teacher and these are the kids who are going to be in your class." I wasn't prepared for her reaction. She fell onto the couch and bawled her eyes out. She said, "Take me out of WSD. Take me back to Seattle. I don't want to be with these kids. I really want to learn. I'm not going to learn here." My husband looked at me and looked at her and stepped outside because he didn't want to cry in front of her. It was the "take me back to Seattle" part that nailed us both. He came back in and explained to her that Mom and Dad are not upset with you. We're upset because you're hurt, and we don't like to see you hurt.

Another set of changes the school made involved the day students. It was decided that day students could no longer be picked up in the cafeteria with the other students following after-school activities. They had to go to the library. They were being segregated out, and the kids were starting to notice it. The day students were also not allowed to eat dinner any more at the school. There had been a few people who took advantage of that, but the majority of us did not. None of this was explained in advance of the decision. The kids thought something was wrong with them. The parents of day students got together and wrote down the positive and negative effects of these decisions. We gave them to the superintendent because WSD doesn't have a school board. We never received a response.

Before I went to my MDT meeting, I specifically called my school district representative and asked her to attend. The school psychologist had done extensive testing on Ashli, including IQ testing. She said:

> Good news, bad news. In areas that deaf students typically score really well, Ashli scored ok. In areas that deaf students typically don't score well, your daughter scored off the charts. She's highly capable in these areas, I might even say gifted. The good news is that she's going to get the English patterns. The bad news is that she may find one way to do something and think that's the only way to do it. She cannot have her schedule changed on her and if it is, don't expect her to accept it. She's going to need to have decisions explained to her in advance.

So one of the things we requested was to know, by the IEP time, what her "time in educational program" was. We wanted it specified on the IEP. We also asked for extra language time for Ashli because by this time, another new decision had been made involving the communication disorders specialist, who was now only allowed to work with the kids on speech, and Ashli wouldn't benefit from speech.

At the IEP meeting, the teacher said that she wanted one-on-one time with Ashli to teach her some reading strategies because Ashli tends to read word for word. I agreed to that. We went over the IEP, and that was it. I quit my job as secretary shortly thereafter. During Christmas vacation, Ashli's teacher became sick. She was gone for quite a while before Ashli told me. I went in to the school because I wanted a copy of the IEP. I asked the supervising teacher to sign the

(continued)

ESSAY 7.1   CONTINUED

IEP as long as we were both there. At this point, with both of our signatures, it became a legally binding contract.

Shortly afterward, we got a letter from the school stating that instead of being dismissed at two o'clock on Fridays, the kids would be getting out at twelve o'clock. Keven called the director of education and asked to talk about it in his role as president of the Parent–Staff Organization. When he showed up for the meeting, the director and all three of the supervising teachers were there. Keven explained that he was at the meeting as a PSO representative and not as Ashli's parent. He asked if they had checked the IEPs to see if they were out of compliance by shortening the school day. One of the supervising teachers said that they would do IEP addendums. Keven expressed the parents' concerns that things were changed in the middle of the year with very little notice. While other parents would need to find day care in this type of situation, parents of deaf children must not only find day care but day care providers who can at least somewhat communicate with our children. In addition, our children will be in day care at a time of day when other school-age children are in school. Not only will they be sitting with people who have very little communication, but they'll be with kids who are four years old.

The school sent out an addendum to the IEP, and we wouldn't sign it. WSD finally called a meeting. Ashli's teacher was just getting back after six weeks of illness. During that time, there had been a variety of substitutes. We asked where Ashli-Marie was with her IEP goals, and they reported that Ashli had not met a single goal. Never before had she had a problem meeting her IEP goals. I know there's no guarantee about passing IEP goals. However, you can reasonably expect her to pass them when she's in fourth grade, she's been in school since she was two and a half, and she's never not passed one. She also hadn't met any of the January benchmarks. The school offered to give us four Fridays when she would have one-on-one instruction from twelve to two P.M. They wanted us to sign the addendum that day because the four Fridays would make up for the lost time on the IEP. We said we wouldn't sign it now but would see if she was making progress after four weeks and if so, we'd come back and sign the addendum. The supervising teacher said that she had to get approval and left the room. At this point, we didn't know that her actions were illegal. Later, we learned that according to the Regulations, the school district was required to send a representative who had full authority to make decisions about anything discussed in the meeting. She came back and said that Ashli could have the four Fridays, and we should sign the addendum. I said no, because as soon as we signed it, we would have no legal recourse to make changes. The supervising teacher said that was all she was authorized to offer. I asked her if she was bribing us, giving Ashli the four Fridays so that we would sign the addendum. Our school district representative then went into the superintendent's office and stayed there for a while. The meeting ended on that note.

The next thing we knew, we received notice from the school that they were going to a due process hearing because we refused to sign the addendum. They also wrote that if we'd rather go through mediation, they would be willing to do that. We originally agreed to mediation. But we also decided to file due process. There were other things that had been going on that we had been documenting. For example, the kids were often left alone with teaching assistants. As my husband was researching how to file due process, he discovered that if you go to mediation, any of the evidence that you use in mediation cannot be used in due process later. At this point, there was no trust between the school and us, so we decided not to go through mediation.

We went ahead with due process. We were scared to death. We couldn't afford a lawyer, but we made just a little too much to get legal assistance. So we were on our own. As a state school, they had the Assistant Attorney General as their lawyer. The first meeting was a phone conference. We brought a friend with us to give us support and take notes. The lawyer started out saying that the state was willing to concede that the school didn't send out notice of the plan to change the schedule. I said, "Your Honor, the issue is not only that. We didn't receive a notice of action for the IEP for the proposed addendum. The only thing we received was an MDT notice and I sent that out myself. And they only had ten days to get that to us because there's a pretty strict time line." We could hear them conferring at the other end of the phone. Then the lawyer said, "Your Honor, we're willing to concede that we did not send out the proper paperwork."

The Judge had told them that they had to make our witnesses available. And if they weren't able to be there within fifteen minutes, he would subpoena them all and they'd sit there for the whole hearing, which meant that the school would have to pay subs for the whole day. The lawyer had stacks of previous cases that they were citing. And we had the most wonderful family and friends behind us. I had friends who helped me organize the papers, come up with the questions, and write my summation. They called all through the hearing, asking how it was going, what was said, what can I do, telling us that we were doing what's right.

Ashli-Marie wanted to testify. We obviously couldn't hide that something was going on, especially when Mom and Dad are all dressed up and showing up at the school two days in a row. We told her that we and the school were talking to a judge about whether Ashli-Marie would get extra practice during the summer before going to fifth grade.

The state presented its case first, so we were able to take our cues from them, like how they started each testimony by asking people their names, experience, and work history. We were able to cross-examine their witnesses. The Judge was really helpful in that he knew we were parents. We had no legal experience. If we made a mistake, he didn't yell at us. He'd say things like, "you can't ask that or you need to ask that in another way." If someone used a legal term, he'd explain it to us. We hit WSD with everything we could think of. We wanted to make sure that we were getting our point across. For example, there's a "Reg" that says if you provide an activity to one segment of your population, you have to provide it to everybody. We felt that was happening to the day students who couldn't participate in certain activities. We were pretty sure we couldn't win this one, but some other parents had asked us to test the waters on this issue because they were thinking of suing the school for discrimination or filing a class action suit.

The first day, the state presented their case, and when they finished, we presented ours. We called in the business office people, who were not exactly thrilled to be testifying. All Keven asked was, "Can you separate money? Does the state give you money separately for dorm students and day students, or is it

(continued)

ESSAY 7.1 CONTINUED

all together?" Of course they said it's all together. We asked the personnel director questions about teacher certification and if the WSD assistants are state certified as assistants. He said they are not. The state said that when assistants were
left in the classroom, teachers checked in with them all the time, and they were
really never left completely alone with the students. We suggested that an assistant be brought over to testify, and the Judge agreed. The assistant said that she
never got support from teachers, never saw them, and didn't have lesson plans.
The state's lawyer asked, "If she needed help, couldn't she have opened her
door and asked for help from the teacher across the hall." And, God bless her,
she was really honest and said, no, she couldn't because the teacher across the
hall had made it clear that she didn't want to be interrupted. When the superintendent testified, we asked if he was ever allowed to deny a service to a child because of budgetary restrictions. Of course he said no though it had been his
policy not to hire subs and to either combine classes or put assistants in classes
alone with children when a teacher was absent. We called many witnesses including the teacher, the director of education for the dorms, who couldn't tell us
how many elementary students were in the dorms or how many staff supervised the elementary students, and the director of education for academics.

It was kind of nice to see the process. It was also really frightening and
emotional. Parents need to be prepared for that. When you go through due process, for good or bad, you're watching your child get dissected. We had brought
a picture of Ashli into court so that we could all remember that our big issue is
Ashli. She's a child. She's not a number or a file. Their most important witness
was the school psychologist, and she basically turned into our witness. She admitted being concerned because during the six weeks when the teacher was ill,
there had been so many different individuals in the classroom. I think we
counted twelve different individuals who had been teaching Ashli during those
six weeks. It also helped for her to say that, knowing what she knew about Ashli
and her capabilities, it was quite reasonable to expect that Ashli would have
passed the goals on her IEP if she'd had consistent teaching.

During the summation, the state pulled out a newspaper article that discussed the importance of families eating dinner together. They said that obviously Ashli-Marie is a bright child with parents who are capable of signing, so
she doesn't have language concerns. But it's not the school's job to raise the
child. I said that I'm not asking the school to raise my child. We moved to Vancouver to have my child in our home, to teach her values that the school can't
and shouldn't teach her. Never in this country have we said that because you
have the right to sit at the front of the bus, you must sit at the front of the bus.
I'm not saying that my child is going to stay for dinner every night. But she has
the right to the access and the choice. My child doesn't go home to a neighborhood with children who can communicate with her. She doesn't get invited to
slumber parties and birthday parties. The only neighborhood she has is this
state school. And that's why we asked for what we have. We're not lawyers or
smooth talking politicians. We're parents, trying to do what's best. We're seeing
our child not reaching her potential.

When it was all over, I went into the parking lot and threw up. And I cried
because it was over. We hadn't asked for much. We didn't ask for money. We

just asked for compensatory education. The judge said that he was impressed by the civility of the proceedings. I told him that we appreciated the time he had spent and the information he had provided to us during the proceedings. He told us that we should be proud of the work we had done here.

The judge ruled in the school's favor on one issue and our favor on the other. He found insufficient evidence to conclude that the administrative changes involving day student access to the dorms amounted to a change in placement. Because Ashli's IEP did not identify evening access to the dorms as part of her educational program, the school was not required to provide notice to the parents or include them in the school's decision to implement the new policy. He also concluded that limiting day students' evening access to the dorms does not amount to a denial of service.

The judge ruled that the school had failed to provide Ashli-Marie with a free and appropriate public education for six weeks. While the school was not responsible for the teacher's absence, it was responsible for the assignment of substitute personnel and could not use difficulty in finding qualified and certificated staff as an excuse. The evidence established a need for compensatory education to recoup the lost educational opportunity. The school was ordered to provide an additional two hours of instruction per week until the end of the school year and at that time, if the IEP team determined that she had not met all goals and objectives, the school must provide instruction during the summer, not to exceed four weeks, Monday through Friday, four hours of one-on-one instruction per day.

Ashli will be in fifth grade next year, but not at the school for the deaf. We toured other schools, and we made our decision as a family. She had the option of going to our neighborhood school, and she almost went. She thought she would get a better education at her neighborhood school, which were her words. But she wasn't ready to say that she wouldn't be around other deaf students. I told her that if she felt she would get a better education in the mainstream, she didn't have to be self-contained. She could go out and back for support. So she's going to a mainstream program for deaf children at the school district next to the one in which we live.

I have one piece of advice for parents that I learned through due process. If it's starting to get sticky with the school and you have questions about it, keep the envelopes because they have the postmarks on them. And don't think you're alone. I had a party at my house the other night and of the four families with deaf children, three had been through due process, all in different places.

Although the academic achievement of deaf students is at variance with the achievement of hearing students, at least when sample populations are compared, the dropout rates for deaf students appear to be no different than those for hearing students. In addition, the causes appear to be the same, including family and community affluence levels, local and regional mores and values with respect to schooling, and individual academic ability (Kluwin & Kelly, 1992a; Kluwin & Stinson, 1993).

Educational placement is intertwined with communication. The language and communication modalities described in Chapter 3 are directly related to the methods of communication used in educational programs. Indeed, educational programs for deaf students tend to be defined according to communication method.

COMMUNICATION METHODS

Three communication methods are used in educational programs for deaf students—oral/aural, bilingual, and total communication.

Oral/Aural Communication Method

Oral/aural methods are characterized by instruction in spoken English, curriculum in speech and aural habilitation, and the expectation that the students will use speech, speechreading, and auditory skills for communication.

The history of deaf education has largely been a history of methodology controversy. For more than a century, the controversy centered on whether oralism or manualism was the better method of communication. Until the 1970s, most deaf children were educated in programs using oral/aural methods. At that time, research into the academic achievement of deaf students, as well as research into sign language, caused a dramatic shift to programs that incorporated sign language. The controversy about methodology, however, continued.

The research into methodology has never shown a distinct advantage for one communication method over another. These investigations are fraught with bias at the outset, with researchers biased toward oralism conducting studies that showed the benefits of oralism and researchers biased toward sign language conducting studies that showed the benefits of sign language.

Clearly not all deaf children can be successful learning language through amplification, auditory training, speechreading, technological aids, and tactile methods only. The children who can learn English orally/aurally are in an advantageous position for reading, writing, and communicating with hearing individuals. These children learn one language and use this language for communicating, thinking, and learning. It is the language of most of the individuals in their environment, and it is the language used for communicating through writing. Some research has shown that deaf children educated orally demonstrate significantly better achievement in reading, writing, and general achievement (Geers & Moog, 1989). Again, it is important to note that the research comparing achievement with communication method has been equivocal.

Cued speech is a method of supplementing oral communication. Developed by Cornett (1967), cued speech employs a set of hand cues to distinguish between patterns of speech seen on the lips of the speaker. Consonants are cued by eight hand configurations and vowels are cued by four hand positions. For example, given that *p, b,* and *m* look identical on the lips, each has a different hand cue. By using the hand cue simultaneously with speech, the deaf child can distinguish between these three consonants and know when the speaker is saying *pay* versus *bay* or *may.*

Cued speech is not a substitute for speech or sign language. Cued speech is designed to make speech unambiguous to the deaf child and by accomplishing this level of accurate input, the deaf child can learn to internalize the rule structure of English just as a hearing child could. Cued speech has never been widely used in educational programs in the United States, though many parents are strong advocates (Calvert, 1986).

Bilingual Communication Method

Bilingual methods are characterized by instruction in ASL, the expectation that the students will use ASL for communication, and the teaching of English through the written form with no or little use of spoken English. Most bilingual programs for deaf students are based on English-as-a-second-language models. ASL is introduced as the child's first language, and English is taught as a second language.

The interest in and advocacy for bilingual programs grew dramatically during the 1990s. These programs are often referred to as bilingual/bicultural or bi/bi programs because they emphasize the attainment of two languages and two cultures—ASL and English, and Deaf culture and hearing culture. Three attributes are considered integral to bilingual programs for deaf children. First, ASL is the child's first language. Second, Deaf individuals play a major role in designing, implementing, and evaluating the educational program. Third, Deaf culture is part of the curriculum.

The English-as-a-second-language, or ESL, models that have been developed for children learning spoken languages have not been easily adapted to children learning one visual–gestural language and one spoken language (Baker, 1996; Cummins, 1987; Romaine, 1989; Trueba, 1979).

1. *Immersion.* In the immersion model, all or most classroom instruction is in the second language. The immersion model looks quite different depending on whether the second language is the language of the majority or minority culture. When the second language is the language of the majority culture, such as English in the United States, children typically are expected to ultimately use the majority language exclusively and be assimilated into the majority culture. When the second language is the language of the minority culture, such as in a French immersion school in the United States, children are typically expected to become bilingual in both languages, be enriched by the culture of the second language but retain their own home culture. When applied to bilingual education for deaf children, the model varies depending on the child's home language and culture. If the deaf child comes to school having developed ASL as a first language, immersion would mean classroom instruction in English with, perhaps, ESL pull-out instruction about English conducted in ASL. If the deaf child comes to school having developed a contact language of sign and English, or pidgin sign, immersion could mean either ASL-only or English-only instruction in the classroom with pull-out instruction in the other language. In either scenario, the deaf child receives most instruction in a language with which they are not proficient. It is unlikely that a deaf child who has developed spoken English as a first language would be placed in an ASL immersion program as a young child, though sometimes this occurs later in the school years. Until these students attain proficiency in ASL, they are submerged in a school language they do not know very well and expected to perform academically, though they have little ability to understand the language of instruction.

2. *Transitional.* In the transitional model, classroom instruction is initially in the child's first language, which is the minority language. The second language is gradually introduced and the goal is to ultimately place the child full-time into classes in which the second language is used exclusively for instruction. The goal is for the child to use only the second language in school and to be assimilated into the majority culture. The transitional model would seem to be inappropriate for deaf children because the goal is monolingualism and not bilingualism.

3. *Maintenance.* In the maintenance model, the child's first language is given equal emphasis as a language of instruction throughout his or her schooling. In one form of this model, the child's first language is used for face-to-face communication. The second language is the language of instruction in the subject areas and is used in reading and writing. In a second form of this model, reading, writing, and subject matter instruction are conducted in both languages, though the second language is used predominantly for all subjects except culture. In a third form of this model, there is an equal balance in the use of both languages. One assumption underlying this model, as well as the other two models, is that children come to school with proficiency in a first language. In the maintenance model, it is assumed that this proficiency can be maintained as the second language is introduced. For most deaf children, this assumption cannot be made because they come to school without proficiency in a first language, either ASL or English. However, some of the strategies used in this model are quite appropriate for classrooms with deaf students. For example, using ASL and English for differential instruction may be quite beneficial to deaf children acquiring both languages. Another strategy within this model is having two teachers who each use one language. In some educational programs, one teacher uses English while a paraprofessional uses ASL or classes are team taught by one teacher using English and another using ASL.

4. *Dual language.* In a dual-language model, both languages have equal status, both languages are taught as languages, the teachers are bilingual and use both languages, and half of the students use a minority language and half use a majority language. The languages are generally compartmentalized so that only one language is used for instruction at any time. Although quite appropriate for bilingual programs for deaf children, this is a difficult model to implement because of the challenge in finding qualified teachers who are proficient in both ASL and English and knowledgeable enough to teach the rule structures of both languages. Also, dual-language programs seem to work less successfully when the children are not initially fluent in any language, which is often the case in classrooms of young deaf children.

Although many educational programs for deaf children have incorporated features of English-as-a-second-language models, there has been a lack of research on the effectiveness of these approaches. The rhetoric has been high, and the literature contains numerous articles and essays supporting bilingual education. But the programs that have been implemented have provided little data to help others know what features are and are not effective (Andrews, Ferguson, Roberts, & Hodges, 1997; Drasgow, 1993; Johnson, 1998; Neuroth-Gimbrone & Logiodice, 1992; Saunders, 1997; Strong, 1995).

Total Communication Method

Total communication is characterized by instruction in simultaneous communication, which is the use of speech with manually coded English. The expectation is that students will use simultaneous communication for academic and social discourse. Total communication also incorporates curriculum in speech and aural habilitation, and sometimes includes curriculum in ASL.

Total communication is an approach that has gone somewhat out of favor. One reason is that the idea of using every communication technique and mode available is unrealistic. Teachers typically emphasize speech and audition at the expense of sign language, or vice versa. And students attend more to one mode than another. A second reason total communication as a method has become controversial is because it was predicated on having the teacher use speech and sign language simultaneously. Given that it is not physically or cognitively possible because the two languages have entirely different rule structures, teachers must use either a manually coded English sign system or pidgin sign. As discussed in Chapter 3, the problems inherent in using either of these has led many educators to believe that total communication is an inappropriate method.

When total communication was introduced as a teaching philosophy in the 1960s, it was conceptualized as communication that would involve all avenues including sign, fingerspelling, speech, audition, speechreading, gesture, facial expression, and writing. The actual implementation of total communication did not often match this philosophical conceptualization. As Stewart (1993a) noted:

> Total communication is often misinterpreted as meaning the simultaneous presentation of English in signs and speech rather than a conscientious selection of modalities based on the communication and education needs of the students. This misinterpretation is partly to blame for much of the criticism against the use of manually coded English. Indeed, this kind of misinterpretation and an overall poor implementation of total communication policies may well have doomed to failure the use of any kind of sign communication system with deaf children. (pp. 332–333)

Recently, programs that use total communication have modified the approach to incorporate language switching. In this approach, the teacher individualizes so that information is presented to some students orally/aurally and to others in simultaneous communication or ASL. Stewart (1992) proposed a reform model of total communication. In this reconceptualization, total communication programs would be explicit about when, how, and why ASL and English are used in the classroom; teachers would be capable of communicating in ASL and efficiently coding English into signs; and ASL and English, in all of its modalities, would be used effectively for instruction.

Although the research has not provided clear-cut benefits to any given communication method, there is some evidence to indicate that students' own perceptions of communication ease in the classroom significantly contribute to academic achievement (Braeges, Stinson, & Long, 1993; Long, Stinson, & Braeges, 1991). When students both understand

and feel understood by the teacher and peers, they are more likely to be engaged in learning and to be academically successful.

Total communication continues to be a popular method with parents and many educators (McCallem, 1994; Meadow-Orlans, Mertens, Sass-Lehrer, & Scott-Olson, 1997). No fail-safe, success-guaranteed method exists for educating deaf children, though periodically through the history of deaf education various methods have been proposed as the pedagogical solution. In the 1960s and 1970s, total communication was considered to be the answer. In the 1980s and 1990s, bilingual education was touted as the solution. With the increase in cochlear implants, greater numbers of children are being educated orally/aurally than a decade ago, and oral/aural approaches have seen renewed interest. Ultimately, the profession may recognize that only a range of approaches can meet the needs of a range of deaf children.

Teaching strategies are not prescribed by communication method, though some strategies are clearly more likely to be used in certain kinds of programs. No one model of instruction, set of materials, or collection of teaching strategies is right for every deaf child. The next section will discuss some of the teaching strategies that have been proven to be particularly effective with deaf students as well as specialized curriculum.

TEACHING STRATEGIES AND CURRICULUM

After the passage of the Education of the Deaf Act in 1986 in the United States, which granted university status to Gallaudet College and established the National Commission on Education of the Deaf to assess the education received by deaf students, leaders in deaf education were brought together for a panel to discuss educational programs for deaf children (Corson et al., 1987). The following principles of quality educational programming were presented:

1. Strong leadership comes from school administrators, teachers, parents, and the Deaf community.
2. Decisions are made based on objective, reliable information.
3. Assessment is ongoing and involves multidisciplinary teams of individuals who are committed to student progress.
4. Lack of progress is not accepted.
5. Programs are implemented with consistency.
6. Professionals continuously develop their knowledge and skills.
7. Partnerships are sustained with parents and the Deaf community.
8. A continuum of programming that supports successful transition from home-based to school-based programs and from school-based to work-based programs is provided.

Noticeably absent from these laudable principles is the core of any educational program, which is teaching and learning. Excellent education is quality teaching, which brings about optimum learning. Five features of quality teaching with deaf students are the involvement of students in experiential activities, building on the students' knowledge and skills, capitalizing on the visual medium, maintaining active student engagement, and creating a need to interact with peers. In Figure 7.1, instructional strategies that incorporate these features are presented.

Quality teaching involves not just the "how" of teaching but the "what" of teaching. Teaching strategies answer the question, "How should deaf students be taught?" Curriculum answers the question, "What should deaf students be taught?"

There are two schools of thought about curriculum for students who are deaf. According to one, these students need a specialized curriculum in all subject areas. According to the other school of thought, deaf students do not need specialized curriculum for content subjects because they have no special learning needs in these areas. They are able to learn as much material and at the same level of complexity as hearing children. The specialized curriculum they do need relates to their special learning and developmental needs.

Both schools of thought recognize the importance of specialized curriculum in the areas of Deaf culture, and speech and aural habilitation. In addition, curriculum in language, reading, and writing are considered essential, whether specialized or modified.

Language, Reading, and Writing

Historically, a curriculum for deaf students in language, reading, and writing was analytical in nature. Deaf students were taught the rules, or grammar, of spoken and written language and given practice in applying the rules. A curriculum in language often consisted of teaching the students English sentence patterns, starting with the basic patterns and moving to increasingly complex structures. Teachers used strategies that focused almost exclusively on English syntax, such as the Fitzgerald Key and Apple Tree (Caniglia, Cole, Howard, Krohn, & Rice, 1975; Fitzgerald, 1949; Pugh, 1955). A curriculum in reading regularly involved using books with relatively simple grammatical structures or basal reading materials that were designed so that sentence patterns increased in difficulty from book to book, such as Reading Milestones (Quigley, King, McAnally, & Rose, 1993). Teachers used strategies that focused almost exclusively on word identification skills and sentence-level understanding. A typical writing curriculum required students to learn the rules for different types of discourse, such as writing essays and paragraphs, and

FIGURE 7.1   Teaching Strategies

Mr. Smith and Ms. Jones are teaching about the food pyramid. Mr. Smith employs teaching strategies that involve the students actively in learning, build on their background knowledge, visually represent information being presented, and engage them in meaningful discussion with their peers. Ms. Jones uses very few appropriate strategies with her deaf students.

MR. SMITH	MS. JONES
Mr. Smith asks the students to keep a log of what they eat for one day.	Ms. Jones explains the foods in the food pyramid. She then gives each student a list of food groups and asks them to write the names of at least two foods for each group.
The next day, he asks the students to work in pairs and compare their food logs. They should decide on what kinds of foods they ate and how much of each kind. After 10 minutes, they have a whole-class discussion during which Mr. Smith writes their findings on the white board. They come to consensus on categories for foods and count how much the class ate in each group.	The next day, she reviews the foods in each food group of the pyramid. The students are asked to add at least two more foods to each group.
The next day, Mr. Smith shows a food pyramid on a chart and explains it to the class. Next to it, he presents a chart of the class's findings from yesterday. He asks them to get together in pairs again and put the food from their daily log onto the food pyramid. He asks them to keep a log of what they eat for one day, from the time they leave school today.	The next day, Ms. Jones gives the students a blank copy of the food pyramid and asks them to fill in the name of each food group in the appropriate place. They swap papers and correct each other's work as a group under Ms. Jones's guidance.
The next day, Mr. Smith asks the students to use their log in figuring out how much food from each group they ate. He then asks them to decide on a diagram that best represents their food intake, such as a circle, rectangle, inverted triangle, or triangle.	The next day, Ms. Jones gives out magazines, scissors, and glue and asks the students to cut out pictures of food and glue them onto their food pyramids in the correct places.
The next day, Mr. Smith asks the students to work in small groups in creating an ideal menu for one day.	The next day, Ms. Jones asks her students to write a paragraph about the food pyramid.

the rules of grammar because these were the most obvious areas with which deaf students had difficulty. Teachers used strategies that focused on the correctness of form through teaching skills and rules, providing students with practice in mastering techniques, and evaluating student progress by the number of errors in completed compositions.

Curriculum in language, reading, and writing today can be best described as a balance of analytical and holistic. In the language curriculum, deaf students are engaged in communicating in spoken English or ASL through conversation and discussion. Grammatical rules are taught but only after the deaf child demonstrates understanding of the grammatical form when used by others or after it appears in the child's own expressive language. Teachers use strategies such as modeling, restating, clarifying, and extending that bring the deaf child's attention to syntax, semantics, pragmatics, and phonology within the context of communication.

In the reading curriculum, as much emphasis is placed on reading comprehension as on word identification and sentence-level understanding. Instruction of skills takes place during the reading of stories and novels that are written for audiences of children, not just deaf children. Deaf children are given lots of time and opportunities to read and to learn about reading through skills instruction. Teachers use strategies that involve teaching students to recognize words automatically, think critically and creatively about what they have read, self-question during reading, predict, summarize, and apply their background knowledge.

In the writing curriculum, emphasis is placed on helping deaf students see that writing is a process rather than a finished product and that writing involves many qualities, of which English grammar is just one. Teachers use strategies that help students understand and use the writing processes of planning, composing, and revising. And they evaluate compositions based on multiple qualities such as ideas, organization, use of details to support main points, word choice, mechanics, and sentence structure.

Deaf Culture

A curriculum in Deaf culture is important for all deaf students regardless of their educational setting, though many educators and members of the Deaf community argue that it is even more important in public school programs because children in these settings typically have relatively little contact with Deaf adults. The following components typically form the nucleus of a Deaf culture curriculum.

- American Sign Language
  Linguistic differences between ASL and English

> How ASL developed as a visual–gestural language of the Deaf community in the United States
> Interaction norms and conversational rules in ASL

- Political activism
  > Movements such as the Deaf President Now protest at Gallaudet University
  > Advocacy activities that have led to the passage of laws and regulations designed to improve education and accessibility for individuals with hearing loss
- History and biography
  > Deaf individuals who have made important contributions to society
  > Contributions from the Deaf community such as the football huddle, originally developed at Gallaudet University by all-deaf football teams
- Theater, art, and literature
  > Groups such as the National Theatre of the Deaf
  > Visual art of Deaf artists
  > Literature of Deaf authors
- Clubs and organizations
  > Information about and participation in the activities of local Deaf clubs, organizations, fraternal orders and sororities, churches and synagogues, and sports such as deaf sport
  > Competitions such as the Deaf Olympics and Miss Deaf America
- Folklore
  > Legends and traditions of the Deaf community
  > Jokes and humorous stories
  > Games and sign play
  > Naming practices
  > Customs, rituals, and celebrations

Speech

A speech curriculum involves teaching the skills involved in producing spoken language, and then in improving speech. Because deaf children do not hear speech or do not hear it without distortion, they can neither figure out how to produce speech nor monitor their own speech without assistance. They not only have difficulty producing individual speech sounds, but they also have problems with volume, pitch, and nasality.

The most widely used curriculum for teaching speech was developed by Ling (1976, 1989). In the Ling approach, sounds are taught auditorally first, and visual and tactile cues are added as needed. Deaf children rely heavily on how each sound feels as speech is produced because they cannot rely solely on how the sounds they produce sound. Speech instruction involves teaching the deaf child breath control, vocalization, voice patterns, and sound production.

The visual cues of speechreading are particularly important for enhancing the deaf child's ability to both understand and produce speech. However, the benefits of instruction in speechreading are questionable. If used without residual hearing, speechreading has limited benefits for many reasons. One reason is that about half of English words have at least one other word that appears the same on the lips. Another reason is that most speakers do not face forward and speak clearly at all times. Speakers move, place items in front of their faces, chew gum, and make sounds that are not words. Also, some speakers have beards and mustaches, hardly move their lips when they speak, or have accents that produce unfamiliar speech patterns.

Not all deaf students benefit from speech instruction. As deaf students become older, their motivation for speech intervention often declines.

Aural Habilitation

An aural habilitation curriculum involves teaching deaf students how to use their residual hearing, through amplification or cochlear implant, and to respond to sound. For some deaf students, response to sound may be simple awareness and for others it is comprehension of the speech being used. Between these two ends of the continuum are localization, discrimination of sound differences, and recognition of sound. The differences between these can be illustrated by the word *dog*.

- *Awareness.* The child hears a dog barking and stops playing for a moment.
- *Localization.* The child hears a dog barking and turns to the fence, where the dog is.
- *Discrimination of sound differences.* The child hears a dog barking and Mom saying, "The mailman must be here." The child looks at the dog and then at Mom.
- *Recognizing the sound.* The child hears a dog barking, looks at Mom, and says, "Elsie is angry," and runs into the living room looking for the dog.
- *Comprehending sounds.* Mom says, "Where's our dog?", and the child says, "Elsie?"

As with speech, not all deaf students benefit from aural habilitation. Learning to respond to sounds, such as a dog barking, is considerably easier than learning to respond to speech sounds. As discussed in Chapter 1, speech sounds are complex and encompass a range of intensities and frequencies.

Two points in the deaf child's life are particularly relevant educationally because they mark the child's transition from home to school and from school to work. Educational programs at these two transition points have goals that do not fully overlap with the goals of what is typically referred to as K–12 or kindergarten through high school education.

TRANSITION

Early Childhood Programs

The 1997 amendments to IDEA (Public Law 105-17) included the following outcomes for early childhood intervention:

1. To enhance the development of infants and toddlers with disabilities and to minimize their potential for developmental delay;
2. To reduce the educational costs to our society, including our Nation's schools, by minimizing the need for special education and related services after infants and toddlers with disabilities reach school age;
3. To minimize the likelihood of institutionalization of individuals with disabilities and maximize the potential for their independently living in society;
4. To enhance the capacity of families to meet the special education needs of their infants and toddlers with disabilities; and
5. To enhance the capacity of State and local agencies and service providers to identify, evaluate, and meet the needs of historically underrepresented populations, particularly minority, low-income, inner-city, and rural populations. (Part C, Sec. 631)

In early childhood, IDEA prescribes an individualized family services plan (IFSP). The IFSP is developed by a multidisciplinary team that includes the child's parents, it is reviewed with the parents every six months, and it is evaluated each year. All IFSPs include the child's present levels of development (physical, cognitive, communication, social or emotional, and adaptive), the family's priorities and concerns, major outcomes, time lines and procedures for services, criteria for evaluating the effectiveness of services, early intervention services, the natural environments in which the services will be provided or why natural environments will not be provided, and the steps that will support transition to preschool or other appropriate services.

According to Meadow-Orlans (1987), the hallmarks of excellence for early intervention programs for deaf children are the following:

- Strong emphasis on parent counseling both within parent groups and individual sessions

- Teachers who are knowledgeable of audiology so that they can ensure that the child is always receiving optimal amplification from hearing aids
- Teachers who are knowledgeable of speech development and committed to encouraging the child to develop oral skills
- Teachers who are knowledgeable of sign language and committed to helping parents learn sign when total communication is the approach used with the child
- Presence of deaf persons in the program as teachers, paraprofessionals, staff, or volunteers

In Essay 7.2, Karen Clark describes the early intervention program of the Dallas Regional Day School Program for the Deaf. The core resource for this program is the SKI*HI Model, which is a comprehensive model for early identification of children with hearing losses and family-centered, home-based intervention (Strong et al., 1994). The model differentiates goals for children and parents. For the children, the goals are to "(a) communicate meaningfully, (b) use residual hearing, (c) develop a communication method (aural/oral, ASL, total communication, or other methods), (d) develop optimal receptive and expressive language levels, (e) be provided with the most appropriate amplification, and (f) be prepared to enter school ready to learn." For the parents, the goals are to "(a) have a warm, positive relationship with the child, (b) provide a stimulating, interactive environment, (c) be able to manage the child's hearing aids, (d) help the child use his or her residual hearing, and (e) provide communication/language and cognitive stimulation" (p. 26).

■ ■ ■ ■ ■ ▬▬▬

ESSAY 7.2

Karen Clark and the Dallas Regional Program

Learning what parents want for their children, and combining that with effective parent education, is the heart of a family-centered program for infants and toddlers who are deaf and hard of hearing. The Dallas Regional Day School Program for the Deaf provides services to more than thirty infants and toddlers from birth to three years of age. The program serves the Dallas Independent School District and eight member school districts. In Texas, general early intervention services, which are mandated by IDEA Part C, are combined with deaf education services, which are mandated by state law. Children, who are initially referred to their local Early Childhood Intervention Program, are in turn referred to the local education agency if a hearing loss is suspected. Professionals from both groups come together in forming an assessment team with the educator of the deaf responsible for guiding the communication portion of the assessment. The assessment is conducted in the child's natural environment, which Part C of IDEA defines as any place the child lives, learns, and plays. With infants and toddlers, the natural environment is most often the child's home.

The parent, educator of the deaf, and at least one other early childhood intervention professional develop the individualized family service plan. The parent or parents share with the team the outcomes they would like for their child. In our experience, the outcomes stated by parents reflect their own knowledge and experience at that particular moment in time. For example, often hearing parents will describe their most desired outcome as having their child talk. This is not the time for educators to provide information concerning the difference between speech and language or to suggest that the parent might consider other outcomes as equally or more important. Instead, this is precisely the time for professionals to listen to the parents' hopes and dreams for their child and to begin planning the strategies and experiences that will bring about the desired outcome. These strategies and experiences will ultimately broaden the parents' understanding of deafness, and they will increasingly be able to see wider varieties of desirable outcomes.

Most families in the family-centered birth-to-three program receive at least weekly home visits from a teacher of the deaf. This person is called a parent advisor. The SKI*HI Model for Home-Based Programs is the core resource. This model involves listening to parents, gathering continuous observational assessment data, sharing resources with parents, and determining the topics that are appropriate as the parents are able to integrate new information and develop new skills. Parent advisors show the parents how to capitalize on the child's interests, incorporate daily routines, such as bath time and mealtime, and use interaction and listening strategies that encourage the development of communication.

Parental choice is central to the program. We have noticed that parents have many questions about communication methodology and issues related to communication. They have often read and heard about American Sign Language, manually coded English, auditory/oral methods, hearing aids, and cochlear implants. It is critical for parent advisors to provide objective information about all areas regardless of personal or professional bias. Parent advisors typically provide written, verbal, and visual information to answer parents' questions, but they also offer a wide variety of resources including access to other parents, adults who are deaf or hard of hearing, and professionals with expertise on specific topics.

In addition to home visits, a range of other support services are available to parents. Audiological services are provided through a contract with the Callier Center for Communication Disorders at the University of Texas at Dallas. The Program for Amplification for Children of Texas, which is part of the Texas Department of Health, provides hearing aids for children who live at or below 150 percentile of the federal poverty level. Sign language classes are offered weekly, including one class each week for families who speak Spanish. At present, the school district is exploring the use of cable television for offering sign language classes through a distance learning medium. The Early Intervention Program, partner to the Dallas Regional Day School Program for the Deaf, coordinates the delivery of the services deemed essential by the individualized family service plan.

(continued)

ESSAY 7.2   CONTINUED

The diverse population of Dallas presents the many challenges inherent to other urban areas. Parent advisors spend considerable time and log substantial mileage on roads and expressways visiting families. Traffic congestion, high crime areas, and other personal safety issues are part of the daily stress involved in a program that places home visits as central to effective early intervention. Parent advisors often combine visits with the services of other professionals so that they are not alone. Although mandated to provide services at times convenient for families, most parent advisors generally restrict their visits to daylight-only. Diverse languages are also a way of life for parent advisors. The current group of four parent advisors can communicate through sign language, two are bilingual in Spanish and English, and one is a certified sign language interpreter. The parent advisors possess the ability and desire to communicate with all parents through any means possible and so use spoken language, sign language, gestures, writing, interpreters, or any combination of these.

All successful programs for families share a common feature—the ability to change to meet current and evolving needs. In Texas, legislation mandating a statewide early hearing detection program has resulted in greater numbers of identified infants. With more than 300,000 births annually, the conservative prevalence figure of two per one thousand infants who are deaf or hard of hearing means that 600 or more children are likely to be identified annually. Meeting the needs of these newborns and their families is one of our greatest challenges. Another challenge involves staying knowledgeable about the research on best practices in working with infants and families, which is published at an ever-increasing rate. Yet we also know that this type of outcome data must be combined with good family-centered practices. We believe that our own experiences with infants must be documented and shared with colleagues. A further challenge has been the growth in the numbers of non-English-speaking families. We must develop better strategies to meet their needs and to do this, we must learn their cultures. We have initiated deaf mentor programs because they offer new resources and opportunities to all families. Our Dallas program looks forward to these challenges and to developing even better ways of meeting the needs of all families.

Reprinted by permission of the author.

High School Transition Programs

According to IDEA, beginning at age 14, the IEP must include the student's transition service needs, such as participation in advanced placement courses or a vocational education program. Beginning at age 16, or earlier if the evaluation team determines that it is appropriate, an individualized transition plan (ITP) must be developed and included as part of the IEP process.

The 1997 amendments to IDEA defined transition services as a coordinated set of activities for a student with a disability that:

(A) is designed within an outcome-oriented process, that promotes movement from school to post-school activities, including postsecondary education, vocational training, integrated employment (including supported
employment), continuing and adult education, adult services, independent
living, or community participation;

(B) is based on the student's needs, taking into account the student's preferences and interests;

(C) includes instruction, related services, community experiences, the development of employment and other post-school objectives, and, when
appropriate, acquisition of daily living skills and functional vocational
evaluation. (Part C, Section 602)

Freeburg, Sendelbaugh, and Bullis (1991) examined school-to-community transition issues for deaf youth and found several barriers to successful transition. The major barrier for both deaf and hard of hearing
students was communication. For deaf students, the other barriers included educational programming that inadequately prepared them for
transition and a shortage of community support services to provide transition assistance. For hard of hearing students, the other barriers involved
personal characteristics such as lack of preparation in self-advocacy and
assertiveness.

Transition programs are designed to assist students in making a
successful transition from high school to postsecondary education or the
workplace. Busby and Danek (1998) noted:

> As we enter the complex global society of the twenty-first century, Americans
> are competing in a high-technology, information-based, transnational econ-
> omy. Fragmented educational and adult service programming will not be suf-
> ficient to prepare deaf and hard of hearing youth to enter this economy. Long
> before students cross the threshold into independence and adulthood, careful
> transition planning in the schools should begin, and individuals from a variety
> of community, service, and business organizations should be involved in a
> partnership with the school to effect a successful transition process. (p. 10)

In addition to the particular educational needs of children at transition points, special programs, curricula, and strategies have been suggested for deaf students with special needs.

STUDENTS WITH SPECIAL NEEDS

The learning characteristics of deaf students changed dramatically during
the past century. At the outset of the twentieth century, postlingual deafness was quite common due to disease and injury. The population of
schoolchildren was a mix of those who were born deaf and those who
became deaf subsequent to learning language. At the outset of the

twenty-first century, postlingual deafness among schoolchildren is considerably less common due to medical advances. Conversely, proportionally more children are born deaf due to conditions and diseases contracted in-utero, and many of these children have additional disabilities. Since the rubella epidemic of the mid-1960s, children often referred to as "vanilla" deaf because their only exceptionality is deafness have become increasingly rare. Researchers and educators have paid specific attention to deaf children with learning disabilities, attention deficit disorder, severe and multiple disabilities, and giftedness.

Learning disabilities in deaf children has been a difficult area to study because the characteristics exhibited by learning disabled hearing students overlap with characteristics exhibited by deaf students, such as a disparity between achievement and ability. There are no precise criteria for identifying deaf students with learning disabilities (Bunch & Melnyk, 1989; Elliott, Powers, & Funderburg, 1988; Laughton, 1989; Mauk & Mauk, 1992). Given the difficulty in identifying these children, there are no reliable prevalence estimates. The importance of appropriately diagnosing a learning disability is essential for providing an appropriate educational program for the deaf child. By using observational techniques, curriculum-based assessment, and standardized instruments, the likelihood for misdiagnosis is diminished (Plapinger & Sikora, 1990; Roth, 1991). Morgan and Vernon (1994) recommended the use of a battery of assessment instruments including a case history, an educational history, two measures of intellectual functioning, a measure of educational achievement, neuropsychological screening, assessment of adaptive behavior functioning and/or classroom behavior, a current audiological evaluation and vision screening, and information on communication and language skills.

Attention deficit disorder (ADD) is characterized by inattentiveness, distractibility, impulsivity, and hyperactivity. Educationally, children with ADD often demonstrate poor academic performance and are considered by their teachers to have behavioral problems that interfere with classroom learning of themselves and other students. There is a dearth of information on prevalence, identification, and treatment with deaf students (Kelly, Forney, Parker-Fisher, & Jones, 1993a, 1993b). As with other children with ADD, there is great controversy regarding the use of medications such as Ritalin, and many educators recommend applied behavior analysis techniques rather than medication. When using applied behavior analysis, the teacher analyzes the new skill or behavior to be learned into subskills or subtasks, directly and frequently measures student performance, provides frequent opportunities for the student to actively respond during instruction, provides immediate and systematic feedback, and provides opportunities for the student to apply the new skill or behavior successfully across settings and over time (Cooper, Heron, & Heward, 1987).

The education of deaf children with severe or multiple disabilities has centered on functional curriculum and issues involved in the transition from school to community. Functional curriculum focuses on the student's work, living, and social needs. The following recommendations have been offered to educational programs in preparing deaf students with severe or multiple disabilities for successful community living and competitive employment (Arkell, 1982; Davis & Bullis, 1990; Reiman, Bullis, Davis, & Cole, 1991):

- Analyze current and possible future living and working environments, and match instructional goals to the skills needed in these environments.
- Before teaching any skill, consider whether the student will be in school long enough to develop proficiency.
- Teach the student skills that can be used in multiple environments.
- Teach adaptive communication methods only when the student cannot learn common communication methods.
- Develop or practice skills in natural environments wherever possible.
- Recognize that parents are the long-term stakeholders in their child's success.

Giftedness has been something of a stepchild in the field of special education because it seems strange to many professionals to regard the needs of gifted children as comparable to the needs of children with disabilities. Although it would seem outlandish for a gifted athlete to train for the Olympics by competing in intramural sports, the corollary of special school services for intellectually gifted students is considered by many educators to be needless. Yet the intellectual or creative gifts of these students are equivalent to the athletic gifts of the individual preparing for the Olympics. Complicating the situation for gifted children is the lack of agreed-upon criteria for giftedness among all children and giftedness among deaf children in particular (Rittenhouse & Blough, 1995). For example, when parents and teachers were asked to identify giftedness among deaf students at a school for the deaf and a public school system, a significant percentage of children with high IQ scores were missed in this nomination process (Yewchuk & Bibby, 1988, 1989; Yewchuk, Bibby, & Fraser, 1989). Rittenhouse and Blough (1995) suggested that educational programs take the following actions to meet the needs of gifted deaf students:

1. Assume that students with hearing impairments in your classroom have unique talents that if developed can improve their overall learning profiles.
2. De-emphasize verbal test scores as indicators of giftedness and more prominently include nonverbal, performance scores, and other nontraditional data.

3. Develop an inventory of unique talents among normal hearing students identified by your local gifted program and evaluate your students with hearing impairments against it.
4. Individualize instruction and subject matter in your classroom, based on the unique talents identified in your students.
5. Create thematic units that incorporate individual activities that draw on the talents of your students. (p. 53)

The teaching strategies, curriculum, and programs described in the previous sections are delivered by professionals and paraprofessionals involved in the educational lives of deaf children and youth.

ROLES AND COMPETENCIES OF PROFESSIONALS

Teachers, interpreters, speech–language specialists, audiologists, school psychologists, school counselors, and other related-service personnel such as residence life personnel and social workers play important roles educationally with deaf students. With the child, parents, and family, these individuals work together in providing an effective education that will enable the child to enjoy a full and independent life in the workplace and community.

Teachers of the Deaf

At present, more than 70 colleges and universities in the United States and Canada offer teacher education programs at the baccalaureate or master's degree level for individuals who want to become teachers of students who are deaf and hard of hearing. The oldest programs were founded in the 1800s—Boston University in 1873, Smith College in 1889, and Lenoir-Rhyne College in 1894. Teachers of the deaf are certified or licensed by individual states through departments of education or state certification/licensure departments. In addition, the Council on Education of the Deaf (CED) offers national certification. CED standards for certification are used by the major national organization for accreditation, National Council for Accreditation of Teacher Education, which in turn is used as the accrediting standards by many states.

Teachers of the deaf work in the continuum of educational placements described earlier in this chapter. They can teach in self-contained classrooms in schools for the deaf or public schools, where they usually teach small groups of six to eight deaf students who represent a relatively restricted span of age and grade levels, though often different ability levels. They can also teach in resource rooms with students from a range of grade levels who spend portions of each day in general education class-rooms. Some resource room teachers split their time between schools, so the numbers of children they serve can be substantial. Increasingly greater numbers of teachers of the deaf are being hired to serve as itinerant or con-sultant teachers. These teachers have a caseload of students from several schools, often covering fairly wide geographic regions. Some of the stu-dents spend one or a few periods of time each week with the itinerant teacher, whereas other students are served indirectly because the consult-ant teacher of the deaf works directly with the classroom teacher.

Teachers of the deaf are expected to possess an impressive array of knowledge and skills about special education in general and deaf educa-tion in particular. The areas of knowledge include the philosophical, his-torical and legal foundations of special education; characteristics of learners; assessment, diagnosis, and evaluation; instructional content and practice; planning and managing the teaching and learning environment; manag-ing student behavior and social interaction skills; communication and col-laborative partnerships; and professionalism and ethical practices (The Council for Exceptional Children, 1995). Given that they are certified to teach all grade levels and all subject areas to deaf and hard of hearing chil-dren with any degree of hearing loss using any method of communication needed by the child within the continuum of educational settings, the re-sponsibilities on each teacher's shoulders are certainly great.

Several issues have emerged as particularly challenging for pro-grams preparing teachers. One of these is the dilemma of recruiting and educating deaf individuals to become teachers at a time when increasing numbers of states require standardized assessment, such as the Praxis series developed by Educational Testing Service, for certification or licen-sure (Kensicki, 1995; Serwatka, Anthony, & Simon, 1986). Included in this issue is the recruitment of teachers from underrrepresented populations, which is crucial given the increase in school enrollments of children from racially and ethnically diverse homes. Andrews and Jordan (1993) sur-veyed professionals in deaf education programs and found that 10.4 per-cent were from nonwhite or minority/ethnic cultural backgrounds, of which 11.7 percent were deaf.

A second issue is the development of assessment instruments that appropriately measure the knowledge essential to teaching deaf students (Rosenfeld, Mounty, Ehringhaus, & Klem, 1993). A third issue is provid-ing a program that enables individuals to gain the competencies needed for the different settings in which they will teach. For example, it has been found that the competencies needed by itinerant and consultant teachers are quite different than those needed by teachers in self-contained class-rooms (Luckner & Miller, 1994; Sass-Lehrer, 1983, 1986a, 1986b). An issue related to teacher competencies for different settings is the fourth issue, communication skills of teachers. Teachers in oral/aural settings need to be highly competent in teaching oral/aural skills, teachers in total communication settings need to be competent in teaching oral/aural skills and proficient signers in simultaneous communication, and teachers in bilingual settings need to be competent in ASL. It is not realistic to expect any teacher education program to ensure all of these communication skills, which is problematic given that when they complete the program, graduates are certified to teach in all types of programs (Clarke, Clarke, & Winzer, 1988; Stewart, Akamatsu, & Bonkowski, 1988; Stewart et al., 1989; White, 1990). A similar problem relates to competency in subject matter, which is a fifth issue. Though teachers of the deaf are certified to teach all subject areas to deaf students, in many states they do not need to have demonstrated competency in subject areas such as science or math (Luckner, 1991a). A sixth issue is the lack of preparation that teachers-in-training typically receive in working with deaf students who have a concomitant disability, such as a behavior disorder, a learning disability, or mental retardation (D'Zamko & Hampton, 1985; Elliott & Powers, 1988).

Professional development programs are crucial for teachers of the deaf. Not only do these programs upgrade teachers' knowledge and skills and keep teachers informed of recent research, but they also reduce the isolation that many teachers experience in their professional lives (Johnson, 1995).

Interpreters

At present, slightly more than 100 community colleges, colleges, and universities in the United States and Canada offer interpreter training programs. The majority of these programs are at the associate's degree level and many programs are nondegree or certificate only. Just thirteen programs, in the same number of states, offer interpreter training at the baccalaureate level and only three offer graduate programs.

Two organizations offer interpreter certification, the National Association of the Deaf (NAD) and the Registry of Interpreters of the Deaf (RID), though these organizations are currently collaborating to develop one certification system. Established in 1964, RID's mission is to provide the three Qs of interpreting—quantity, qualifications, and quality through the following three activities:

- Training of new interpreters and professional development of practicing interpreters
- Certification of interpreters
- Self-regulation through a national ethical practices system

Through the RID National Testing System, individuals can seek certification as interpreters and transliterators in a broad range of settings including community, educational, legal, medical, and performing arts.
Interpretation involves interpreting between ASL and spoken English and
transliteration involves transliterating between English-based sign language and spoken English, both sign-to-voice and voice-to-sign. A separate certificate is offered for oral transliterators who transliterate the spoken
message from a person who hears to a person who is deaf or hard of hearing by using speech and mouth movements. In addition, certification is
available to individuals who are deaf or hard of hearing to work in settings
in which a deaf or hard of hearing interpreter would be beneficial.

The educational interpreter's purpose is to facilitate communication and equalize learning opportunities. As increasing numbers of deaf
children are educated in public school classrooms with hearing students
and no teacher of the deaf, it has become important to professionalize the
role of the educational interpreter. In the early years of educational interpreting, these individuals were often the mothers of deaf children who
had learned sign language to communicate with their child and generally had adequate though not proficient signing abilities. The following
issues are at the forefront of educational interpreting today (Elliott &
Powers, 1995; Hayes, 1993; Kluwin, 1994b; Salend & Longo, 1994;
Shroyer & Compton, 1994; Wilcox, Schroeder, & Martinez, 1990):

■ *Role of the educational interpreter.* As a team member with the classroom teacher, teacher of the deaf, and other professionals, the educational interpreter is often expected to take on responsibilities such as
classroom aiding, tutoring, and assessing the child's performance. Issues
of confidentiality are often less than clear-cut when the interpreter is
sharing information that has been observed in the classroom, through
one-to-one interactions with the child, or from interpreting between
peers. For the interpreter in an educational setting, the role of consultant
and collaborator is distinct from any other interpreting setting.

■ *Knowledge and skills.* Not only is the educational interpreter expected to be a skilled communicator in the manually coded English sign
system being used in the school and ASL, but he or she also must understand the language levels, comprehension abilities, and learning differences of deaf children, as well as have knowledge of the variety of subject
matter and subject vocabulary.

■ *Certification.* Many states require educational interpreters to be certified, which is designed to promote higher quality interpreting. The dilemma is the differential between the numbers of certified interpreters and
the numbers of children who need educational interpreters. Compounding

this dilemma is the reality that interpreters in educational settings are often not paid as well as either freelance interpreters or other professionals in the educational setting.

Other Professionals

In addition to teachers and interpreters, other professionals provide important educational services to deaf children. These include speech–language specialists, audiologists, school psychologists, and school counselors.

Speech–language specialists and audiologists are certified by the American Speech-Language-Hearing Association (ASHA). The relationship between teachers of the deaf and speech–language specialists has often been prickly because of differing perspectives on language development. Whereas teachers of the deaf view the language acquisition of deaf children within a developmental perspective, speech–language specialists view language development within a clinical/medical perspective. Teachers of the deaf consider that deaf children will be challenged in developing language but have the same cognitive abilities to learn language as hearing children. Speech–language specialists consider that deaf children have a communication disorder and need remediation in order to develop language. In recent years, the trend has been to delegate speech development to the speech–language specialist, typically during pull-out periods of time, and language development to the teacher of the deaf (Otis-Wilborn, 1992).

School psychologists are licensed by the American Psychological Association (APA) and the National Association of School Psychologists (NASP), and school counselors are licensed by the Council for Accreditation of Counseling and Related Educational Programs (CACREP). Few programs exist for preparing school psychologists and school counselors to work specifically with deaf children. In comparing school psychological services for deaf and hard of hearing students in the mid-1970s and the mid-1990s, Weaver and Bradley-Johnson (1993) found that the majority lacked training in working with deaf and hard of hearing students, though more school psychologists in the 1990s reported having some type of special training than their counterparts in the 1970s.

SUMMARY AND CONCLUDING THOUGHTS

This chapter discussed the educational placement options available to deaf students, how placement decisions are made, the components of effective placements, and factors involved in the academic achievement of deaf students. It also presented the range of communication methods used with deaf students in educational programs. In addition, it provided a description of the special teaching strategies and curriculum used by teachers of the deaf, the transition points of early childhood-to-school and high school-to-community, and deaf students with special needs.

It seems appropriate to conclude this chapter with a vision statement developed from a survey of more than 2,500 deaf students between ages 8 and 18 nationwide in the United States attending schools for the deaf and public school programs, conducted by students at Gallaudet University (Page, 1996):

- American Sign Language is accepted and widely used even within the hearing community.
- Our families have a greater understanding, acceptance, and involvement in our educational, emotional, and communication development.
- The standard and quality of our education is greatly improved. We have better teachers, more deaf teachers, more challenging courses, greater communication, improved reading skills, and education on par with hearing students.
- We have frequent opportunities to interact with, learn from, and look up to deaf and hard of hearing role models.
- We have greater access to advances in technology, such as computers, captioned media, TTYs, hearing aids, and assistive devices.
- We have the same opportunities to participate in extracurricular activities in school and in the community as do hearing students.
- America has a greater awareness of deaf and hard of hearing people and our diverse cultures.
- We are allowed to use the form of communication best suited to our individual needs, which may be speech, sign language, or any other means of effective communication. (p. 10)

CHAPTER EIGHT

ECONOMIC AND OCCUPATIONAL OPPORTUNITIES

FOCUS QUESTIONS

- What impact has ADA had on access to higher education for deaf individuals?
- What are the major challenges faced by deaf students in community college, college, and university classes?
- How have employment trends changed since the early twentieth century?
- Why do unemployment and underemployment continue to characterize the employment status of deaf individuals?
- In what ways can health care situations better accommodate the communication needs of deaf patients?

In the mid-1980s, a group of leaders in education, vocational rehabilitation, and government were brought together to discuss the lifelong spectrum of learning, from infancy through adulthood, and employment for deaf individuals. Melton summarized the situation at the time as the following:

- Deaf and severely hard of hearing students generally do not possess the personal and interpersonal skills needed for successful interaction with co-workers and supervisors;
- Often, they display poor work behavior and habits, they do not understand the value of work and they are unaware of most career fields and occupations;
- For many, lack of language and reading skills limit their opportunities for successful training and job placements;
- A lack of exposure to those experiences which enhance independent living, personal responsibility and survival skills, including appropriate use

of leisure time, is often a primary problem in helping them adjust to the community and postsecondary or job training. (1987, p. 315)

This chapter will explore whether the situation described by Melton exists currently. It will discuss postsecondary education, employment status, and quality-of-life issues as they are impacted by the economic and occupational opportunities available to deaf individuals.

POSTSECONDARY EDUCATION

According to the National Center for Education Statistics (1999), of the students with a hearing loss who exited the educational system in 1994–1995, just over 40 percent earned a diploma and almost 9 percent earned a certificate. An estimated 23,860 students with a hearing loss were enrolled at two-year and four-year postsecondary education institutions during 1996–1997 or 1997–1998 (institutions were asked to provide data for the 1996–1997 school year but if it was not available, they could provide data for the 1997–1998 school year), which was an increase of 16 percent from 1992–1993. More than half were enrolled in two-year institutions. Of the thousand institutions surveyed, 48 percent reported enrolling students with a hearing loss. The size of the institution was directly related to enrollment, with only one-third of institutions with less than 3,000 students enrolling students with a hearing loss compared to 100 percent of institutions with more than 10,000 students. Institutional type also was related to enrollment. Whereas less than one-third of private two-year and four-year institutions enrolled students with a hearing loss, 83 percent of public two-year and 91 percent of public four-year institutions enrolled students with a hearing loss.

Kasen, Ouellette, and Cohen (1990) examined the postsecondary educational status of a group of young deaf adults who had become deaf as a result of the mid-1960s rubella epidemic. They found that higher levels of mainstreaming in elementary and secondary schools were associated with higher levels of postsecondary education; however, individuals who were previously mainstreamed primarily chose postsecondary programs for the deaf such as the National Technical Institute for the Deaf. They also found that minority deaf young adults had low levels of postsecondary education. Attrition is particularly high among deaf postsecondary students. Walter and his associates found that between 70 and 75 percent of deaf college students withdraw without graduating, which is considerably above the 50 percent rate typically estimated for hearing students (Stinson & Walter, 1992; Walter, 1987; Walter & Welsh, 1986).

In the United States, Congress has shown particular interest in the postsecondary education of deaf students, and there has been a history of providing funding to postsecondary institutions to serve deaf adults that is unique among minority populations.

Postsecondary Institutions

Originally named the National Deaf Mute College, Gallaudet College was established by the U.S. Congress in 1864 as the first liberal arts college for the deaf in the world. One hundred years later, Congress authorized the establishment of the National Technical Institute for the Deaf, and in 1968, it opened as part of the Rochester Institute of Technology. At the same time, four federally funded institutions were selected to provide regional postsecondary educational opportunities for deaf individuals. These colleges were Lee College in Texas, Seattle Community College in Washington, Delgado College in Louisiana, and St. Paul Institute in Minnesota.

Subsequently, programs were established in institutions of higher education throughout the United States and Canada. With the increase in mainstreaming during elementary and secondary years, greater numbers of deaf students began attending institutions not offering special programs for deaf students beyond the support services needed for access. The passage of the Americans with Disabilities Act in 1990 accelerated the growth in demand for educational services within institutions that had previously not enrolled deaf students. Deaf students now choose institutions for a complexity of reasons including academic reputation, excellence in programs of study, and geographic location, as well as opportunities for socialization. However, they no longer have to choose institutions based on support services.

Support Services

During the 1996–1997 or 1997–1998 academic years, 45 percent of two-year and four-year postsecondary educational institutions provided sign language interpreters and 69 percent provided classsroom note takers (National Center for Educational Statistics, 1999), the two most widely used support services by adult deaf students.

The other services that are often provided include preferential seating, tutoring, assistive listening devices, and, increasingly, real-time graphic display. With real-time graphic display, notes can be generated subsequent to class that are considerably more detailed than the average note taker can take. For the older deaf adult with an adventitious hearing loss who does not know sign language, real-time graphic display moderates the communication problems they would otherwise experience (Schmidt & Haydu, 1992).

In addition to these services, ADA guidelines include several other types of auxiliary aids for addressing the communication needs of deaf and hard of hearing individuals. These include transcription services, written materials, telephone handset amplifiers, telephones compatible with hearing aids, closed-caption decoders, open and closed captioning, text telephones, and videotext displays or other types of visual representation of material presented aurally.

Little research has yet been conducted on the benefits and drawbacks of these services, and the relationship to academic success. Several problems inherent in the use of sign language interpreting within an environment in which the discourse is complex and abstract are expressed by Lynn Woolsey in Essay 1.1 and Gary Rollins in Essay 8.1.

■ ■ ■ ■ ■ ▬▬▬▬▬▬▬▬▬▬▬▬▬▬▬▬▬▬▬▬▬▬▬▬▬▬▬▬▬▬▬▬▬▬▬▬▬

ESSAY 8.1

Gary Rollins

I was a welder for fourteen years before becoming an interpreter. During the last nine of those years I worked for a company that periodically hired deaf men to come in and do odd jobs. It was seasonal work for most of us, but it was particularly seasonal for them. Being the last hired, they were always the first laid off when business slowed. The next year the same person wasn't always available, so the company would hire someone else. In the course of time, I worked with three or four different deaf men. At each break or lunch period, whoever was working with us at the time always ended up sitting off in the corner of the shop area alone, since no one could sign with them. In the lunchroom, the rest of use would often comment that someone should learn sign language so they could join us. For a long time nobody did. Eventually I decided I would. I asked the deaf man who was working with us at the time if he would help me. He was pretty shocked at first that someone would bother, but agreed that he would.

I started taking sign language classes at the local community college extension center. My teacher was a very sweet woman, though she could not actually sign very well. Each week she would go through the book, a page or so each class. She'd make a sign, we'd practice it, and then we'd talk. As I recall, the classes were mostly chatting sessions. During the next week, the deaf man and I would sit in a corner of the lunch room at break times, and he would show me how to make the signs correctly. Over time, I learned enough to be able to carry on simple conversations with him.

Eventually, my next door neighbor heard I was studying sign language and informed me that she was an interpreter. Until then, I had no idea there was such a profession. We talked about what it was like to be an interpreter. I found out where she had gotten her training years before. The more we talked, and the more I thought about it, the more fascinated I became. One day, I took a day off from work to check out the interpreter training program my neighbor had attended. As it turned out, I arrived on registration day. The more I talked with people in the program, and the more I thought about it, the more I wanted to enroll. By the end of the day, the program director and her colleagues had excused me from satisfying the long list of prerequisites, and admitted me into the program. It was quite a remarkable day.

I drove home that night, quit my job, and started school the next day. It was probably the most frightening thing I've ever done. Every day, I wondered about the sanity of it. I couldn't have made it without determination and the support of friends. During that year in school, I would sometimes visit the deaf man who had helped me learn to sign. I think the abruptness of my becoming an interpreter surprised him, but he always said he thought I had a natural ability.

The thing that comes to my mind first when I think about being an interpreter is communication. As an interpreter, I feel I'm in a unique position to appreciate people who communicate well, both deaf and hearing. When people have a hard time expressing themselves, it definitely makes the job of interpreting more difficult. There are a lot of decisions an interpreter must make that in anyone's book would often seem presumptuous. An interpreter must listen to a person speak or watch a person sign, decide what they mean, and communicate that to someone else. Even if someone is a clear, concise communicator, taking that message and translating it into a second language is tricky. If the person who initiates the communication isn't very clear in the first place, it can get scary. The interpreter must make decisions about what the speaker really means. Sometimes, if the message is too vague, the interpreter simply must interrupt the process and say things like, "I'm sorry. I don't get that." "What did you say after you said such-and-such?" "What was your point?" "What did you mean?"

I think language itself is a poor tool for communication. It's fraught with difficulties. Unfortunately, it's the only tool we have given that we're not telepathic yet. That anybody understands anyone else is bordering on the miraculous. Adding an interpreter, a third person, inserts even more variables into the process. It's humbling. At the same time, if you get too serious, you lose your flexibility and your ability to chuckle at your mistakes. An old joke comes to mind. How many interpreters does it take to screw in a light bulb? It takes ten. One to screw it in and nine to say they wouldn't have done it that way. There are so many decisions that have to be made during the interpreting process. Two interpreters will almost never interpret something in exactly the same way.

There are all kinds of horror stories about interpreters who try to cover their mistakes because they were too embarrassed to admit they made one. An interpreter can't let that happen. The more serious the event, the more important it is to get it right. I know it's humbling and frightening, yet an interpreter must be able to say, "Oops, I did that wrong." And try again.

Physical space has a lot of impact on the dynamics of interpreting. If the setting is an auditorium, for example, and the interpreters are placed down on the floor, really close to the deaf consumer, you might as well be miles from the speaker. In that situation, the interpreter can easily relate to the deaf consumer, but not to the speaker on the platform. Standing up during the presentation and saying, "I'm sorry, I didn't hear that," isn't an option. Your only option lies with the deaf consumer. The interpreter has to be willing to say something like, "I didn't get that." If the interpreters are placed on the stage, however, the dynamics change in the other direction. In that case, it's easier to interrupt the speaker, although on a platform that's pretty dicey anytime. Interpreters must make those kinds of judgments as they go along. Some speakers don't want interpreters anywhere near them. Either they feel the stage is theirs and don't want

(continued)

anyone else there, or they don't want the distraction of someone waving their arms nearby. People are often uncomfortable with having somebody interpret what they say. Maybe it's intimidating. They don't want to deal with the visual evidence of what they've just said. I can't count how many times people have said, "Oh, you don't have to sign that."

An interpreter must be tactful and have nerve as well. I typically do not ask permission for much when I'm interpreting. I just do what I think needs to be done. Being confident and acting as if you know what you're doing will take you a long way. Of course, actually knowing what you're doing is a big plus. For example, I typically don't ask if I can be on stage. I'll say something like, "I understand you're the speaker. My name is Gary Rollins. I'm going to be your sign language interpreter. I'm going to be standing right over here. I just want you to know who I am. Don't let this distract you." I typically don't say, "Do you mind if I stand over here?" If they say no, I'm stuck.

The more time goes by, the more people become familiar with ADA, the more you find people who have experience working with interpreters. I was interpreting at a workshop recently, and the presenter said, "I've worked with interpreters before and they did such-and-such. What are you going to do?" I said, "That's exactly what I'm going to be doing." This person was particularly fun to work with. It is a joy to work with someone who not only has experience working with interpreters, but a positive experience, and has a great outlook on life. That presenter felt free to be relaxed and to move the interpreters around from one place to another to accommodate the presentation. When presenters are intimidated, they don't know what to do, and that makes everything more uncomfortable. The more experience people have, the greater their comfort level, the easier the job of interpreting becomes.

When I first began as an interpreter ten years ago, it wasn't uncommon to work with people who had never used an interpreter. Now, greater numbers of deaf students are in public schools where they experience interpreters. That experience, coupled with the effects of laws like the ADA, have raised awareness in the Deaf and hearing communities both. People are beginning to have a better understanding of what they should expect from an interpreter. As an interpreter, I walk into a situation and try to ascertain how much experience the individuals have and how much they know. More and more the comfort level of everybody is increasing among both deaf and hearing individuals.

Another issue for interpreters is being privy to sensitive information. Socializing with people in the Deaf community sometimes can be uncomfortable, depending on the participants. Interpreters who work in sensitive areas such as medical, mental health, and legal settings sometimes know things about people that are sensitive and private. In social situations, interpreters may well find themselves in the company of former or current clients. I suspect that interpreters who can't figure out how to handle their knowledge of sensitive, personal, difficult information don't survive very long as interpreters.

The deaf client in turn has to be comfortable with that interpreter. It's not just an issue of confidentiality. It's difficult for some people to know that someone else knows their personal and private things. This doesn't happen often with hearing people because the hearing community is so much larger. Typically when an interpreter is called into a situation, the sensitive information is primarily about a deaf client, as opposed to a hearing client. It's not often that an interpreter gets called in to interpret, for example, in a mental health situation involving a deaf counselor and a hearing client. When interpreters start socializing in the Deaf community, which in any locale is relatively small, one is bound to run into clients. Interpreters have to recognize that some clients may just be uncomfortable having someone in the room who knows that much about them. If this happens, one's social contact can become limited.

Sometimes it seems as if the Deaf community has a love-hate relationship with interpreters. For some things interpreters are really necessary. But no one really wants to have an impartial third party privy to sensitive information. Interpreters sometimes know things about people that no one else really should ever know. Historically, I think this has been a sensitive issue.

Confidentiality is a critical part of this issue of knowing personal information. An interpreter can't just go home and talk about the tough time they had at work that day. Another part of this issue is dealing with the personal information you know. Anyone who has been in the field very long has been in a situation in which you recognize that something just isn't right. There's a strong human element that makes you want to correct it. People who become interpreters tend to be people who like to help, and that's not always healthy. Professional interpreters follow a Code of Ethics that not only requires confidentiality but also requires that we aid in the process of communication but not intervene in it. Interpreters can be enablers as much as they can be helpers. Often there's a tendency to want to contribute. That's why we got into the profession. It's really interesting to think that the thing that draws us to a profession could be the reason you can't do this job. There is a huge red boundary that can't be crossed. An interpreter can't offer to help. It's important for me to remember that there is my "stuff" and their "stuff," and this "stuff" that's going through my head and going through my fingers or coming in my eyes and going out my mouth is theirs and not mine. One has to care but not too much. I work hard to remember this.

I had an interesting experience as an interpreter just this last spring. I was interpreting in a class at the university, and someone asked a question toward the end of the session. Nobody knew the answer. As the class ended, the professor said, "I'll check this out and try to bring you this information next week." I knew that piece of information. After the students left, I casually said, "As it turns out, I happen to know this." I told him the answer. He said, "Very interesting. Thank you very much." The next week, at the beginning of class, he came up to me and said, "Would you mind telling the class what you told me last week?" I felt stuck, but I checked with the other interpreter and with the deaf consumers. They all said, "Fine, go ahead." I was one of a team of two interpreters, so I was sitting off to the side waiting for my turn to interpret when the professor said, "Gary happens to know the answer to the question that was asked last week. He's agreed to answer it for you." I went ahead and briefly shared the information with them. It took maybe two or three minutes and then it was done. I wasn't sure if I had stepped over the line, but at least I had the approval of the participants.

Another issue for interpreters is relationships with deaf clients. I think some people probably raise their eyebrows when interpreters become involved with deaf or hard of hearing individuals, and some people probably don't care. I

(continued)

ESSAY 8.1   CONTINUED

feel the interpreter doesn't really have the same role as a counselor, doctor, or psychiatrist, for example, so the barbed wire rules about relationships don't apply. In reality, any deaf or hard of hearing person with whom you become involved is a potential client. As it turns out, I'm in a relationship with a former client. I don't discuss my work with Lynn, though if she were particularly snoopy, it wouldn't be too difficult to find out where I'm going when I work. She has a lot of respect for the interpreter's role. She doesn't snoop into my calendar and see where I'm going, and doesn't ask me any questions when I get back. It would be easy for some other member of the Deaf community to assume that she knows everything I know, but we work to make sure that doesn't happen.

When I think about giving advice to someone who will be working with deaf individuals, I think more about individuals who will be using interpreters than interpreters themselves. I would like to say to them, "Pay attention to the difference in language." One of my pet peeves is that educators often forget that bridging the language gap imposes restrictions on the communication process. You can't do the same things linguistically, if there's a deaf participant using an interpreter, that you would do if all participants were hearing. There are timing issues. It takes more time when an interpreter is involved because there's a delay between when the speaker says something and the interpreter signs it, and another delay while the deaf participant processes it. It simply takes longer to communicate through an interpreter. Also, be visual; the more visual, the better. Allow time periodically for visual transitions. Recognize that if the deaf participants are looking away at visual aids, they are not watching the interpreter, which means in effect they're no longer "hearing" the presentation. Wait a moment for them to look back, if possible, before beginning again.

One final note to "would be" or new interpreters. Enjoy the privilege of doing this work. Help without enabling. Have fun without being silly. Take your responsibility seriously without being morbid. And most of all, remember to breathe! Do the best you can and don't lose sleep at night over what you can't do. Remember that your clients survived just fine before you arrived on the scene, and they'll undoubtedly do just fine when you're gone.

Reprinted by permission of the author.

Johnson (1991) examined the miscommunication and confusion that can occur in university classrooms between deaf individuals and sign language interpreters. She found the following major problems:

1. High percentage of fingerspelled words because of the likelihood within university courses for instructors to use proper names and highly technical terminology
2. Differences in word order between English and ASL

3. Discrepancies between facial expression used to express English and ASL
4. Time lag between the instructor and the interpreter
5. Divided attention between the interpreter and the visual diagram, written description, exhibit, or example that the instructor is using
6. Unfamiliarity with the subject by the interpreter

She also found that the adult deaf student might not be aware that the information received in class was inaccurate or incomplete. She noted that deaf students need to resolve areas of confusion rather than assume that their difficulties originate in limitations within their own abilities.

Kalivoda, Higbee, and Brenner (1997) noted, "It is imperative that faculty members understand that they bear the responsibility for insuring that students with hearing impairments have equal access to the information presented in their classrooms" (p. 16). However, deaf postsecondary students bear the responsibility to request accommodations. This may be particularly difficult for older deaf students with late-onset hearing loss who may not be as knowlegeable about requesting services that will enable them to receive maximum benefit from classroom instruction (Patterson & Berry, 1987).

Support services alone can certainly not ensure a good educational experience. The quality of postsecondary programs varies as greatly as the quality of elementary and secondary programs. It is important, therefore, to examine the components of quality postsecondary programs.

Components of Quality Postsecondary Education

Deaf individuals often enter postsecondary educational programs, including degree programs and adult basic education programs, with significant gaps in their skills and knowledge (Khan, 1991). Yet deaf students are assuredly able to succeed beyond high school. After two decades of enrolling deaf students at California State University at Northridge, Jones (1986) reported, "(a) qualified deaf students can successfully compete with hearing students in a wide range of vocational and academic classes; (b) deaf students can successfully complete vocational certificates, associate arts, bachelor's, master's, and doctorate degrees; and (c) after graduation, deaf students can be competitively employed in fields for which they have trained" (p. 48).

In postsecondary programs, the following strategies, techniques, and approaches have been found to be particulary effective for deaf students (Bateman, 1987; Cummins, 1992; Foster & Elliot, 1986; Jones, 1986;

Khan, 1991; Lieberth, 1992; Martin & Jonas, 1989; Saur & Stinson, 1986; Stinson, Liu, Saur, & Long, 1995; Tebo, 1984):

- Emphasis on the applied more than the theoretical
- Use of experiential techniques such as discussion, problem solving, dramatization, and hands-on activities; avoidance of lecture format only
- Development of literacy skills through focused instruction and embedded within other courses
- Class size that allows for ample teacher–student and student–student interaction
- Reading materials that are not too difficult to comprehend
- Instruction that promotes higher-order thinking
- Pacing that enables all students to understand the information and participate
- Encouragement of personal control and responsibility
- Clear and complete communication

One of the major roadblocks to success at the postsecondary level for deaf individuals has been their difficulty with English syntax. Berent (1993) found that deaf college students can benefit from explicit grammar instruction in English and that those with the lowest proficiency may actually benefit more than those with higher abilities. He suggested that improving knowledge of English syntax should have a concomitantly positive effect on ability to read college-level material.

Quality of instruction is an obviously important component of quality postsecondary education. Studies of faculty development programs for college and university instructors rated highly by students have found that the following are characteristic of effective postsecondary instruction (Lang & Conner, 1988; Lang, Dowaliby, & Anderson, 1994; Sass-Lehrer, Cohen-Silver, & Bodner-Johnson, 1990):

- *Teacher affect.* Demonstrates flexibility, willingness to help, warmth and friendliness; understands deafness
- *Teaching strategies.* Uses a variety of strategies, reinforcement and feedback, visual aids; involves students in learning activities; provides clear lectures and explanations, real-life applications of information
- *Communication.* Is sensitive to diverse communication preferences; uses clear signs enhanced by facial expression, body language, gesture, and mime
- *Course management.* Has clear expectations; is fair and equitable in treatment of students
- *Knowledge.* Knows subject and discipline well

Whether individuals choose postsecondary education or not, ultimately they seek employment. The importance of satisfying employment can hardly be overstated given the relationship between work, self-esteem, and socioeconomic status.

EMPLOYMENT

Historically, deaf individuals were trained for a narrow range of jobs. At the beginning of the nineteenth century, it was common for deaf men to be working as printers and deaf women as seamstresses. My own grandmother, who was deaf, worked in a factory making Gibson blouses until she married, and subsequently sewed linings for many of the fur coats that my grandfather made. At the outset of the twenty-first century, printing is a highly technical field that depends on the knowledge and skill of individuals trained to use complex computer technology. And much of the work of seamstresses is now done by women, men, and children earning extremely low wages in underdeveloped countries. The employment opportunities for deaf individuals are not limited by deafness but are certainly limited by education in a knowledge-based society.

Schildroth, Rawlings, and Allen (1991) found that employment issues for deaf students revolve around the following factors:

- *Academic development.* The low level of academic achievement, particularly in reading and math, places many deaf individuals at a great disadvantage within competitive job markets.
- *Minority status.* The number of deaf individuals from ethnic and racial minority backgrounds has increased commensurate with the increase within the general population. Deaf minority individuals face a double jeopardy in obtaining positions within managerial, technical, and professional fields.
- *School enrollment patterns.* The number of graduates from schools for the deaf has declined as the number from public schools has increased. Until the last quarter of the twentieth century, schools for the deaf played a major role in preparing deaf students vocationally. With advances in technology and smaller budgets, schools for the deaf can no longer provide comprehensive vocational training. In addition, public schools typically do not have the same strong relationship with state departments of vocational rehabilitation that schools for the deaf maintain, which diminishes opportunities for deaf students during the transition process of school to work. Conversely, public schools can offer opportunities through relationships with other schools, local agencies, and industry such as on-the-job

training, apprenticeship, job sampling, alternative education centers, job coaching, and supported employment.

■ *Vocational versus academic preparation.* The question of whether and when deaf students should be encouraged to pursue vocational or academic preparation is an open one.

Placement in vocational courses reduces the proportion of instructional time available for academic instruction. Thus, as many deaf students arrive at high school with reading levels comparable to those of hearing students in the third grade, the reduced emphasis on academic instruction implies that substantially increasing the literacy levels of deaf youth is not possible. The jobs of the near future in the United States will require higher levels of literacy and mathematics. Therefore, placing students in vocational tracks where reading and mathematics are deemphasized may impose barriers to these students by limiting their opportunities to acquire important academic skills. At the same time, a basic tenet of vocational education is that schools have a responsibility to contribute to a student's preparation for the workplace, often by providing training in specific areas. (p. 43)

■ *Graduation rates.* As noted earlier, graduation rates for deaf students are considerably lower than the national average for hearing students. Gender, ethnicity, and additional disability status are related to graduation. Males, white non-Hispanics, with no additional disability are more likely to receive diplomas than females, individuals with minority background, and those with additional disabilities.

(In Essay 8.2, Tina Harrison describes her frustration with a school system intent on pigeonholing her into a vocational track.)

■ ■ ■ ■ ■ ▬▬▬▬▬▬▬▬▬▬▬▬▬▬▬▬▬▬▬▬▬▬▬▬▬▬▬▬▬

ESSAY 8.2

Tina Harrison

I am a teacher of the deaf. I am hard of hearing. And I've worked hard since the day I was told that I'd be sweeping the streets.

My hearing loss was diagnosed when I entered kindergarten. My teacher was frightened of me. In her twenty-five years of teaching, she had never had a child with a hearing loss in her classroom. I struggled for two years in the school close to my home before my parents realized that a neighboring school district offered a self-contained program for deaf and hard of hearing children.

For the first time, I felt accepted among my peers and teachers. With pride, I wore the hearing aid strapped to my chest. My reading and math scores skyrocketed. Alas, after two successful years in the program my parents relocated. Between the ages of nine and eighteen, I lived in four different states. In most of the places, I was only provided with itinerant and audiological services for hard of hearing children.

From the third grade until middle school, I was served by itinerant teachers. Some were trained to work with deaf students and others were not. They met with me an average of one hour each week. For the remainder of each school day, I was placed in either special education resource rooms or I was mainstreamed into a regular education classroom. My classmates in the resource rooms had a range of disabilities, from severe mental retardation to behavior disorders. There were very few deaf and hard of hearing students. Often, I was the only hard of hearing student in the school. I felt isolated. My self-esteem and my grades plummeted.

Then we moved to a small, rural California town. My parents were poor. While I was in my first year of high school, we lived in a travel trailer. My bedroom consisted of a mattress pushed up against a metal wall. Every morning, I awoke thinking that this would be my future unless I took steps to change my life.

I always wanted to go to college, so I dug out my self-esteem and focused on my grades. I told my special education teacher, who was a trained teacher of the deaf, about my future plans. She said, "Now, Tina, remember that you need to set realistic goals for yourself. You are a special education student. If you get a job sweeping the streets, you should be happy with that." Stuck in the remedial track in high school, I couldn't see how to attain the training that would allow me to do much else besides sweeping the streets. I was spending a good part of my school life in low-level classes, trapped in a succession of rote learning exercises and meaningless worksheets.

Despite my constant protests, begging, and pleading, my case manager refused to let me register for college preparatory courses. She used the excuse that I did not have the background to tackle such advanced classes. I felt trapped in a vicious cycle.

My parents eventually moved to another state with even fewer services for the deaf and hard of hearing. This was my chance to escape the confines of special education. Upon arriving at my new high school, I refused services. Of course, many meetings and a lot of paperwork followed my refusal. Eventually, I was released from my IEP and special services. Even without a case manager determining the classes I would be allowed to take, I still had to prove to the staff at my new high school that I was capable of succeeding in college preparatory courses without having the background knowledge the other students had. I was required to undergo interviews with the teachers and provide samples of my work; none of this was required of other students who wanted to take college prep courses.

It was hard, but I worked hard. It took me twice as long to complete assignments because all I had previously been required to do in school was fill in blanks on worksheets. I had to teach myself all of the basic skills that the other students had acquired years earlier. I had math tutoring every afternoon and carried a dictionary with me to help fill the gaps in my vocabulary.

My goal was to study psychology and education. I wanted to attend the University of Washington because it had an excellent psychology program. My high school counselor warned me that the university would never accept me because I had not taken the appropriate high school coursework. She suggested that I apply to the local state college because the requirements were not as rigor-

(continued)

ESSAY 8.2   CONTINUED

ous as those for the university. I started at Adams State College in Alamosa, Colorado, where I spent three days before packing my bags and heading to Seattle. Once there, I registered at the local community college. I acquired an A.A. degree in two years and then transferred to the University of Washington. I graduated with a 3.45 grade point average and a B.A. degree in psychology and a post-B.A. in elementary education. I went to graduate school at Lewis & Clark College, where I graduated with a 3.9 grade point average and a master's degree in education of the deaf. From there, I went on to teach deaf children in itinerant, resource room, and residential school settings.

As a teacher and case manager, I utilized my personal and academic experiences for the betterment of children in special education. Currently, I am a graduate student pursuing a Ph.D. degree in special education at The Ohio State University. I hope that my doctoral studies will enable me to continue my quest to improve special education for deaf students and initiate positive change in the educational system.

I have gone back to that small town in California a few times. Each time, I have left notes for my former case manager, letting her know that I'm not sweeping the streets. She has never written back.

Never underestimate the potential of a special education student.

Reprinted by permission of the author.

In order to understand fully the impact of these factors on the work lives of deaf individuals, it is crucial to examine their employment status.

Employment Status

Unemployment and underemployment have characterized the status of deaf individuals for as long as statistics have been kept (Kasen, Ouellette, & Cohen, 1990; Passmore, 1982). Unemployment is the major issue for deaf individuals who are routinely referred to as low functioning or traditionally underserved (Danek, Seay, & Collier, 1989; Long, 1992). Underemployment is the major issue for deaf individuals with a postsecondary educational background.

Deaf individuals have been found to spend less time in each job, earn lower wages, work slightly longer hours than hearing individuals, and have less job mobility and advancement (Bullis, Bull, Johnson, & Peters, 1995; Myers & Danek, 1990). Deaf women and men tend to experience similar levels of unemployment in their twenties, but beyond mid-thirties, deaf women tend to be unemployed at higher rates than deaf men in spite of attaining similar levels of education (MacLeod-Gallinger, 1992).

Factors Contributing to Employment Status

Some of the external and personal factors that contribute to employment status are occupational stereotyping, career education, employment discrimination, vocational training, self-awareness of aptitudes and interests, self-expectations, and the work disincentive of Supplemental Security Income (Myers & Danek, 1990).

The role of Supplemental Security Income (SSI) and Supplemental Security Disability Income (SSDI) as work disincentives has received substantial attention from professionals in vocational rehabilitation. El-Khiami (1993) examined the vocational experiences of almost 500 deaf and hard of hearing individuals during the five years following exit from a postsecondary program and obtained results contrary to the myths "that substantial numbers of deaf youths rely exclusively on SSI benefits as a source of income or that they require multiple job placements before their employment status stabilizes. This may have applied in the past, but times have changed and the expansion in education and rehabilitation services for youths with hearing loss has truly paid off" (p. 365). In another study of deaf adults who were three to four years out of high school, Bullis, Davis, Bull, and Johnson (1995) found that individuals receiving SSI/SSDI were less likely to be working or enrolled in postsecondary educational programs but more likely to be living independently than individuals not receiving this support.

The major factor in the successful employment of deaf individuals is postsecondary education, and successful employment has a concomitantly positive effect on socioeconomic status (Brown, 1987; Welsh & Walter, 1988). MacLeod-Gallinger (1992) observed the following about the career status of deaf individuals:

> Having a postsecondary degree plays a large role in the attainments of deaf adults. Yet, it is clear that numerous other factors intervene in their overall labor force and occupational patterns: sex-role stereotyping, inadequate science curriculums and weak academic preparation generally; limited career education and guidance; a narrow range of career options; communication difficulties and the resulting isolation from information; and ultimately, job discrimination based on deafness. The cumulative effects of these factors can result in what amounts to career-arrested development. Relative to the hearing population, deaf adults as a group are less well educated, experience more unemployment, are often underemployed, and have lower incomes. And these effects appear to be compounded for deaf women. (p. 323)

Other factors that serve to enhance or impede the deaf person's ability to succeed on the job include work habits, interpersonal skills, understanding and becoming part of the culture of the workplace, awareness of appropriate behavior, making clear requests for accommodations, and adapting to change (Compton, 1993; Foster, 1991; Johnson, 1993). Walter (1993) noted that adapting to change is the most important of these. "Retraining will be the challenge of education and rehabilitation in the twenty-first century. A collaborative partnership between education, rehabilitation, and industry must be forged in order that deaf and hard of hearing persons can access the rapidly changing technologies that will determine their mobility in the workplace" (p. 420).

Attitudes of hearing employers also play an important role in the job success of deaf individuals. Legislation such as ADA that prohibits discrimination against individuals with disabilities cannot mandate positive attitudes toward the hiring of deaf individuals. Zahn and Kelly (1995) used videotapes of deaf individuals performing tasks within eight occupations as a method for changing the attitudes of prospective employers. They found that attitudes shifted from neutral to positive as hearing individuals developed a broader understanding of the capabilities of deaf workers.

Skills for Successful Employment

When deaf individuals have been asked about their employment experiences, researchers have found the following commonalities (Backenroth, 1995, 1997; Foster, 1987a; Mowry & Anderson, 1993):

- Communication skills in one-to-one situations are crucial for success in the workplace, particularly with supervisors. Although most deaf individuals report that their communication skills are functional for one-to-one situations, they are not adequate for the informal communication networks that exist in most workplaces.
- Career goals tend to be modest among deaf employees, who often do not report aspiring to managerial or supervisory positions. Opportunities for empowerment are more likely in work environments with more than one deaf employee, but these opportunities also brought stress and role conflicts.
- Well-being in the workplace is largely dependent on cooperation, social relationships, positive attitude, openness, and equality.

Bullis and Reiman (1989) found the following 12 skills to be critical for deaf individuals to live and work successfully in the community:

1. Accept criticism from supervisors at work.
2. Obtain training opportunities.
3. Evaluate and identify one's own job interests.

4. Demonstrate appropriate procedures for quitting a job.
5. Develop awareness of legal rights in getting a job and advancing within a job.
6. Evaluate and establish long-term career goals.
7. Become aware of the language and terminology used in the job application and interviewing process.
8. Respond to and ask appropriate questions in a job interview.
9. Display appropriate assertiveness on the job with coworkers.
10. Display appropriate assertiveness in searching for a job.
11. Demonstrate skills in writing resumes and completing job applications.
12. Demonstrate job-related reading skills.

Role of Career Planning and Vocational Rehabilitation

Career awareness and career planning are key variables to success in career paths. Bullis, Davis, Bull, and Johnson (1997) found that deaf adolescents are less likely than hearing adolescents to develop a career plan, and those who do are less likely to follow it after high school. They concluded "that adolescents who are deaf may either not plan to work and, for some reason, end up working after high school, or the reverse. It is not too farfetched to believe that employment secured without planning and preparation may pay less and lead to a less upwardly mobile career than jobs that are secured after careful planning" (p. 262). Schroedel (1991) observed significant differences between deaf high school seniors who had vocational training with those who did not. Seniors with vocational training were more knowledgeable about their vocational aptitudes and the skills needed in their chosen career, more likely to consider several career paths before choosing one, and more motivated to pursue postsecondary education in order to achieve their career goals.

Parents play a particularly crucial role in the career development of their children. Schroedel and Carnahan (1991) found that parents considered themselves most helpful in preparing their deaf adolescents for post-secondary education or the workplace through the following activities:

- Pressing their children to continue their education beyond high school
- Understanding deafness and holding high expectations for individuals who are deaf
- Teaching values and encouraging self-reliance and independence in their children
- Teaching work values and assisting their children in obtaining part-time and summer jobs

- Helping their children to set career goals and understand how to attain these goals
- Seeking assistance from professionals and other parents to meet the needs of their children

Every state in the United States is mandated to provide vocational rehabilitation services designed to change individuals with disabilities from unskilled workers into successful employees who are functioning to their maximum potential. The process involves several steps, the first of which is an evaluation that typically includes medical, psychological, and vocational testing. If eligibility is established because the assessment shows that the individual's hearing loss is a substantial barrier to employment and that vocational rehabilitation services will enable the individual to secure employment consistent with abilities, a rehabilitation plan is developed and carried out. The plan might involve counseling, training, postsecondary education, medical treatment, or provision of devices to assist the deaf individual, such as hearing aids and text telephones.

Vocational rehabilitation counselors work with employers as well as clients to ensure successful employment, though a number of issues can impede the process, including counselors who cannot communicate effectively with deaf individuals, size of the counselor's caseload, financial resources, pressure to close cases successfully, limitations in the knowledge and skill of the counselor, and nature of the partnership between the deaf client and the counselor (Caccamise, Newell, Fennell, & Carr, 1988; McCrone, 1984; Phillippe & Auvenshine, 1985; Warner, 1987; Wax, 1993). The specialized nature of vocational rehabilitation with deaf individuals is evident in the professional journals that are devoted to this endeavor including the *Journal of Rehabilitation of the Deaf* and *JADARA* (formerly the *Journal of the American Deafness and Rehabilitation Association*).

Special Circumstances of Adventitiously Deaf and Older Deaf Adults

Two populations of deaf individuals are particularly vulnerable to changes in employment status—individuals with adult-onset hearing loss and older deaf adults. Glass and Elliott (1993) studied more than 1,000 persons between ages 18 and 65 who were working at the time they became hard of hearing or deaf. The following were unexpected findings because they were counter to prevailing beliefs about the lives of adventitiously deaf adults.

- Few sought vocational rehabilitation services; most were unaware of these services.
- Most continued successfully in their jobs, were promoted, or did not change occupations. Individuals with prior success in their jobs

reported feeling as competent, successful, and appreciated as they felt before their hearing loss.

- Most experienced initial difficulties in coping, but the hearing loss did not irretrievably impair their ability to work successfully.
- Most reported believing that their earning power had been diminished.
- Relatively few shared information about their hearing loss with supervisors or coworkers.
- Relatively few received accommodations at work such as amplified telephones, note takers for meetings, and assistive listening devices.

In Essay 8.3, Wendy Woods describes her life from the day she woke up with a hearing loss.

ESSAY 8.3

Wendy Woods

I woke up one day and was deaf. Some would identify my hearing loss at the time as moderate. To me, personally, it was of a magnitude that was incomprehensible. It seemed to have occurred overnight. I woke up one day with tinnitus. It was the same ringing in the ear that hearing people sometimes experience after a loud concert, only mine has never stopped. I could not mask the ringing with loud music, the television, or conversation. I lasted about four hours before I went to an eye, ear, nose, and throat specialist, without an appointment, which was only acceptable because it was someone with whom I had previously worked. The results were not what I had anticipated. I was twenty-three years old, and I was diagnosed with a permanent hearing loss.

In hindsight, it may have taken months for my hearing loss to occur because most people are not aware of a gradual onset. It was the tinnitus that brought me to the doctor's office and on a road that I would never have imagined. That was eighteen years ago. Today I have a severe to profound loss. If I take my hearing aids out, I cannot hear someone screaming at me. Many changes have taken place during these eighteen years that I would like to share.

At times I feel my experience is different from many because my age of onset is unique. Most people who lose their hearing are either relatively young or elderly adults. I have yet to find a large number of people who lost their hearing as young adults. I have met many culturally Deaf individuals who would not want to "fix" their deafness, and I understand that being Deaf is part of their identity. I, on the other hand, would "fix" my deafness tomorrow because I see myself as a hearing person who lost part of my identity—my hearing. For several years, when my hearing loss was moderate, I felt "stuck" in the middle of worlds between the hearing and the deaf.

I went through a rough time at first. I felt that something was taken away from me, and I grieved that loss as if it were a death. My doctor sent me to a

(continued)

ESSAY 8.3 CONTINUED

specialist who told me I needed hearing aids. I was devastated. I thought those were for old people, and I told the doctor so. His response (because I'm sure he didn't know what to do with an emotional Italian who was losing her hearing) was, "It's like anything else, as we get older things wear out." I screamed, "I'm only twenty-three!" His final reply was, "It's just like people who wear glasses!" I said I had glasses, and they don't bother me! It was not a great entry into a new world.

I know that my family and friends noticed a distinct difference in my personality shortly after my diagnosis. I lost my spontaneity, my confidence, and a natural openness that I had with people. Not until my best friend made an appointment for me to see a psychologist did I launch down the road to accepting my life changes. I stayed in counseling for about a year, but after three months, I rarely talked about my hearing loss. I was just enjoying the counseling! I had decided to move on and be myself once again.

Without any prior knowledge of deafness, I tried to find out as much as possible during the early years after my diagnosis. I read about the types and the prognosis. Needless to say, I was not happy with the information I gathered because I quickly learned that sensorineural hearing losses, such as mine, are permanent and not correctable with surgery. I was working in a factory making medical/surgical tubing at the time of my loss, trying to earn money to pay for college. It became more and more apparent that I could not hear in that work environment. I remember at the time that my Bureau of Vocational Rehabilitation counselor encouraged me to go into the computer field because "deaf people like yourself won't have to talk to people, you can just work on computers." I explained again and again how much I love working with people and reiterated that I could not possibly envision myself working at a computer all day. I now sometimes tease myself by saying that I would love the money I would be making today if I had listened to that counselor. But I'm sure I wouldn't be having as much fun as I am now.

After much debate, I convinced the Bureau of Vocational Rehabilitation that I needed to be around people and I went to college to study sociology. I encountered challenges that I hadn't anticipated. For a sociology degree, I was required to take twelve hours of a foreign language. I knew I would not be able to hear all the sounds expressed in a foreign language so I quickly switched my major to general studies. I still took all the sociology courses and I felt just as satisfied with myself because I was successfully completing a college degree. One day my sociology professor asked me why I wasn't pursuing a sociology degree given that I had all A's in my coursework. I explained my foreign language dilemma. The professor replied, "It seems unfair that because of your hearing loss you would be unable to get a sociology degree." My professor learned that there was a process for waiving the foreign language requirement. I wrote a letter explaining why I couldn't meet the foreign language requirement and supplied medical information verifying my inability to hear speech sounds. I submitted a one-page synopsis that I thought was wonderful and to the point. It was rejected by the first person who read it. That person responded, "What you are doing here is begging, and you need to do two or three more pages of it!" I was devastated. I didn't feel that I should have to beg. Being informative should be sufficient. I didn't rewrite that letter for almost three months, at which point it was two months prior to graduation. The tone was more personal, touched with a little anger. The Foreign Language Waiver Committee Board of unknown, unseen individuals accepted my second letter, and I went on to graduate with a degree in sociology.

While I was earning my degree, I took two classes related to deafness for my own interest. They changed my life. One course was sign language, though it was titled Manual Communication and was not accepted as a foreign language at that time. The other course was titled Nature and Needs of the Hearing Impaired, which explored the etiologies of deafness and the history of deaf education. The professors for both of these classes encouraged me to continue in deaf education studies. Their reasoning was that "we need more positive role models for the deaf." I told them I was interested but had already received an assistantship in sociology to pursue a master's degree. If they wanted to consider giving me an assistantship to obtain a master's in deaf education, I would consider it. I received a full-time assistantship in deaf education at Kent State University in Kent, Ohio.

Since I had no education courses, my course of study consisted of 63 graduate hours of study, in comparison to the usual 32. It took me two years to complete, which was enough time for me to become comfortable with my hearing loss. As a matter of fact, I began to use it to my advantage.

Shortly after graduation I was hired as a teacher in a large deaf education program of an urban school district. I firmly believed that the most important thing I could teach my deaf students was to have high expectations of themselves, higher than many people would have of them. I also felt that it was crucial for me to be a source of strength for parents by letting them know that their children could achieve their dreams. I made a strong commitment to teach my students to learn about and understand their own hearing losses so that they would be able to confidently explain their hearing loss to others.

I began by teaching kindergarten. It was a wonderful experience from the very first day. I loved teaching. I loved watching my students learn, discover, and explore. For the first time, I felt that my hearing loss had meaning. This is where I belonged. Yet in spite of the joy I experienced in teaching young children, I knew that I wouldn't be satisfied unless I also taught adults about the intricacies of deafness. I began teaching part-time at the university where I had earned my degree in deaf education. I started with two classes, the same two that I had originally taken for my own interest—Manual Communication and Nature and Needs of the Hearing Impaired! These classes are now American Sign Language and Introduction to Deaf Studies. I have been teaching at the university part-time ever since, focusing on special education courses at the undergraduate and graduate levels. Through my teaching, I feel that I have the best of both worlds. I teach kindergarten children, who are like sponges. They love to be at school and they want to learn. And I teach university students, which keeps me current on all related issues in special education. While these adult students aren't exactly sponges, they want to be in school to learn as much as possible. One of my greatest strengths with my adult students is sharing my experiences, both personal and professional. I am able to give them insight into the world of deafness, and help them to appreciate our cultural diversity.

(continued)

ESSAY 8.3   CONTINUED

I recently started a new position. I now work as a supplemental service teacher of children with a range of disabilities who are mainstreamed full-time in their neighborhood schools. My role is student advocate and educator/supporter for the regular education teacher. I make sure that all accommodations are being provided to ensure that the special education students have the opportunity to be successful in the regular classroom.

I have continued to lose my hearing over the past eighteen years. I take advantage of the technology that helps make my life more independent. I have sound/alert monitors at home for the phone, doorbell, and my children when they cry. I do not rent movies or watch television without using closed captions. I do not use the phone without a volume control with people I know, and when the voice is unfamiliar, my partner interprets for me. I use an interpreter for staff meetings, workshops, and conferences. At the university, I rely on the students to find ways for communicating effectively with me. I make the argument that if they don't feel comfortable communicating with me here, then I would not want them to be a teacher of our special needs population. Although I believe I'm an excellent lipreader and have great success as long as I know the topic, it is essential that my students also do their part in ensuring successful communication interactions. I need to take responsibility, but they do, too. They are taking these classes to become teachers of exceptional children, so they should feel comfortable, but I also feel it's my job to make them feel comfortable as well. I want them to have the insight necessary to see our special needs population for who they are—people, just like me, capable of achieving success as well as the next person.

My hearing loss changed my life and enabled me to be who I am today.

Reprinted by permission of the author.

Older deaf adults are also vulnerable to changes in the workplace. Whereas the changes for adventitiously deaf adults are internal, the changes for older deaf adults are external as a result of differences in workplace needs and demands. Older deaf adults who had never been trained for technically oriented jobs are finding themselves in weak positions within the current and projected job market. Emerton, Foster, and Royer (1987) noted that older deaf workers need assistance with understanding how technology will affect their job positions both directly and indirectly, and with support in finding methods for coping with changes due to technology. However, professionals assisting older deaf adults must recognize that they are more likely to respond positively to low-risk solutions that enable them to maintain the status quo in their work lives.

Postsecondary education is the strongest predictor of employment status, and employment status is the major factor in the socioeconomic status of deaf adults. Although socioeconomic status can bring material comforts, health is at least as important to the deaf individual's quality of life.

HEALTH CARE

Access to health care has been a serious concern for decades. In 1981, DiPietro, Knight, and Sams observed:

> Specialties have evolved within the health care system to identify and diagnose deafness, offer therapy for remedial conditions of the ear, conduct hearing aid evaluations, develop and implement programs for the prevention of hearing loss, and provide special education and rehabilitation to deaf and hard of hearing people. Such specialties deal principally with only one component of health care delivery to the deaf patient—the ear and its dysfunction. However, the health care system is most frequently called upon to provide care for the deaf patient when that patient's complaint is unrelated to deafness. It is here that the system has the most difficulty adapting. (p. 106)

Communication has posed the greatest barrier to health care access for deaf individuals given the central importance of communication in attaining precise and accurate diagnosis and treatment.

The research has been clear in demonstrating the need for effective communication between health care professionals and deaf patients and the recognition that communication barriers are not broken down simply through the use of interpreters (Ludders, 1987; Wood, 1987). Consider the following situation experienced by a deaf man in his mid-40s.

> Jacques has been admitted to the hospital because he has had a stroke. The left half of his body is paralyzed. He is dazed and disoriented. He is unable to sign and has great difficulty writing because of the paralysis. With his glasses on the table next to his bed, he has limited visual ability to see the interpreter let alone speechread the doctor.

In order to ameliorate communication difficulties, programs have been aimed at sensitizing physicians, medical students, and health care and hospice workers to the unique issues faced by deaf patients. Smith and Hasnip (1991) developed an experiential program that helped medical students recognize the limitations of verbal communication, realize how language can be used as a tool of power and control, understand deafness from the deaf person's perspective, and recognize their own biases about the relationship between verbal ability, intelligence, and competence. Salladay and San Agustin (1984) created the following list of "do's" and "don'ts" for hospice and hospital personnel working with critically ill deaf patients.

Do's

1. Determine the patient's verbal ability, capacity to understand communication skills, to lipread, or to use sign language.

2. Be certain that the patient is looking directly at you when you attempt to communicate by speech, gesture, or other means. Establish eye contact and watch the patient's facial expression for confirmation.

3. A hand gently placed on the person's forearm or shoulder will gain attention but be careful to avoid sensitive areas where patient may be receiving radiation therapy, etc.

4. Speak slowly and distinctly, using simple words and phrases. Do not exaggerate your mouth movements, as this confuses those who read lips. Be sure your mouth is clearly visible at all times while conversing. Keep your hands away from your face.

5. Make a list of common expressions such as "How are you feeling?", "What kind of pain do you have?", "Take a walk?", etc. Use pictures and diagrams to help patients understand any procedure for which informed consent and signatures are required. Use marker type pens to write large on an erasable memo-board. Always keep paper and pen by the bedside.

6. Make sure 24-hour services of a skilled pool of interpreters are available and that these people are introduced to the patient before a "crisis" situation arises.

7. Always supplement your speech. Write important words, even if the patient lipreads well.

8. Stand in a well-lighted area so you can be readily observed. Approach the patient so he or she can see you coming. Approaching from behind may startle the deaf person.

9. Learn a few simple signs. Observing patients will help you pick these up quickly if he or she can speak, too.

10. Keep eyeglasses readily available if a patient needs them. The deaf person is dependent on vision for communication. If the patient wore a hearing aid, she or he should have it on whenever it is feasible to wear it.

11. Alert the staff to the patient's special needs by making some signs and tags reading "patient reads lips" or "please write." Sign must be placed at the end of the bed, above the name on the door of the patient's room, and on the chart cover. Request the patient's help in following these procedures, so it is clear that such techniques are not labels or stereotypes intended to harm.

12. It is advisable to put the patient where she or he can see what is going on. The room opposite the nurses' station is ideal. The patient cannot hear the usual commotion, so all he or she has to do to rest is shut the eyes. But when patients are awake, they are visually involved.

Don'ts

1. Do not expect to communicate via intercom.
2. Do not cover your mouth with your hands. Do not talk with your back to a lighted window because it casts a shadow over your face, which makes it difficult to lipread.
3. Do not turn away in the middle of a sentence. (This is rude even to a hearing patient.)
4. Do not keep the patient in complete darkness. A deaf person relies on sight and is completely isolated in the dark. Use a night light unless a patient specifically requests otherwise.
5. Do not shout. If the patient is hard of hearing but has a hearing aid, shouting will cause the hearing aid to vibrate, a painful sensation.
6. Do not insist that a patient remove a hearing aid at night. Some persons normally wear them at night to avoid the isolation of a silent world. (pp. 267–268)

From Special needs of the deaf dying patient, *Death Education, 8*, 257–269, S. Salladay & T. San Agustin, Taylor & Francis, Philadelphia, PA. Reproduced with permission. All rights reserved.

SUMMARY AND CONCLUDING THOUGHTS

The beginning of this chapter quoted a group of leaders from the mid-1980s who described the limited economic and occupational opportunities available to deaf individuals because of inadequate interpersonal skills, poor work behavior and habits, unawareness of career possibilities, lack of language and reading skills, and circumscribed experiences. Although the opportunities available to deaf individuals presently are considerably greater than they were even twenty years ago, it is obvious that economic and occupational parity with the hearing population, and the concomitant quality of life these bring, has not yet been achieved. Changes to this picture will occur with the young deaf people who are currently in school.

Predictions about the knowledge and skills needed for well-paying, secure, and satisfying jobs in the future ring a cautionary bell to the professionals involved in the lives of deaf children, youth, and adults. As Allen, Rawlings, and Schildroth (1989) commented, these predictions present special challenges.

To the educators, they present the challenge of bringing the reading, mathematics, and reasoning skills of their deaf students to a level sufficient for competing in the job market. To rehabilitation personnel, the data challenge them to provide adequate vocational counseling, job training, placement, and follow-up—even the development of job areas—for their deaf clients. To employers, they present the challenge of keeping their minds and businesses open to the possibility of hiring qualified deaf workers. To deaf students, these data challenge them to achieve their maximum potential and to plan for their postsecondary careers. (p. 234)

CHAPTER NINE

ASSESSMENT

- What kinds of assessment information do the various stakeholders want?
- How has the Stanford Achievement Test been used with deaf students since the first special edition was developed?
- What are the benefits and drawbacks of using an interpreter during testing?
- Why are special norms developed for deaf individuals helpful for some tests but not helpful for others?
- What is the best approach for choosing a test or other assessment technique?

Assessment, diagnosis, measurement, and evaluation are terms that are used to describe the process of gathering information about an individual's abilities or knowledge and using this information to make judgments about instruction, intervention, training, or rehabilitation. The kinds of assessment conducted and the purposes for the assessment depend on the stakeholders who want the information. Some of the stakeholders include the following:

- *Public policymakers, the general public, and the press.* These stakeholders want information related to groups of individuals to determine if publicly supported programs are effective. For example, they are interested in assessment that indicates if the schools are doing a good job, accountable to standards of performance, and meeting state and national goals.

- *Program administrators.* These stakeholders want information that helps them judge the effectiveness of the programs they direct within schools or agencies. For example, school administrators are interested in information about the quality of curriculum, materials, and instruction.

■ *Direct service providers.* These stakeholders want information that enables them to monitor the deaf person's growth in the attainment of individual goals. For example, teachers are interested in monitoring the learning of each student and using assessment information to make instructional decisions.

■ *Parents and family members.* These stakeholders want information that helps them determine whether their deaf family member is making good progress within the current program. For example, parents are interested in comparing their child's progress to other children so they can determine if the educational program is appropriate and meeting their child's needs.

■ *Deaf persons.* These stakeholders want information about their own strengths and needs so that they can decide where to place their energies. For example, deaf students are interested in the match between the expectations of their teachers and their own abilities and interests.

The reason for the array of assessment instruments, techniques, and approaches is the differing needs of the stakeholders. This chapter will discuss the primary types of assessment and the major issues involved in the assessment of deaf individuals.

SOURCES OF INFORMATION

There are six major sources of assessment information—observations, recollections, tests, artifacts, extant information, and professional judgments (Choate, Enright, Miller, Poteet, & Rakes, 1995; Cohen & Spenciner, 1998; Salvia & Ysseldyke, 1998; Taylor, 1997).

1. *Observations.* In informal observations, the observer watches the deaf individual in a natural environment and notes behaviors, characteristics, and interactions. These observations are considered to be anecdotal, subjective, and unreplicable. An example of informal observations is the "kidwatching" that teachers do while deaf students are engaged in a learning activity. In systematic observations, the observer predetermines the behaviors and activities to observe as well as how to record the observations. An example of systematic observations is the Praxis III developed by Educational Testing Service, which is an assessment of first-year teachers. In this test, teacher behaviors are categorized in four domains and nineteen criteria, and assessors are trained to carry out the procedure reliably.

2. *Recollections.* In recollections, deaf individuals or people familiar with the deaf person are asked to provide information from memory. This source of data is gathered from interviews or rating scales. The most common type of rating scales use Likert-like options such as "agree strongly" to "disagree strongly" in response to a statement. An example of interviews is the research conducted with deaf adults asking about their public or residential school experiences that was discussed in Chapter 8. In some of these studies, the researchers used a combination of open-ended interviews and rating scales to obtain as much information as possible about the deaf individual's feelings and beliefs.

3. *Tests.* A test is simply a set of questions or tasks. The questions or tasks are predetermined, and the results are scored in a consistent manner across all test takers based on predetermined criteria and standardized scoring procedures. In one type of standardized scoring procedure, normative standards are used. In these norm-referenced tests, the individual's performance is compared to the performance of a group of individuals considered to be peers. For example, in the Gates-MacGinitie reading test, the deaf child's results are compared to the norms established from a group of 65,000 hearing students who were representative of the U.S. population on a number of variables but not deafness. If it is important to determine how well the deaf child reads in comparison to hearing peers, then the norms are valuable. However, if it is only important how well the deaf child reads in comparison to other deaf children, then the norms established for the Gates-MacGinitie would not be considered valuable for deaf children. In a second type of standardized scoring procedure, absolute standards are used. In these criterion-referenced tests, the individual's performance is compared to a predetermined level of mastery. When the deaf child takes an end-of-chapter test, the teacher is using criterion-referenced testing. Curriculum-based assessment, which involves the assessment of specific curriculum skills within actual course content, is a derivative of criterion-referenced testing. For example, if the deaf child's curriculum in reading includes learning the 220 Dolch basic sight words, then the deaf child would be presented with each of the words and asked to read them. The words that the child could not identify automatically would be targeted for instruction.

4. *Artifacts.* Artifacts are a collection of items that reflect the deaf individual's strengths, weaknesses, growth, and goals. Artifacts are a major component of portfolio assessment, which is a system for gathering student work over time to reflect changes in skills and knowledge. For example, samples of compositions can be gathered periodically during the school year to demonstrate progress in the deaf student's writing ability.

5. *Extant information.* Information that has been previously gathered and is available to be reviewed is typically in the form of school, medical, or personnel records. For example, cumulative school records regularly include IEPs, report cards, results of standardized tests, attendance records, developmental milestones, relevant medical history, audiological information, reports from specialists such as speech–language pathologists and school psychologists, and multidisciplinary team evaluations. Extant information may also be found in the anecdotal records kept by teachers and counselors. For example, teachers often keep a log of student behaviors in order to figure out appropriate interventions.

6. *Professional judgments.* All of the assessment information is interpreted by an individual who exerts professional judgment about its meaning and importance. The assessment information gathered through the first five sources is as valuable as the professional is skilled. As Salvia and Ysseldyke (1998) observed, "Judgments represent both the best and the worst of assessment data. Judgments made by conscientious, capable, and objective individuals can be invaluable aids in the assessment process. Inaccurate, biased, and subjective judgments can be misleading at best and harmful at worst" (p. 37).

Much of the research on the assessment of deaf persons has centered on formal measures used to assess areas such as academic achievement, intelligence, personality, language, reading, school subjects such as mathematics, vocational aptitude and interests, and sensory abilities. Other important areas have received considerably less attention including written expression, problem behavior and emotional status, perceptual–motor skills, adaptive behavior, and instructional ecology (i.e., the relationship between the student and the classroom context).

AREAS OF ASSESSMENT

Achievement

Achievement tests are designed to assess academic accomplishment by comparing the student's knowledge and understanding of specific curricular areas with other students at the same age or grade level. Achievement tests are the most popular tests in educational settings. The stakeholders who have the greatest interest in achievement tests are school administrators who want to know how well the students in their district or school compare to other students. Public policymakers and the public used to be very interested in achievement tests, but in recent years, their interest has shifted to state proficiency tests, which measure how well students at specific grade levels are able to perform in key subject areas such as reading and math.

Most achievement tests are actually batteries of tests measuring skill development in multiple academic areas. The four most widely used group-administered tests are the California Achievement Tests, the Iowa Tests of Basic Skills, the Metropolitan Achievement Tests, and the Stanford Achievement Test Series. Three of the most widely used individually administered tests are the Kaufman Test of Educational Achievement, the Peabody Individual Achievement Test, and the Wide Range Achievement Test. Of these, the Stanford Achievement Test (SAT) is overwhelmingly used with deaf students because normative data for deaf students has been developed. In the 1970s, the Office of Demographic Studies at Gallaudet developed a special edition of the SAT, which was referred to as the SAT-HI or Special Edition of the Stanford Achievement Test for Hearing-Impaired Students. The reasons underlying the development of this special edition for the sixth and seventh editions of the SAT included the following (Allen, White, & Karchmer, 1983):

- Achievement test batteries are typically set up according to traditional school grade levels and tend to be of equivalent difficulty across content areas. Given the wide range of ability levels among deaf students at any given grade level and their uneven development of abilities, with reading and language falling behind areas such as math, the assignment of deaf students on the basis of grade level is troublesome.
- Instructions are difficult to carry out in sign language without altering standardized language and procedures, which are essential to the reliability of the test.
- Items, and even entire subtests, are often biased against individuals with a hearing loss.

Some of the concerns ultimately raised about the SAT-HI included questionable test bias, validity, and reliability (French, 1987; Wolk & Ziezula, 1985). In subsequent editions of the SAT, the special edition was dropped although special norms continued to be developed for deaf students. These norms enable educators and parents to compare the academic achievement of deaf students with deaf peers. The general norms continue to provide information for comparing the academic achievement of deaf students with hearing students at similar grade levels.

Intelligence

Intelligence tests are designed to measure a set of behaviors thought to be part of intelligence. In the complete domain of behaviors that arguably should be assessed, any given test assesses a relatively small sample. The current tests of intelligence measure different samples of behaviors, and although there is overlap, no two tests evaluate identical kinds of behaviors. The stakeholders most interested in intelligence tests are teachers and parents because unlike achievement tests, which assess what has already been learned, intelligence tests are supposed to assess the child's capacity to learn. For example, if a deaf child is assessed as intellectually gifted and is achieving only at grade level, the parents might logically argue that the child is not achieving to capacity and would, therefore, benefit from a change in instructional approaches because an intellectually gifted child, deaf or hearing, should be achieving above grade level.

The most widely used intelligence tests, the Stanford–Binet Intelligence Scale and the Wechsler Scales, are designed to be individually administered by professionals who are formally trained to administer, score, and interpret the tests. The three Wechlser scales are the most popular—Wechsler Adult Intelligence Scale, Wechsler Intelligence Scale for Children, and Wechsler Preschool and Primary Scale of Intelligence.

Tests that can be administered by teachers and other nonpsychologists have also been developed, though these tests are not considered to be as valid or reliable as the Stanford–Binet or Wechsler. Two of these individually administered tests are the Slosson Intelligence Test and the Detroit Tests of Learning Aptitude. The most widely used nonverbal intelligence tests include the Test of Nonverbal Intelligence, the Leiter International Performance Scale, the Raven's Progressive Matrices, and the Peabody Picture Vocabulary Test, which is not precisely an intelligence test because it measures only one sample of behaviors, receptive vocabulary. The Hiskey–Nebraska Test of Learning Aptitude was developed specifically to assess the intelligence of deaf children. Two other commonly used tests, the Woodcock–Johnson Psychoeducational Battery and the Kaufman Assessment Battery for Children, also measure aspects of intelligence, but the tests themselves are diagnostic systems rather than intelligence tests per se.

When Braden (1992) reviewed the published literature on the intellectual assessment of deaf and hard of hearing people, he found support for the following conclusions:

■ Recommended practice is the use of nonverbal tests, or performance subtests. Verbal tests yield substantially lower IQ scores than nonverbal tests and should not be used with deaf and hard of hearing individuals.

■ Tests should be administered by psychologists who are proficient in the language systems used by deaf persons. Psychologists should not rely on oral, written, or gestural directions, or directions interpreted by a sign language interpreter.

> Psychologists who administer tests to deaf and hard of hearing children with an interpreter do so without knowing what, if any, effects the interpreter may have on the deaf or hard of hearing child's test scores. Psychologists who do not have communication skills for serving deaf people should develop arrangements with other psychologists, districts, or regional centers serving deaf and hard of hearing children in order to obtain the services of a psychologist with appropriate skills and experience for assessing deaf and hard of hearing children. (p. 92)

■ The question of using deviation IQs based on normative samples from the deaf population is still open, but the research tends to support arguments against the use of special norms. In other words, comparing deaf individuals exclusively to the performance of other deaf individuals is not considered best practice.

■ The research regarding intelligence of deaf and hard of hearing people has shown a slow rate of growth and is isolated from mainstream psychological research. "The net effects of this journalistic isolation are that psychologists who do not read journals related to deafness and hearing disorders are unlikely to be familiar with the research, and the field of deafness is unlikely to attract high-quality psychological researchers because of the low visibility of research about deafness and hearing disorders" (p. 90).

Controversies, differing viewpoints, and conflicting research will undoubtedly continue to characterize discussions about intelligence testing with deaf persons. For example, Sullivan and Montoya (1997) found no differences in IQ scores resulting from signed administration versus interpreted administration. The tests of intelligence listed above have all been studied by researchers in deafness and found to have strengths and weaknesses (for example, Blennerhassett, Strohmeier, & Hibbitt, 1994; Boyd & Shapiro, 1986; Braden, 1989a; Gibbons, 1989; Maller, 1997; Maller & Ferron, 1997; Phelps & Branyan, 1988). The choice of tests and interpretation of results should be considered in light of the following three considerations offered by Salvia and Yssledyke (1998):

> First, intelligence tests are usually administered for the purpose of making a prediction about future academic performance. In selecting an intelligence test, test givers must always ask, "What is the relationship between the kind(s) of behavior sampled by the test and the kind(s) of behavior I am trying to predict?" The closer the relationship, the better the prediction.

Second, test givers must always consider what behaviors or attributes are being assessed by intelligence-test items. In particular, when different kinds of intelligence tests are used to assess students with disabilities, it is very important to be aware of the stimulus and response demands of the items. When we assess students' intelligence, we want the test results to reflect intelligence, not sensory dysfunction.

Third, it is important to remember that intelligence is not a fixed thing that we measure. Rather, it is an inferred entity, one that is understood best by evaluating the ways in which individuals who have different kinds of acculturation perform several different kinds of tasks. Intelligence tests differ markedly; individuals differ markedly. Evaluations of the intelligence of an individual must be understood as a function of the interaction between the skills and characteristics the individual brings to a test setting and the behaviors sampled by the test. (p. 386)

Personality

Personality tests are designed to evaluate the state of an individual's mental health and provide diagnostic information relevant to mental disorder. The stakeholders most interested in personality tests are deaf individuals because these tests provide assessment information that is used to determine eligibility to receive mental health services as well as the nature of the counseling or therapy the individual will receive. However, personality tests have been particularly problematic when used with deaf individuals for the following reasons (Cates & Lapham, 1991; Freeman, 1989; Heller & Harris, 1987):

- High dependence on verbal skill in English of most tests
- Inappropriate test items that are based on the assumption that the individual can hear
- Unfamiliarity of psychologists and other mental health professionals with deafness and Deaf culture
- Lack of communication skills of psychologists or other diagnosticians
- Inadequate training and experience with the deaf population
- Paucity of theory and research on deaf personality assessment

Personality inventories, a standard part of the battery of tests administered by psychologists, pose a considerable challenge because of the language and reading level required. The Minnesota Multiphasic Personality Inventory (MMPI) is the most widely used personality inventory, and there has been an effort to develop deaf norms (Briccetti, 1994). Brauer found that it was possible to adequately translate the MMPI into ASL, though recognized that assuring linguistic equivalence is not identical to assuring psychological and conceptual equivalence (1992, 1993). Most of the research on the personality assessment of deaf individuals has focused on the Sixteen Personality Factor test, which has been used most successfully with deaf individuals of high academic ability (Bannowsky, 1983; Jacobs, 1987).

Projective tests have been suggested as more appropriate for deaf individuals than self-report tests such as the MMPI because they are less reliant on English language skills. Projective drawing tests are often used because they utilize the visual rather than verbal modality, although little empirical support for these instruments is available. Indeed, the research indicates that these tests have questionable validity and reliability (Briccetti, 1994; Cates, 1991a; Johnson, 1989; Ouellette, 1988; Zwiebel & Wolff, 1988). The most popular of these tests are the Draw–a–Person and House–Tree–Person tests. The other types of projective tests that are frequently used include the Thematic Apperception Test (TAT) and the Rorschach Inkblot test, though it is recommended that they be used only with deaf individuals who have fluent language skills and administered by psychologists who are knowledgeable about deafness (Cates & Lapham, 1991; Schwartz, Mebane, & Malony, 1990).

A number of self-concept tests have been studied with deaf individuals including the Tennessee Self-Concept Scale, Self-Concept Scale for the Hearing Impaired, and the Self-Description Questionnaire. Although each of these tests has proponents, limited evidence for reliability and validity have been found (Gibson-Harman & Austin, 1985; Oblowitz, Green, & de V. Heyns, 1991; van Gurp, 1996).

The Meadow–Kendall Social–Emotional Inventory was designed to be used by teachers or others with lengthy and extensive opportunities to observe the behavior of deaf children (Meadow, 1983; Meadow, Karchmer, Petersen, & Rudner, 1980). It is not intended as a diagnostic test but rather as an aid for identifying children experiencing social or emotional difficulties. The Meadow–Kendall is used widely in educational programs for deaf children.

Language and Literacy

The purpose of assessing the language and literacy abilities of deaf individuals is to provide information that teachers, parents, and deaf individuals themselves can use in promoting language and literacy growth and development. Special needs in the areas of language and literacy constitute the fundamental reason that deaf children are entitled to individualized education programs.

Language

When the language abilities of hearing children are assessed, this area is typically referred to as oral language, to distinguish it from written language. Given the visual–gestural modality of the language of many deaf individuals, it is more appropriate to refer to this area as face-to-face language.

Assessment of face-to-face language involves the four major components of syntax, semantics, pragmatics, and phonology. When the stakeholders are school administrators, the assessment is likely to include predominantly standardized tests of language. Examples include the Test of Early Language Development as a screening instrument; the Word Test to assess vocabulary knowledge; the Clinical Evaluation of Language Fundamentals, Test of Language Development—Primary and Intermediate, and the Test of Adolescent Language to assess syntax and semantics; and the Goldman–Fristoe Test of Articulation and the Wepman Auditory Discrimination Test to assess phonology and phonemic awareness. These tests are typically administered by speech–language specialists.

When the stakeholders are teachers, the assessment is likely to include predominantly informal measures of language. The most common informal measure is language sampling. A language sample is a segment of a deaf child's language performance regarded as representative of his or her linguistic ability. The language sample is obtained from a naturalistic setting, for instance child–child or teacher–child interactions, and analyzed according to protocols such as the Framework of Language Development (Schirmer, 2000).

Standardized language tests offer several advantages including ease of administration and consistency of usage. However, they measure the deaf child's comprehension or use of decontextualized language (that is, outside of the context of conversation or other natural communication milieu), and most of the tests have limited or poor validity. Informal assessment techniques offer the advantage of providing information about the deaf child's understanding and use of language within natural communicative settings and, therefore, have the best potential for providing a link between assessment and instruction. However, the accuracy and completeness of information gathered about the child's language abilities depend heavily on the skill of the teacher. A limitation of both approaches is the lack of currently available instruments for assessing the acquisition of ASL.

Literacy

Assessment of reading involves the four major areas of comprehension, word recognition skills, fluency, and vocabulary. Emergent readers are assessed on their knowledge of literacy concepts, conventions of written language, recognition of letters and simple words, and phonemic awareness. Assessment of writing involves areas such as writing traits (examples include ideas, organization, word choice, sentence structure, and mechanics), writing process (the child's engagement in planning, composing, and revising), and kinds of writing (the child's ability to utilize a variety of forms, such as essays, stories, and reports).

There is a fair amount of discussion by professionals regarding the usefulness of standardized tests to measure literacy ability and growth. The information provided by achievement tests about reading is extremely limited and the accuracy is highly questionable. Diagnostic reading tests offer somewhat more complete and accurate information, but in most of these tests, there is a heavy focus on isolated reading skills such as phonic analysis and structural analysis of words, comprehension is measured with relatively short passages unrelated to one another, and knowledge of vocabulary is often assessed with words that are out of context. Several of the most widely used diagnostic reading tests are the Gates–MacGinitie Reading Tests, Gray Oral Reading Test, and the Woodcock Diagnostic Reading Battery. Teachers also frequently use informal reading inventories such as the Analytical Reading Inventory and the Standardized Reading Inventory. Standardized instruments to assess writing are relatively recent, and one that is considered to have good reliability is the Test of Written Language. Many teachers use analytical writing scoring techniques as informal measures of writing. Two examples are the Writing Assessment Rubric (Schirmer, Bailey, & Fitzgerald, 1999) and the Six-Trait Analytical Scale (Spandel & Stiggins, 1997).

Given the importance of reading proficiency and the general low reading achievement among deaf students, some educators have recommended the development of deaf norms for current tests and the creation of new tests of reading exclusively designed for deaf children and youth. Conversely, many educators have argued that deaf norms and special tests are misleading and potentially damaging because they lead stakeholders to believe that deaf individuals are incapable of becoming literate in the written language of the broader society in which they live. Figure 9.1 illustrates the assumptions about the literacy capabilities of deaf individuals on which testing is based.

Vocational Aptitude and Interest

The purpose of vocational assessment is to identify aptitudes and interests. Once aptitudes and interests are identified, training and education can be determined, with the ultimate goal of employment that enables the deaf person to meet his or her potential. The stakeholders most interested in vocational assessment are direct service providers such as teachers and vocational rehabilitation counselors, parents of deaf youth, and deaf individuals, although certainly public policymakers have been the force behind legislation related to vocational education, rehabilitation,

FIGURE 9.1   Assumptions about Literacy within Kinds of Tests

	KIND OF TEST	
ASSUMPTIONS ABOUT LITERACY CAPABILITY OF DEAF INDIVIDUALS	*General Test/ Hearing Norms*	*Special Test/ Deaf Norms*
The reading process		
is different for deaf readers.		x
is similar/no different for deaf and hearing readers.	x	
Deaf readers can be expected to read		
no higher than the fourth/fifth grade level.		x
as well as hearing readers.	x	
Reading materials for deaf children and youth		
should be contrived to adjust for English sentence structure difficulty.		x
should be identical to reading materials for hearing children and youth.	x	
Reading skills involved in proficient reading are		
dependent on degree of hearing.		x
not dependent on degree of hearing.	x	

and special education that has driven recent interest in vocational assessment. (The reader is encouraged to review examples of selected U.S. federal legislation in the Appendix.)

Work sample evaluation has been the most prevalent approach for assessing vocational skills. According to Elrod, Tesolowski, and Devlin (1998), virtually thousands of noncommercial work samples have been developed and dozens of commercial ones. Work samples are essentially simulations of a work activity designed to represent as closely as possible actual tasks, materials, technology, and tools of a given job or cluster of jobs. Recent high-technology work simulators are able to assess "vocational interests and values, career awareness, physical skills, functional academic skills, aptitudes and worker traits, specific vocational skills, work behaviors and attitudes, learning style, related functional living skills, career decision-making skills, job-seeking skills, and personal understanding of oneself and the world of work" (p. 426).

Two instruments have been developed specifically with the deaf population in mind. The National Independent Living Skills Screening

Instrument (NILS), which is designed to measure an individual's ability to engage in employment and function independently in their family and community, has been found to be a viable assessment tool with deaf individuals 16 years of age or older as well as with deaf adolescents and adults who have concomitant disabilities (Dunlap, 1987; Sands, 1992).

The Transition Competence Battery for Deaf Adolescents and Young Adults (TCB) assesses vocational and independent living skills. It is administered in sign language, and therefore is considered language-appropriate for deaf individuals, and assesses the particular skills necessary for deaf individuals to work and live successfully in the community, and therefore is viewed as content-relevant for deaf individuals. These two qualities, language appropriateness and content relevance, make this test unique among vocational assessment instruments. The TCB is available as a full battery and mini-screening test on videodisk, and CD-ROM is being developed (Bullis & Reiman, 1992; Bullis, Reiman, Davis & Reid, 1997; Bullis, Reiman, Davis, & Thorkildsen, 1994).

SUMMARY AND CONCLUDING THOUGHTS

This chapter discussed the purposes of assessment, the stakeholders for assessment results, and the kinds of assessment conducted with deaf children, youth, and adults. It also discussed the issues involved in assessing deaf persons, particularly the limitations of standardized tests.

Assessment at the outset of the twenty-first century is a huge industry. The beliefs about the truth value and scientific accuracy embodied by published tests that greeted educators, parents, and legislators at the beginning of the twentieth century are held just as strongly 100 years later. Certainly, we have no other explanation for the preponderance of what is referred to as "high stakes assessment" in which one standardized test can be the deciding factor for promotion from one grade to another, graduation with a degree from high school, certification or licensure for teachers, and accreditation of schools. The stakes are definitely high and based on boundless belief in the capacity of any given test to assess the depth and breadth of relevant knowledge and skill.

Assessment of deaf individuals is fraught with all of the problems associated with testing in general, along with the confounding factors of English proficiency, communication compatibilities between the deaf person and the individual administering the test, and culturally relevant experiential differences between the deaf person and the population on which the test was normed (Gordon, Stump, & Glaser, 1996). Accommodations, such as modifications of tests and adaptations to the delivery of instructions, may only serve to invalidate results. The development of tests or norms specifically for deaf individuals may only serve to isolate deaf individuals from the opportunities within the broader educational and economic community because of the assumptions about capability on which they are based.

I would like to end this chapter, and this book, with a vignette about my own family because it illustrates the potential power of assessment. One evening my parents went to a parent–teacher conference at Post Road Junior High School in White Plains, New York, to meet with my brother's teachers and counselor. When they came home, my mother said that his counselor had told them that Stephen's test scores weren't very good, and his grades weren't very good either. The counselor suggested that Stephen pursue a vocational career. My mother, the daughter of a deaf woman, knew a lot about expectations. She related to my brother and me that she said to the counselor, "I'm sure he is at least capable of becoming a teacher!" And with that statement, she and my dad walked out. My parents had not attended college, but they knew that their children would. My mother didn't feel particularly negative about teaching, she just felt that her son was at least as smart as the counselor, who clearly had earned a degree in education. Today, my brother is a professor of laboratory medicine and internal medicine and director of the clinical microbiology laboratory at Yale University. The counselor at Post Road Junior High School had a lot of power to effect change in my brother's life. But on that one night, he did not, because one parent said to herself, "These results don't make sense."

I hope that each professional and future professional reading this book will remember that he or she has the power to effect positive change in the lives of the deaf individuals they touch. Assessment is the starting place.

RESOURCES

ORGANIZATIONS, CENTERS, AND RESOURCES

ADARA: Professionals Networking for Excellence in Service Delivery with Individuals Who Are Deaf or Hard of Hearing, formerly known as the *American Deafness and Rehabilitation Association,* promotes quality human service delivery to deaf and hard of hearing persons through agencies and individuals. Founded in 1966, ADARA publishes a professional journal (*JADARA*), a newsletter, monographs, and special publications. [P.O. Box 727, Lusby, MD 20657 / www.adara.org]

Alexander Graham Bell Association for the Deaf promotes communication of deaf and hard of hearing persons through maximizing hearing/listening potential, speechreading, speech and language skills. Established in 1890, the organization publishes journals (*The Volta Review* and *Volta Voices*), books, and other materials. [3417 NW Volta Place, Washington, DC 20007-2778 / www.agbell.org]

American Academy of Audiology provides professional development, supports research, and promotes increased public awareness of hearing disorders and audiologic services. The organization publishes a newsletter, a magazine, and the *Journal of the American Academy of Audiology.* [8300 Greensboro Drive, Suite 750, McLean, VA 22102 / www.audiology.org]

American Society for Deaf Children advocates for deaf or hard of hearing children's total quality participation in education, the family, and the community. Founded in 1967 as an organization for parents and families, it publishes a newsletter, holds an annual conference, has a speaker's bureau, and sponsors a parent-to-parent network. [P.O. Box 3355, Gettysburg, PA 17325 / www.deafchildren.org]

American Speech-Language-Hearing Association (ASHA) is the professional and scientific association for speech–language pathologists, audiologists, and speech, language, and hearing scientists. ASHA publishes materials, monographs, and several journals including the *American Journal of Audiology, American Journal of Speech-Language Pathology, Journal of Speech, Language, and Hearing Research,* and *Language, Speech, and Hearing Services in Schools.* [10801 Rockville Pike, Rockville, MD 20852 / www.asha.org]

American Tinnitus Association promotes the relief, prevention, and the eventual cure of tinnitus. Founded in 1971, the association provides the latest information about research and medical advances, school and workplace hearing protection programs, seed grants for tinnitus researchers, access to support groups, and publications, including the journal *Tinnitus Today.* [P.O. Box 5, Portland, OR 97207-0005 / www.ata.org]

Association of Late-Deafened Adults serves the needs of individuals who have become deaf, rather than born deaf; it provides resources, information, advocacy, and awareness. [1145 Westgate Street, Suite 206, Oak Park, IL 60301 / www.alda.org]

Better Hearing Institute provides information about hearing loss and available help through medicine, surgery, amplification, and other rehabilitation. Established in 1973, it donates public service announcements and distributes free educational booklets, hearing help films, technical information, and news and human-interest features. [5021-B Backlick Road, Annandale, VA 22003 / www.betterhearing.org]

The Caption Center serves as a resource to caption consumers and captions nearly 100 hours per week of programming from all segments of the television industry. As the world's first captioning agency and a nonprofit service of the WGBH Educational Foundation, the Caption Center played an instrumental role in the creation and passage of the Television Decoder Circuitry Act of 1990, which requires built-in caption decoder circuitry in most new televisions. [125 Western Avenue, Boston, MA 02134 / www.wgbh.org]

Captioned Media Program provides free-loan, open-captioned media to deaf and hard of hearing individuals, teachers, parents, and others. Formerly the Captioned Films/ Videos Program, it is funded by the U.S. Department of Education and administered by the National Association of the Deaf. The program makes over 4,000 educational and general-interest titles available, and approximately 300 titles are added each year. [1447 East Main Street, Spartanburg, SC 29307 / www.cfv.org]

Center for Assessment and Demographic Studies investigates the deaf and hard of hearing population in the United States and adapts tests so that they are more valid when administered to deaf and hard of hearing students. [Gallaudet Research Institute, Gallaudet University, 800 Florida Avenue, NE, Washington, DC 20002 / www.gallaudet.edu/~teallen/maincads.html]

Children of Deaf Adults was founded in 1983 for the adult hearing sons and daughters of deaf parents. Yearly activities include an international conference, Mother Father Deaf Day, and local retreats. [www.coda-international.org]

Conference of Educational Administrators of Schools and Programs for the Deaf (CEASD) provides leadership for the improvement and advancement of a continuum of educational opportunities that promote the general welfare of the deaf and encourages the efficient management and operations of schools, programs, program service centers, and governmental units providing for the needs of the deaf. [P.O. Box 1778, St. Augustine, FL 32085-1778 / www.educ.kent.edu/deafed]

Convention of American Instructors of the Deaf is a resource for classroom teachers, a clearinghouse for information on deafness, and a forum for educational developments and research findings in the field. Founded in 1850, it publishes the *American Annals of the Deaf*, which is considered the oldest educational journal in the United States. [P.O. Box 377, Bedford, TX 76095-0377 / www.caid.org]

Council for Exceptional Children is dedicated to improving the educational outcomes for individuals with exceptionalities. It advocates for appropriate governmental policies, sets professional standards, provides continual professional development, advocates for newly and historically underserved individuals with exceptionalities, and helps professionals obtain conditions and resources necessary for effective professional practice. Founded in 1922 as the International Council for the Education of Exceptional Children, CEC publishes books, materials, a newsletter, and the journals *Exceptional Children* and *Teaching Exceptional Children*. [1920 Association Drive, Reston, VA 20191 / www.cec.sped.org]

Council on Education of the Deaf sets standards for the certification of teachers of the deaf and accreditation of college and university programs preparing teachers of the deaf. [www.educ.kent.edu/deafed]

Deaf World Web is a deaf-related Web site that provides comprehensive resources around the world. [www.deafworldweb.org]

Dogs for the Deaf rescues and professionally trains dogs to assist people who are deaf or hard of hearing. [10175 Wheeler Road, Central Point, OR 97502 / www.dogsforthedeaf. org]

The EAR Foundation provides the general public with support services promoting the integration of the hearing and balance impaired into mainstream society; provides practicing ear specialists with continuing medical education courses and related programs specifically regarding rehabilitation and hearing preservation; educates young people and adults about hearing preservation and early detection of hearing loss, enabling them to prevent early age hearing and balance disorders. Founded in 1971, it offers online support groups, free information and referral, and continuing medical education. [1817 Patterson Street, Nashville, TN 37203-2110 / www.theearfound.org]

HandsOn is dedicated to providing greater accessibility to arts and cultural events for the Deaf and hard of hearing community. Founded in 1982, its mission is to bring the performing and fine arts to deaf people of all ages. [57 East 11th Street, 9th Floor, New York, NY 10003-4605 / www.handson.org]

House Ear Institute is dedicated to developing knowledge about hearing and related disorders and to sharing that knowledge so that the lives of individuals with hearing loss may be improved. [2100 West 3rd Street, Los Angeles, CA 90057 / www.hei.org]

John Tracy Clinic provides, worldwide and without charge, parent-centered services to young children with a hearing loss and services to aid the professional community in understanding how to work with deaf children. [806 West Adams Boulevard, Los Angeles, CA 90007 / www.johntracyclinic.org]

Laurent Clerc National Deaf Education Center, Info to Go, formerly the National Information Center on Deafness, provides information on topics dealing with deafness, hearing loss, and services and programs related to the age group of birth to 21. [Gallaudet University, 800 Florida Avenue, NE, Washington, DC 20002 / www.gallaudet. edu:80/~nicd]

League for the Hard of Hearing is a rehabilitation agency for infants, children, and adults who are hard of hearing and deaf. The League provides hearing rehabilitation and human service programs for people who are hard of hearing and deaf and their families, regardless of age or mode of communication. Founded in 1910, the League also promotes hearing conservation and provides public education about hearing. [71 West 23rd Street, New York, NY 10010-4162 / www.lhh.org]

National Association of the Deaf represents deaf and hard of hearing Americans in areas including education, employment, health care and social services, and telecommunications. Programs and activities include grassroots advocacy and empowerment, captioned media, certification of sign language interpreters, deafness-related information and publications, legal assistance, policy development and research, public aware-ness, and youth leadership development. [814 Thayer Avenue, Silver Spring, MD 20910-4500 / www.nad.org]

National Captioning Institute is committed to increasing the quality and quantity of closed-captioned television programming for deaf and hard of hearing individuals. [1900 Gallows Road, Suite 3000, Vienna, VA 22182 / www.ncicap.org]

The National Information Center for Children and Youth with Disabilities (NICHCY) pro-vides information on disabilities and disability-related issues for families, educators, and other professionals, with a special focus on children and youth between birth and age 22. [P.O. Box 1492, Washington, DC 20013 / www.nichcy.org]

National Institute on Deafness and Other Communication Disorders conducts and supports basic and clinical research and research training in the normal and disordered pro-cesses of hearing, balance, smell, taste, voice, speech, and language. [National Institutes of Health, 31 Center Drive, MSC 2320, Bethesda, MD 20892-2320 / www.nih.gov/ nidcd]

The National Rehabilitation Information Center collects and disseminates the results of federally funded research projects. Founded in 1979, NARIC's literature collection also includes commercially published books, journal articles, and audiovisuals. [1010 Wayne Avenue, Suite 800, Silver Spring, MD 20910 / www.naric.com]

National Theatre of the Deaf is a professional acting company made up of deaf and hearing actors. Established in 1967, the theatre's signature style is a combination of sign language and spoken words. It was the first theatre company to perform in all fifty states, has toured every continent including Antarctica, and won a Tony Award for theatrical excellence in 1977. [5 West Main Street, P.O. Box 659, Chester, CT 06412 / www.ntd.org]

Office of Special Education and Rehabilitative Services supports programs that assist in educating children with special needs, provides for the rehabilitation of youth and adults with disabilities, and supports research to improve the lives of individuals with disabilities. OSERS consists of three program-related components—the Office of Special Education Programs, Rehabilitation Administration, and National Institute on Disability and Rehabilitation Research. [U.S. Department of Education, 400 Mary-land Avenue, SW, Washington, DC 20202-0498 / www.ed.gov/offices/OSERS]

Rainbow Alliance of the Deaf is a society of Deaf gays and lesbians. Established in 1977, the organization fosters fellowship and promotes educational, economic, and social welfare. [www.rad.org]

Registry of Interpreters for the Deaf provides forums and an organizational structure for the continued growth and development of the professions of interpretation and transliteration of American Sign Language and English. Founded in 1964, RID trains and certifies interpreters and transliterators. [8630 Fenton Street, Suite 324, Silver Spring, MD 20910 / www.rid.org]

Self-Help for Hard of Hearing People (SHHH) promotes the improved quality of hard of hearing people's lives through education, advocacy, and self-help. [7910 Woodmont Avenue, Suite 1200, Bethesda, MD 20814 / www.shhh.org]

Telecommunications for the Deaf is a national advocacy organization promoting equal access issues in telecommunications and media for people who are deaf, hard of hear-ing, late deafened, and deaf blind. TDI was established in 1968 to promote the distribution of TTYs in the Deaf community and to publish an annual national directory of TTY numbers. [8630 Fenton Street, Suite 604, Silver Spring, MD 20910-3803 / www.tdi-online.org]

USA Deaf Sports Federation provides deaf and hard of hearing children and adults with the opportunity to compete with their peers as well as the larger society of athletes worldwide. Established in 1945 as the American Athletic Union of the Deaf, the organization provides year-round training and competition for developing and elite athletes and assists them in developing physical fitness, sportsmanship, and self-esteem. [3607 Washington Boulevard #4, Ogden, UT 84403-1737 / www.usadsf.org]

BOOKS

Alandra's Lilacs by Tressa Bowers, published in 1999 by Gallaudet University Press. This book is the story of a mother and her deaf daughter from the moment, in 1968, when Tressa Bowers learned that her baby daughter was deaf, to the present time, in which Alandra is married to a deaf man and the mother of three deaf children.

The Cry of the Gull by Emmanuelle Laborit, published in 1998 by Gallaudet University Press. This book is the memoir of a 20-year-old deaf woman who had recently won the Molière Award for best new acting talent. Emmanuelle Laborit chose the title for her autobiography from the the the nickname she was given as a child, "Mouette," because in French, *mouette* means *seagull* and Emmanuelle's efforts to talk sounded to her parents like the piercing cries of a seagull.

The Deaf Mute Howls by Albert Ballin, published in 1998 by Gallaudet University Press. Originally published in 1931, this book is an autobiography of the author in which he details his experiences and those of other deaf individuals at a late nineteenth-century residential school for the deaf.

Everyone Here Spoke Sign Language: Hereditary Deafness on Martha's Vineyard by Nora Ellen Groce, published in 1985 by Harvard University Press. This book is a historical look at the towns of West Tisbury and Chilmark on Martha's Vineyard, which experienced a high incidence of hereditary deafness for more than two centuries. From the memories of older residents and archival material, the author describes the extraordinary integration of deaf individuals into the daily life of the island when sign language was used by virtually all deaf and hearing residents.

Forbidden Signs: American Culture and the Campaign against Sign Language by Douglas C. Baynton, published in 1996 by The University of Chicago Press. In this book, the author examines the history of sign language from the midnineteenth century to 1920, a period of time in which sign language went from great popularity to disrepute among hearing American educators.

Listening with My Heart by Heather Whitestone, published in 1997 by Doubleday. In this autobiography, Heather Whitestone, who became deaf at the age of 18 months, describes her journey to Atlantic City in 1995, where she was crowned Miss America.

Movers and Shakers: Deaf People Who Changed the World by Cathryn Carroll and Susan M. Mather, published in 1997 by Dawn Sign Press. This book is a collection of biographies of deaf, hard of hearing, and deaf–blind individuals, some who are famous and some who are not.

Shall I Say a Kiss? The Courtship Letters of a Deaf Couple, 1936–1938 by Lennard J. Davis, published in 1999 by Gallaudet University Press. This book is the correspondence between Morris Davis, a deaf man living in Brooklyn, and Eva Weintrobe, a deaf woman living in Liverpool, during the two years before Eva traveled to the United States to marry Morris in 1938.

Silence of the Spheres: The Deaf Experience in the History of Science by Harry G. Lang, published in 1994 by Bergin and Garvey Press. This book is a history of science from the perspective of the lives and work of deaf scientists.

Sounds like Home: Growing Up Black and Deaf in the South by Mary Herring Wright, published in 1999 by Gallaudet University Press. In this book, the author, an African American woman, describes her transition from being a hearing 8-year-old to a deaf 10-year-old child in North Carolina during the Depression and the outset of World War II.

Train Go Sorry: Inside a Deaf World by Leah Hager Cohen, published in 1994 by Houghton Mifflin. The author chose the title, which is equivalent to the English expression "missed the boat," as a metaphor for the missed connections between the Deaf and hearing worlds. In this book, Leah Hager Cohen presents issues facing Deaf culture from the personal perspective of students, teachers, administrators, and her own family members at the Lexington School for the Deaf.

Wired for Sound: A Journey into Hearing by Beverly Biderman, published in 1998 by Trifolium Books. In this book, the author describes how she became deaf, the impact on her family as she was growing up, how she decided to get a cochlear implant, the testing and surgery involved, and her experiences post-implant.

SELECTED U.S. FEDERAL EDUCATION LEGISLATION

1867   *Department of Education Act* authorized the establishment of the U.S. Department of Education.

1917   *Smith-Hughes Act* provided for grants to states for support of vocational rehabilitation.

1918   *Vocational Rehabilitation Act* provided for grants for rehabilitation through training of World War I veterans.

1943   *Vocational Rehabilitation Act* (Public Law 78-16) provided assistance to disabled veterans.

1958   *Captioned Films for the Deaf Act* (Public Law 85-905) authorized a loan service of captioned films for the deaf.

Education of Mentally Retarded Children Act (Public Law 85-926) authorized federal assistance for training teachers of the handicapped.

1963   *Vocational Education Act of 1963* (Part of Public Law 88-210) increased federal support of vocational education schools; vocational work-study programs; and research, training, and demonstrations in vocational education.

1965   *National Technical Institute for the Deaf Act* (Public Law 89-36) provided for the establishment, construction, equipping, and operation of a residential school for postsecondary education and technical training of the deaf.

1966   *Model Secondary School for the Deaf Act* (Public Law 89-694) authorized the establishment and operation, by Gallaudet College, of a model secondary school for the deaf.

1968   *Handicapped Children's Early Education Assistance Act* (Public Law 90-538) authorized preschool and early education programs for handicapped children.

   Vocational Education Amendments of 1968 (Public Law 90-576) modified existing programs and provided for a National Advisory Council on Vocational Education and collection and dissemination of information for programs administered by the Commission of Education.

1970   *Kendall Demonstration Elementary School Act* (Public Law 91-587) transformed the historic Kendall School, which was founded as a school for deaf and blind children in 1857, into a demonstration elementary school, expanding its role to include research and dissemination.

1973   *Rehabilitation Act, Section 504*, as amended in 1974 (Public Law 93-112), provided that no qualified handicapped individual could, by reason of handicap, be excluded from the participation in any program of activity receiving federal financial assistance.

1975   *Education for All Handicapped Children Act* (Public Law 94-142) provided that all handicapped children have available to them a free appropriate education designed to meet their unique needs.

1983   *Education of the Handicapped Act Amendments of 1983* (Public Law 98-199) added the Architectural Barrier amendment and clarified participation of handicapped children in private schools.

1984   *Carl D. Perkins Vocational Education Act* (Public Law 98-524) continued federal assistance for vocational education through fiscal year 1989. The act replaced the Vocational Education Act of 1983. It provided aid to the states to make vocational education programs accessible to all persons, including handicapped and disadvantaged, single parents and homemakers, and the incarcerated.

1985   *Handicapped Children's Protection Act* (Public Law 99-372) allowed parents of handicapped children to collect attorneys' fees in cases brought under the Education of the Handicapped Act and provided that the Education of the Handicapped Act does not preempt other laws, such as Section 504 of the Rehabilitation Act.

1986   *Amendments to the Education for All Handicapped Children Act* (Public Law 99-457) extended all rights and protections of P.L. 94-142 to preschoolers with disabilities.

1988   *Technology-Related Assistance for Individuals with Disabilities Act of 1988* (Public Law 100-407) provided financial assistance to states to develop and implement consumer-responsive statewide programs of technology-related assistance for persons of all ages with disabilities.

1989   *Children with Disabilities Temporary Care Reauthorization Act of 1989* (Public Law 101-127) revised and extended the programs established in the Temporary Child Care for Handicapped Children and Crises Nurseries Act of 1986.

1990   *Americans with Disabilities Act of 1990* (Public Law 101-336) prohibited discrimination against persons with disabilities.

Individuals with Disabilities Education Act (Public Law 101-476) reauthorized Public Law 94-142 and renamed it to reflect contemporary practice by replacing references to "handicapped children" with "children with disabilities." The law added two new disability categories, autism and traumatic brain injury, and a comprehensive definition of transition services.

1991   *Civil Rights Act of 1991* (Public Law 102-166) amended the Civil Rights Act of 1964, the Age Discrimination in Employment Act of 1967, and the Americans with Disabilities Act of 1990, with regard to employment discrimination. Established the Technical Assistance Training Institute.

1994   *Goals 2000: Educate America Act* (Public Law 103-227) established a new federal partnership through a system of grants to states and local communities to reform the nation's education system. The Act formalized the national education goals and established the National Education Goals Panel. It also created a National Education Standards and Improvement Council to provide voluntary national certification of state and local education standards and assessments and established the National Skill Standards Board to develop voluntary national skill standards.

School-to-Work Opportunities Act of 1994 (Public Law 103-239) established a national framework within which states and communities can develop School-to-Work Opportunities systems to prepare young people for first jobs and continuing education. The Act also provided money to states and communities to develop a system of programs that include work-based learning, school-based learning, and connecting activities components. School-to-work programs will provide students with a high school diploma or its equivalent, a nationally recognized skill certificate, or an associate degree, if appropriate, and may lead to a first job or further education.

1997   *Individuals with Disabilities Education Act Amendments of 1997* (Public Law 105-17) amended the Individuals with Disabilities Education Act (IDEA) to revise its provisions and extend through fiscal year 2002 the authorization of appropriations for IDEA programs. New provisions included regular teacher involvement on IEP teams, inclusion of children with disabilities in general state and districtwide assessments, greater emphasis on involvement of students with disabilities in the general curriculum, and assessment of children's troubling behavior and development of positive behavioral interventions. Attention Deficit Disorder and Attention Deficit Hyperactivity Disorder were added as a separate disability category.

1998   *Amendments to the Higher Education Act of 1965* (Public Law 105-244) amended the Education of the Deaf Act of 1986 (which continued Gallaudet College as Gallaudet University) to authorize a national study on the education of the deaf for the purpose of identifying education-related barriers to successful postsecondary education experiences and employment for individuals who are deaf.

REFERENCES

Acredolo, L., & Goodwyn, S. (1988). Symbolic gesturing in normal infants. *Child Development, 59,* 450–466.

Adams, J. W., & Tidwell, R. (1988). Parents' perceptions regarding the discipline of their hearing-impaired children. *Child Care, Health, and Development, 14,* 265–273.

Adams, J. W., & Tidwell, R. (1989). An instructional guide for reducing the stress of hearing parents of hearing-impaired children. *American Annals of the Deaf, 134,* 323–328.

Akamatsu, C. T. (1988). Summarizing stories: The role of instruction in text structure in learning to write. *American Annals of the Deaf, 133,* 294–302.

Allen, T. (1986). Patterns of academic achievement among hearing impaired students: 1974 and 1983. In A. N. Schildroth & M. A. Karchmer (Eds.), *Deaf children in America* (pp. 161–206). San Diego: Little, Brown.

Allen, T. E. (1992). Subgroup differences in educational placement for deaf and hard of hearing students. *American Annals of the Deaf, 137,* 381–388.

Allen, T. E., & Osborn, T. I. (1984). Academic integration of hearing-impaired students: Demographic, handicapping, and achievement factors. *American Annals of the Deaf, 129,* 100–113.

Allen, T. E., Rawlings, B. W., & Schildroth, A. N. (1989). *Deaf students and the school-to-work transition.* Baltimore: Paul H. Brookes.

Allen, T. E., White, C. S., & Karchmer, M. A. (1983). Issues in the development of a special edition for hearing-impaired students of the seventh edition of the Stanford Achievement Test. *American Annals of the Deaf, 128,* 34–39.

Allen, T. E., & Woodward, J. (1987). Teacher characteristics and the degree to which teachers incorporate features of English in their sign communication with hearing impaired students. *American Annals of the Deaf, 132,* 61–67.

Altshuler, K. Z. (1971). Studies of the deaf: Relevance to psychiatric theory. *American Journal of Psychiatry, 127,* 1521–1526.

Altshuler, K. Z. (1978). Toward a psychology of deafness. *Journal of Communication Disorders, 11,* 159–167.

Altshuler, K. Z. (1986). Perceptual handicap and mental illness, with special reference to early profound deafness. *The American Journal of Social Psychiatry, 6,* 125–128.

Altshuler, K. Z., Deming, W. E., Vollenweider, J., Rainer, J. D., & Tendler, R. (1976). Impulsivity and profound early deafness: A cross-cultural inquiry. *American Annals of the Deaf, 121,* 331–345.

American Annals of the Deaf. (1999). Educational programs for deaf students. *American Annals of the Deaf, 144,* 79–147.

American Speech-Language-Hearing Association. (1999). [www.asha.org]

Anderson, G. B., & Grace, C. A. (1991). Black deaf adolescents: A diverse and underserved population. *The Volta Review, 93,* 73–86.

Andrews, J. F., Ferguson, C., Roberts, S., & Hodges, P. (1997). What's up, Billy Jo? Deaf children and bilingual-bicultural instruction in east-central Texas. *American Annals of the Deaf, 142,* 16–25.

Andrews, J. F., & Jordan, D. L. (1993). Minority and minority-deaf professionals: How many and where are they? *American Annals of the Deaf, 138,* 388–396.

Andrews, J. F., Winograd, P., & DeVille, G. (1994). Deaf children reading fables: Using ASL summaries to improve reading comprehension. *American Annals of the Deaf, 139,* 378–386.

Andrews, J. F., Winograd, P., & DeVille, G. (1996). Using sign language summaries during prereading lessons. *Teaching Exceptional Children, 28,* 30–34.

Anthony, D. (1971). *Seeing essential English.* Anaheim, CA: Educational Services Division, Anaheim Union School District.

Antia, S. (1985). Social integration of hearing-impaired children: Fact or fiction? *The Volta Review, 87,* 279–289.

Antia, S. (1994). Strategies to develop peer interaction in young hearing-impaired children. *The Volta Review, 96,* 277–290.

Antia, S., & Kreimeyer, K. (1987). The effect of social skills training on the peer interaction of preschool hearing-impaired children. *Journal of the Division for Early Childhood, 11,* 206–216.

Antia, S., & Kreimeyer, K. (1988). Maintenance of positive peer interaction in preschool hearing-impaired children. *The Volta Review, 90,* 325–337.

Antia, S., Kreimeyer, K., & Eldredge, N. (1994). Promoting social interaction between young children with hearing impairments and their peers. *Exceptional Children, 60,* 262–275.

Antia, S. D. (1982). Social interaction of partially mainstreamed hearing-impaired children. *American Annals of the Deaf, 127,* 18–25.

Antia, S. D., & Dittillo, D. A. (1998). A comparison of the peer social behavior of children who are deaf/hard of hearing and hearing. *Journal of Children's Communication Development, 19*(2), 1–10.

Antia, S. D., & Kreimeyer, K. H. (1991). Social competence intervention for young children with hearing impairments. In S. Odom, S. R. McConnell, & M. A. McEvoy (Eds.), *Social competence intervention for young children with disabilities* (pp. 135–164). Baltimore: Paul H. Brookes.

Antia, S. D., & Kreimeyer, K. H. (1994–1995). Full inclusion of deaf and hard of hearing children in public schools—When is it possible? In *The Dean's forum for the advancement of knowledge and practice in education* (pp. 39–41). Tucson: University of Arizona.

Antia, S. D., & Kreimeyer, K. H. (1997). The generalization and maintenance of the peer social behaviors of young children who are deaf or hard of hearing. *Language, Speech, and Hearing Services in Schools, 28,* 59–69.

Antia, S. D., & Kreimeyer, K. H. (1998). Social interaction and acceptance of deaf or hard-of-hearing children and their peers: A comparison of social-skills and familiarity-based interventions. *The Volta Review, 98,* 157–180.

Aplin, D. Y. (1987). Social and emotional adjustment of hearing-impaired children in ordinary and special schools. *Educational Research, 29,* 56–64.

Arkell, C. (1982). Functional curriculum development for multiply involved hearing-impaired students. *The Volta Review, 84,* 198–208.

Arnold, P. (1993). The sociomoral reasoning and behaviour of deaf children. *Journal of Moral Education, 22,* 157–166.

Arnos, K. S., Israel, J., & Cunningham, M. (1991). Genetic counseling of the deaf: Medical and cultural considerations. In R. J. Ruben, T. R. Van De Water, & K. P. Steel (Eds.), *Genetics of hearing impairment* (pp. 212–222). New York: The New York Academy of Sciences.

Atkins, D. V. (1987). Siblings of the hearing impaired: Perspectives for parents. *The Volta Review, 89,* 32–45.

Bachara, G. H., Raphael, J., & Phelan, W. J. (1980). Empathy development in deaf pre-adolescents. *American Annals of the Deaf, 125,* 38–41.

Backenroth, G. A. M. (1992). Resources and shortcomings in deaf clients' social network. *International Journal of Rehabilitation Research, 15,* 355–359.

Backenroth, G. A. M. (1993). Loneliness in the deaf community: A personal or an enforced choice? *International Journal of Rehabilitation Research, 16,* 331–336.

Backenroth, G. A. M. (1995). Deaf people's perception of social interaction in working life. *International Journal of Rehabilitation Research, 18,* 76–81.

Backenroth, G. A. M. (1997). Deaf employees' empowerment in two different communication environments. *International Journal of Rehabilitation Research, 20,* 417–419.

Baker, C. (1996). *Foundations of bilingual education and bilingualism.* Clevedon, England: Multilingual Matters.

Bannowsky, A. W. (1983). Issues in assessing vocationally relevant personality factors of prelingually deaf adults utilizing the 16PF-E. *Journal of Rehabilitation of the Deaf, 17*(3), 21–24.

Barrett, M. E. (1986). Self-image and social adjustment change in deaf adolescents participating in a social living class. *Journal of Group Psychotherapy, Psychodrama, and Sociometry, 39,* 3–11.

Barrett, T. C. (1976). Taxonomy of reading comprehension. In R. Smith & T. C. Barrett (Eds.), *Teaching reading in the middle grades* (pp. 51–58). Reading, MA: Addison-Wesley-Longman.

Bat-Chava, Y. (1993). Antecedents of self-esteem in deaf people: A meta-analytic review. *Rehabilitation Psychology, 38,* 221–234.

Bat-Chava, Y. (1994). Group identification and self-esteem of deaf adults. *Personality and Social Psychology Bulletin, 20,* 494–502.

Bateman, G. (1987). *Adult learning and development and the adult deaf learner.* (ERIC Document Reproduction Service No. Ed 296 124)

Bates, E., Thal, D., Whitesell, K., Fenson, L., & Oakes, L. (1989). Integrating language and gesture in infancy. *Developmental Psychology, 25,* 1004–1019.

Bebko, J. M. (1984). Memory and rehearsal characteristics of profoundly deaf children. *Journal of Experimental Child Psychology, 38,* 415–428.

Bebko, J. M. (1998). Learning, language, memory, and reading: The role of language automization and its impact on complex cognitive activities. *Journal of Deaf Studies and Deaf Education, 3,* 4–14.

Bebko, J. M., Lacasse, M. A., Turk, H., & Oyen, A. (1992). Recall performance on a central-incidental memory task by profoundly deaf children. *American Annals of the Deaf, 137,* 271–277.

Bebko, J. M., & McKinnon, E. E. (1990). The language experience of deaf children: Its relation to spontaneous rehearsal in a memory task. *Child Development, 61,* 1744–1752.

Beck, B. (1988). Self-assessment of selected interpersonal abilities in hard of hearing and deaf adolescents. *Rehabilitation Research, 11,* 343–349.

Beck, I. L. (1989). Improving practice through understanding reading. In L. B. Resnick & L. E. Klopfer (Eds.), *Toward the thinking curriculum: Current cognitive research* (pp. 40–58). Alexandria, VA: Association for Supervision and Curriculum Development.

Bender, R. E. (1970). *The conquest of deafness.* Cleveland: Case Western Reserve.

Bennett, A. T. (1988). Gateways to powerlessness: Incorporating Hispanic deaf children and families into formal schooling. *Disability, Handicap and Society, 3,* 119–151.

Berent, G. P. (1993). Improvements in the English syntax of deaf college students. *American Annals of the Deaf, 138,* 55–61.

Bess, F. H., & Humes, L. E. (1995). *Audiology: The fundamentals* (2nd ed.). Baltimore: Williams and Wilkins.

Blachowicz, C. L. Z. (1984). Reading and remembering: A constructivist perspective on reading comprehension and its disorders. *Visible Language, 18,* 391–403.

Blennerhassett, L., Strohmeier, S. J., & Hibbett, C. (1994). Criterion-related validity of Raven's Progressive Matrices with deaf residential school students. *American Annals of the Deaf, 139,* 104–110.

Bloom, B. S., Engelhart, M. D., Furst, E. J., Hill, W. H., & Krathwohl, D. R. (1956). *Taxonomy of educational objectives: The classification of educational goals. Handbook I: Cognitive domain.* New York: David McKay.

Blum, E. J., Fields, B. C., Scharfman, H., & Silber, D. (1994). Development of symbolic play in deaf children aged 1 to 3. In A. Slade & D. P. Wolf (Eds.), *Children at play: Clinical and developmental approaches to meaning and representation* (pp. 238–260). New York: Oxford University.

Bodner-Johnson, B. (1982). Describing the home as a learning environment for hearing-impaired children. *The Volta Review, 84,* 329–337.

Bodner-Johnson, B. (1985). Families that work for the hearing-impaired child. *The Volta Review, 87,* 131–137.

Bodner-Johnson, B. (1986). The family environment and achievement of deaf students: A discriminant analysis. *Exceptional Children, 52,* 443–449.

Bodner-Johnson, B. (1991). Family conversation style: Its effect on the deaf child's participation. *Exceptional Children, 57,* 502–509.

Boison, K. B. (1987). Diagnosis of deafness: A study of family responses and needs. *International Journal of Rehabilitation Research, 10,* 220–224.

Bond, G. G. (1987). An assessment of cognitive abilities in hearing and hearing-impaired preschool children. *Journal of Speech and Hearing Disorders, 52,* 319–323.

Bornstein, H., Hamilton, L., & Saulnier, K. (1975). *The Signed English dictionary.* Washington, DC: Gallaudet University.

Bornstein, H., Saulnier, K. L., & Hamilton, L. B. (1980). Signed English: A first evaluation. *American Annals of the Deaf, 125,* 467–481.

Bowlby, J. (1969). *Attachment and loss; Volume 1, Attachment.* New York: Basic.

Bowman, E. S., & Coons, P. M. (1990). The use of hypnosis in a deaf patient with multiple personality disorder. *American Journal of Clinical Hypnosis, 33,* 99–104.

Boyd, J., & Shapiro, A. H. (1986). A comparison of the Leiter-International Performance Scale to WPPSI performance with preschool deaf and hearing impaired children. *Journal of Rehabilitation of the Deaf, 20*(1), 23–26.

Brackett, D., & Henniges, M. (1976). Communicative interaction of preschool hearing impaired children in an integrated setting. *The Volta Review, 78,* 276–285.

Braden, J. P. (1984). The factorial similarity of the WISC-R Performance Scale in deaf and hearing samples. *Journal of Personality and Individual Differences, 5,* 403–409.

Braden, J. P. (1985a). The structure of nonverbal intelligence in deaf and hearing subjects. *American Annals of the Deaf, 130,* 496–501.

Braden, J. P. (1985b). WISC-R deaf norms reconsidered. *Journal of School Psychology, 23,* 375–382.

Braden, J. P. (1987). An explanation of the superior performance IQs of deaf children of deaf parents. *American Annals of the Deaf, 132,* 263–266.

Braden, J. P. (1989a). The criterion-related validity of the WISC-R Performance Scale and other nonverbal IQ tests for deaf children. *American Annals of the Deaf, 134,* 329–332.

Braden, J. P. (1989b). Fact or artifact? An empirical test of Spearman's hypothesis. *Intelligence, 13,* 149–155.

Braden, J. P. (1992). Intellectual assessment of deaf and hard-of-hearing people: A quantitative and qualitative research synthesis. *School Psychology Review, 21,* 82–94.

Braden, J. P. (1994). *Deafness, deprivation, and IQ.* New York: Plenum.

Braden, J. P., Maller, S. J., & Paquin, M. M. (1993). The effects of residential versus day placement on the performance IQs of children with hearing impairment. *Journal of Special Education, 26,* 423–433.

Braeges, J., Stinson, J. S., & Long, G. (1993). Teachers' and deaf students' perceptions of communication ease and engagement. *Rehabilitation Psychology, 38,* 235–246.

Brauer, B. A. (1992). The signer effect on MMPI performance of deaf respondents. *Journal of Personality Assessment, 58,* 380–388.

Brauer, B. A. (1993). Adequacy of a translation of the MMPI into American Sign Language for use with deaf individuals: Linguistic equivalency issues. *Rehabilitation Psychology, 38,* 247–260.

Briccetti, K. A. (1987). Mental health services for deaf students in California. *American Annals of the Deaf, 132,* 280–282.

Briccetti, K. A. (1988). Treatment needs of emotionally disturbed deaf youths: A California perspective. *American Annals of the Deaf, 133,* 276–279.

Briccetti, K. A. (1994). Emotional indicators of deaf children on the Draw-A-Person test. *American Annals of the Deaf, 139,* 500–505.

Brice, P. J. (1985). A comparison of levels of tolerance for ambiguity in deaf and hearing school children. *American Annals of the Deaf, 130,* 226–230.

Brooks, C. R., & Riggs, S. T. (1980). WISC-R, WISC, and reading achievement relationships among hearing-impaired children attending public schools. *The Volta Review, 82,* 96–102.

Brooks, H. C., & Ellis, G. J. (1982). Self-esteem of hearing-impaired adolescents: Effects of labelling. *Youth and Society, 14,* 59–80.

Brown, P. M., & Brewer, L. C. (1996). Cognitive processes of deaf and hearing skilled and less skilled readers. *Journal of Deaf Studies and Deaf Education, 1,* 263–270.

Brown, P. M., & Foster, S. B. (1991). Integrating hearing and deaf students on a college campus: Successes and barriers as perceived by hearing students. *American Annals of the Deaf, 136,* 21–27.

Brown, R. (1973). *A first language: The early stages.* Cambridge, MA: Harvard University.

Brown, S. C. (1987). Predictors of income variance among a group of deaf former college students. *Journal of Rehabilitation of the Deaf, 20*(4), 20–30.

Bryant, J. D., & Roberts, S. D. (1992). Bibliotherapy: An adjunct to audiologic counseling. *Journal of the Academy of Rehabilitative Audiology, 25,* 51–67.

Buchino, M. A. (1993). Perceptions of the oldest hearing child of deaf parents on interpreting, communication, feelings, and role reversal. *American Annals of the Deaf, 138,* 40–45.

Bullis, M., Bull, B., Johnson, B., & Peters, D. (1995). The school-to-community transition experiences of hearing young adults and young adults who are deaf. *The Journal of Special Education, 28,* 405–423.

Bullis, M., Davis, C., Bull, B., & Johnson, B. (1995). Transition achievement among young adults with deafness: What variables relate to success? *Rehabilitation Counseling Bulletin, 39,* 130–148.

Bullis, M., Davis, C., Bull, B., & Johnson, B. (1997). Expectations versus realities: Examination of the transition plans and experiences of adolescents who are deaf and adolescents who are hearing. *Rehabilitation Counseling Bulletin, 40,* 251–264.

Bullis, M., & Reiman, J. W. (1989). Survey of professional opinion on critical transition skills for adolescents and young adults who are deaf. *Rehabilitation Counseling Bulletin, 32,* 231–242.

Bullis, M., & Reiman, J. W. (1992). Development and preliminary psychometric properties of the Transition Competence Battery for Deaf Adolescents and Young Adults. *Exceptional Children, 59,* 12–26.

Bullis, M., Reiman, J. W., Davis, C., & Reid, C. (1997). National field testing of the "mini" version of the Transition Competence Battery for Adolescents and Young Adults Who Are Deaf. *The Journal of Special Education, 31,* 347–361.

Bullis, M., Reiman, J. W., Davis, C., & Thorkildsen, R. (1994). Structure and videodisc adaptation of the Transition Competence Battery (TCB) for Deaf Adolescents and Young Adults. *Exceptional Children, 61,* 159–173.

Bunch, G. O., & Melnyk, T. (1989). A review of the evidence for a learning-disabled, hearing-impaired sub-group. *American Annals of the Deaf, 134,* 297–300.

Burnes, S., Seabolt, D., & Vreeland, J. (1992). Deaf culturally affirmative programming for children with emotional and behavioral problems. *Journal of the American Deafness and Rehabilitation Association, 26*(2), 12–17.

Busby, H. R., & Danek, M. M. (1998). Transition: Principles, policy, and premises. *Perspectives in Education and Deafness, 16*(5), 8–11.

Caccamise, F., Newell, W., Fennell, D., & Carr, N. (1988). The Georgia and New York state programs for assessing and developing sign communication skills of rehabilitation personnel. *Journal of Rehabilitation of the Deaf, 21*(4), 1–14.

Calderon, R., & Greenberg, M. T. (1999). Stress and coping in hearing mothers of children with hearing loss: Factors affecting mother and child adjustment. *American Annals of the Deaf, 144,* 7–18.

Calvert, D. R. (1986). Speech in perspective. In D. M. Luterman (Ed.), *Deafness in perspective* (pp. 167–191). San Diego: College-Hill.

Cambra, C. (1994). An instructional program approach to improve hearing-impaired adolescents' narratives: A pilot study. *The Volta Review, 96,* 237–245.

Caniglia, J., Cole, N. J., Howard, W., Krohn, E., & Rice, M. (1975). *Apple Tree.* Beaverton, OR: Dormac.

Cappelli, M., Daniels, T., Durieux-Smith, A., McGrath, P. J., & Neuss, D. (1995). Social development of children with hearing impairments who are integrated into general education classrooms. *The Volta Review, 97,* 197–208.

Card, K. J., & Schmider, L. (1995). Group work with members who have hearing impairments. *The Journal for Specialists, 20,* 83–90.

Carroll, J. J., & Gibson, E. J. (1986). Infant perception of gestural contrasts: Prerequisites for the acquisition of a visually specified language. *Journal of Child Language, 13,* 31–49.

Cartledge, G., Cochran, L., & Paul, P. (1996). Social skill self-assessments by adolescents with hearing impairment in residential and public schools. *Remedial and Special Education, 17,* 30–36.

Cartledge, G., Paul, P. V., Jackson, D., & Cochran, L. L. (1991). Teachers' perceptions of the social skills of adolescents with hearing impairment in residential and public school settings. *Remedial and Special Education, 12*(2), 34–39, 47.

Casby, M. W., & McCormick, S. M. (1985). Symbolic play and early communication development in hearing impaired children. *Journal of Communication Disorders, 18,* 67–78.

Casby, M. W., & Ruder, K. F. (1983). Symbolic play and early language development in normal and mentally retarded children. *Journal of Speech and Hearing Research, 26,* 404–411.

Caselli, M. C. (1983). Communication to language: Deaf children's and hearing children's development compared. *Sign Language Studies, 39,* 133–144.

Cates, D. S., & Shontz, F. C. (1990a). Role-taking ability and social behavior in deaf school children. *American Annals of the Deaf, 135,* 217–221.

Cates, D. S., & Shontz, F. C. (1990b). Social and nonsocial decentration in hearing-impaired and normal hearing children. *Journal of Childhood Communication Disorders, 13,* 167–180.

Cates, J. A. (1991a). Comparison of human figure drawings by hearing and hearing-impaired children. *The Volta Review, 93,* 31–39.

Cates, J. A. (1991b). Self-concept in hearing and prelingual, profoundly deaf students. *American Annals of the Deaf, 136,* 354–359.

Cates, J. A., & Lapham, R. F. (1991). Personality assessment of the prelingual, profoundly deaf child or adolescent. *Journal of Personality Assessment, 56,* 118–129.

Cazden, C. B. (1988). *Classroom discourse: The language of teaching and learning.* Portsmouth, NH: Heinemann.

Center for Assessment and Demographic Studies. (1998). *1996–97 Annual survey of deaf and hard of hearing children and youth.* Washington, DC: Gallaudet University.

Chan, L. M., & Lui, B. (1990). Self-concept among hearing Chinese children of deaf parents. *American Annals of the Deaf, 135,* 299–305.

Chang, B. L., & Gonzales, B. R. (1987). A study of conservation abilities between hearing-impaired and normal hearing students in Taiwan. *Journal of Childhood Communication Disorders, 10,* 173–184.

Charlson, E. S. (1990, November). *Hearing children of the deaf.* Paper presented at the annual conference of the National Council on Family Relations, Seattle, Washington. (ERIC Document Reproduction Service No. ED 334 804)

Charlson, E. S., Strong, M., & Gold, R. (1992). How successful deaf teenagers experience and cope with isolation. *American Annals of the Deaf, 137,* 261–270.

Charrow, V., & Fletcher, D. (1974). English as the second language of deaf children. *Developmental Psychology, 10,* 463–470.

Chess, S., & Fernandez, P. (1980). Neurologic damage and behavior disorder in rubella children. *American Annals of the Deaf, 125,* 998–1001.

Choate, J. C., Enright, B. E., Miller, L. J., Poteet, J. A., & Rakes, T. A. (1995). *Curriculum-based assessment and programming* (3rd ed.). Boston: Allyn and Bacon.

Chovan, J. D., Waldron, M. B., & Rose, W. (1988). Response latency measurements to visual cognitive tasks by normal hearing and deaf subjects. *Perceptual and Motor Skills, 67,* 179–184.

Chovan, W. L., & Roberts, K. (1993). Deaf students' self-appraisals, achievement outcomes, and teachers' inferences about social-emotional adjustment in academic settings. *Perceptual and Motor Skills, 77,* 1021–1022.

Christiansen, J. B., & Barnartt, S. N. (1995). *Deaf President Now! The 1988 revolution at Gallaudet University.* Washington, DC: Gallaudet University.

Clapham, J. A., & Teller, H. (1997). Using video to communicate with parents. *Rural Special Education Quarterly, 16,* 42–43.

Clark, R. A., & Sachs, M. L. (1991). Challenges and opportunities in psychological skills training in deaf athletes. *The Sport Psychologist, 5,* 392–398.

Clarke, K. C., Clarke, B. R., & Winzer, M. A. (1988). Teacher competencies related to communications modes: A study of Canadian teachers of the hearing impaired. *Canadian Journal of Special Education, 4,* 101–113.

Clayton, L., & Robinson, L. D. (1971). Psychodrama with deaf people. *American Annals of the Deaf, 116,* 415–419.

Clymer, E. C. (1995). The psychology of deafness: Enhancing self-concept in the deaf and hearing-impaired. *Family Therapy, 22,* 112–120.

Cochlear Corporation. (1999). [www.cochlear.com]

Cohen, L. G., & Spenciner, L. J. (1998). *Assessment of children and youth.* New York: Longman.

Cohen, O. P. (1991). At-risk deaf adolescents. *The Volta Review, 93,* 57–72.

Cohen, O. P., Fischgrund, J. E., & Redding, R. (1990). Deaf children from ethnic, linguistic and racial minority backgrounds: An overview. *American Annals of the Deaf, 135,* 67–73.

Cohene, S., & Cohene, L. S. (1989). Art therapy and writing with deaf children. *Journal of Independent Social Work, 4*(2), 21–46.

Cole, E. B., & Shade, M. (1985). Social-emotional adjustment of integrated hearing impaired adolescents. *ACEHI, 11*(2), 82–91.

Cole, S. H., & Edelmann, R. J. (1991). Identity patterns and self- and teacher-perceptions of problems for deaf adolescents: A research note. *Journal of Child Psychology and Psychiatry and Allied Disciplines, 32,* 1159–1165.

Commission on Education of the Deaf. (1988). *Toward equality: Education of the deaf.* Washington, DC: U.S. Government Printing Office.

Compton, C. (1993). Status of deaf employees in the federal government. *The Volta Review, 95,* 379–390.

Conrad, R., & Weiskrantz, B. C. (1981). On the cognitive ability of deaf children with deaf parents. *American Annals of the Deaf, 126,* 995–1003.

Conway, D. (1985). Children (re)creating writing: A preliminary look at the purposes of free-choice writing of hearing-impaired kindergartners. *The Volta Review, 87,* 91–126.

Conway, D. F. (1990). Semantic relationships in the word meanings of hearing-impaired children. *The Volta Review, 92,* 339–349.

Cook, J. A., Graham, K. K., & Razzano, L. (1993). Psychosocial rehabilitation of deaf persons with severe mental illness: A multivariate model of residential outcomes. *Rehabilitation Psychology, 38,* 261–274.

Cooper, J. O., Heron, T. E., & Heward, W. L. (1987). *Applied behavior analysis.* Upper Saddle River, NJ: Merrill/Prentice Hall.

Cornelius, G., & Hornett, D. (1990). The play behavior of hearing-impaired kindergarten children. *American Annals of the Deaf, 135,* 316–321.

Cornelius, G., & Sanders, D. (1987). *The social and cognitive play behaviors of hearing impaired preschool children.* (ERIC Document Reproduction Service No. ED 300 141)

Cornett, R. O. (1967). Cued speech. *American Annals of the Deaf, 112,* 3–13.

Corson, H. J., Marlowe, J., Brownley, J., Lowell, E. L., Watson, D., & Gjerdingen, D. (1987). Quality educational programming. *American Annals of the Deaf, 132,* 335–350.

Coryell, J., & Holcomb, T. K. (1997). The use of sign language and sign systems in facilitating the language acquisition and communication of deaf students. *Language, Speech, and Hearing Services in Schools, 28,* 384–394.

Coryell, J., Holcomb, T. K., & Scherer, M. (1992). Attitudes toward deafness: A collegiate perspective. *American Annals of the Deaf, 137,* 299–302.

Council for Exceptional Children. (1995). *What every special educator must know: The international standards for the preparation and certification of special education teachers.* Reston, VA: Author.

Cox, L. R., Cooper, W. A., & McDade, H. L. (1989). Teachers' perceptions of adolescent girls who wear hearing aids. *Language, Speech, and Hearing Services in Schools, 20,* 372–380.

Coyner, L. (1993). Academic success, self-concept, social acceptance and perceived social acceptance for hearing, hard of hearing and deaf students in a mainstream setting. *Journal of the American Deafness and Rehabilitation Association, 27*(2), 13–20.

Crittenden, J. B., Waterbury, C. A., & Ricker, L. H. (1985). Adoptive parents of hearing impaired children: Concerns for counseling. *ACEHI, 11*(2), 106–110.

Crittenden, P. M., & Bonvillian, J. D. (1984). The relationship between maternal risk status and maternal sensitivity. *American Journal of Orthopsychiatry, 54,* 250–262.

Crowson, K. (1994). Errors made by deaf children acquiring sign language. *Early Child Development and Care, 99,* 63–78.

Cumming, C. E., & Rodda, M. (1989). Advocacy, prejudice, and role modeling in the deaf community. *Journal of Social Psychology, 129,* 5–12.

Cummins, J. (1984). *Bilingualism and special education: Issues in assessment and pedagogy.* Clevedon, England: Multilingual Matters.

Cummins, J. (1987). Bilingualism, language proficiency, and metalinguistic development. In P. Homel, M. Palil, & D. Aronson (Eds.), *Childhood bilingualism: Aspects of linguistic, cognitive, and social development* (pp. 57–73). Mahwah, NJ: Erlbaum.

Cummins, R. A. (1992). Adult literacy and basic education for deaf and hearing-impaired people: Service provider perspectives. *Australian Journal of Adult and Community Education, 32,* 22–30.

Curl, R. M., Rowbury, T. G., & Baer, D. M. (1985). The facilitation of children's social interaction by a picture-cue training program. *Child and Family Behavior Therapy, 7*(2), 11–39.

Curtiss, S., Prutting, C. A., & Lowell, E. L. (1979). Pragmatic and semantic development in young children with impaired hearing. *Journal of Speech and Hearing Research, 22,* 534–552.

Dampier, K., Dancer, J., & Keiser, H. (1985). Changing attitudes toward older persons with hearing loss: Comparison of two audiotapes. *American Annals of the Deaf, 130,* 267–271.

Danek, M. M., Seay, P. C., & Collier, M. L. (1989). Supported employment and deaf people: Current practices and emerging issues. *Journal of Applied Rehabilitation Counseling, 20*(3), 34–43.

Darbyshire, J. P. (1977). Play patterns in young children with impaired hearing. *The Volta Review, 79,* 19–26.

Das, J. P., Naglieri, J. A., & Kirby, J. R. (1994). *Assessment of cognitive processes: The PASS theory of intelligence.* New York: Allyn and Bacon.

Davey, B., & King, S. (1990). Acquisition of word meanings from context by deaf readers. *American Annals of the Deaf, 135,* 227–234.

David, M., & Trehub, S. E. (1989). Perspectives on deafened adults. *American Annals of the Deaf, 134,* 200–204.

Davis, C., & Bullis, M. (1990). The school-to-community transition of hearing-impaired persons with developmental disabilities: A review of the empirical literature. *American Annals of the Deaf, 135,* 352–363.

de Klerk, A. (1998). Deaf identity in adolescence. In A. Weisel (Ed.), *Issues unresolved: New perspectives on language and deaf education* (pp. 206–214). Washington, DC: Gallaudet University.

Delgado, G. L. (1982). Beyond the norm—social maturity and deafness. *American Annals of the Deaf, 127,* 356–360.

Delgado, G. L. (Ed.). (1984). *The Hispanic Deaf: Issues and challenges for bilingual special education.* Washington, DC: Gallaudet College.

Denmark, J. C. (1994). *Deafness and mental health.* London: Jessica Kingsley.

DePaulo, B. M., & Bonvillian, J. D. (1978). The effect on language development of the special characteristics of speech addressed to children. *Journal of Psycholinguistic Research, 7,* 189–211.

Desselle, D. D. (1994). Self-esteem, family climate, and communication patterns in relation to deafness. *American Annals of the Deaf, 139,* 322–328.

Desselle, D. D., & Pearlmutter, L. (1997). Navigating two cultures: Deaf children, self-esteem, and parents' communication patterns. *Social Work in Education, 19,* 23–30.

deVilliers, P. A., & Pomerantz, S. B. (1992). Hearing-impaired students learning new words from written context. *Applied Psycholinguistics, 13,* 409–431.

Deyo, D. A. (1994). A review of AIDS policies at schools for deaf and hard of hearing students. *American Annals of the Deaf, 139,* 86–95.

Dickert, J. (1988). Examination of bias in mental health evaluation of deaf patients. *Social Work, 33,* 273–274.

Diefendorf, A. O. (1999). Screening for hearing loss in infants. *The Volta Review Monograph, 99*(5), 43–61.

DiPietro, L. J., Knight, C. H., & Sams, J. S. (1981). Health care delivery for deaf patients: The provider's role. *American Annals of the Deaf, 126,* 106–112.

Dolby, K. (1992). An investigation of the sign language community of the deaf: Can anyone join? *ACEHI, 18*(2/3), 80–92.

Dolman, D. (1983). A study of the relationship between syntactic development and concrete operations in deaf children. *American Annals of the Deaf, 128,* 813–819.

Dolnick, E. (1993, September). Deafness as culture. *The Atlantic Monthly, 272*(3), 37–40, 43, 46–48, 50–53.

Donin, J., Doehring, D. B., & Browns, F. (1991). Text comprehension and reading achievement in orally educated hearing-impaired children. *Discourse Processes, 14,* 307–337.

Dowaliby, F. J., Burke, N. E., & McKee, B. G. (1983). A comparison of hearing-impaired and normally hearing students on locus of control, people orientation, and study habits and attitudes. *American Annals of the Deaf, 128,* 53–59.

Drasgow, E. (1993). Bilingual/bicultural deaf education: An overview. *Sign Language Studies, 80,* 243–266.

Drasgow, E. (1998). American Sign Language as a pathway to linguistic competence. *Exceptional Children, 64,* 329–342.

Dreher, M. J., & Singer, H. (1989). The teacher's role in students' success. *The Reading Teacher, 42*, 612–617.

Dubow, S. (1989). "Into the turbulent mainstream"—A legal perspective on the weight to be given to the least restrictive environment in placement decisions for deaf children. *Journal of Law and Education, 18*, 215–228.

Dugan, E., & Kivett, V. R. (1994). The importance of emotional and social isolation to loneliness among very old rural adults. *The Gerontologist, 34*, 340–346.

Dunlap, W. R. (1987). A functional classification for independent living for the hearing impaired. *American Annals of the Deaf, 132*, 283–288.

Dunst, C. J., Trivette, C. M., Boyd, K., & Brookfield, J. (1994). Helpgiving practices and the self-efficacy appraisals of parents. In C. J. Dunst, C. M. Trivette, & A. G. Deal (Eds.), *Supporting and strengthening families (Vol. 1): Methods, strategies and practices* (pp. 212–220). Cambridge, MA: Brookline.

D'Zamko, M. E., & Hampton, I. (1985). Personnel preparation for multihandicapped hearing-impaired students: A review of the literature. *American Annals of the Deaf, 130*, 9–14.

Edmunds, G. A., Rodda, M., Cumming, C., & Fox, G. (1992). Descriptions of deaf individuals' personality structures: Is it more than a coincidence that these descriptions parallel those of the written language of the deaf? *ACEHI, 18*(2/3), 102–109.

Egley, L. C. (1982). Domestic abuse and deaf people: One community's approach. *Victomology, 7*, 24–34.

Eldredge, N. M. (1993). Culturally affirmative counseling with American Indians who are deaf. *Journal of the American Deafness and Rehabilitation Association, 26*(4), 1–18.

Eldredge, N. M., & Carrigan, J. (1992). Where do my kindred dwell?… Using art and storytelling to understand the transition of young Indian men who are deaf. *The Arts in Pyschotherapy, 19*, 29–38.

El-Khiami, A. (1993). Employment transitions and establishing careers by postsecondary alumni with hearing loss. *The Volta Review, 95*, 357–366.

Elliott, R. N., & Powers, A. R. (1988). Preparing teachers to serve the learning disabled hearing impaired. *The Volta Review, 90*, 13–18.

Elliott, R. N., & Powers, A. R. (1995). Preparing intepreters to serve in educational settings. *ACEHI, 21*(2/3), 132–140.

Elliott, R. N., Powers, A. R., & Funderburg, R. (1988). Learning disabled hearing-impaired students: Teacher survey. *The Volta Review, 90*, 277–286.

Elrod, G. F., Tesolowski, D. G., & Devlin, S. D. (1998). Vocational assessment of special needs learners. In H. B. Vance (Ed.), *Psychological assessment of children* (2nd ed.) (pp. 418–453). New York: John Wiley.

Emerton, R. G., Foster, S., & Royer, H. (1987). The impact of changing technology on the employment of a group of older deaf workers. *Journal of Rehabilitation of the Deaf, 21*(2), 6–18.

Ensor, A., & Phelps, L. (1989). Gender differences on the WAIS-R performance scale with young deaf adults. *Journal of the American Deafness and Rehabilitation Association, 22*(3), 48–52.

Epstein, S. (1999). Tinnitus—current concepts in diagnosis and management. *The Volta Review Monograph, 88*(5), 119–127.

Erickson, M. E. (1987). Deaf readers reading beyond the literal. *American Annals of the Deaf, 132*, 291–294.

Esposito, B. G., & Koorland, M. A. (1989). Play behavior of hearing impaired children: Integrated and segregated settings. *Exceptional Children, 55,* 412–419.

Fairweather, J. S., & Shaver, D. M. (1991). Making the transition to postsecondary education and training. *Exceptional Children, 57,* 264–270.

Feinstein, C. B. (1983). Early adolescent deaf boys: A biopsychosocial approach. *Adolescent Psychiatry, 11,* 147–162.

Feinstein, C. B., & Lytle, R. (1987). Observations from clinical work with high school aged, deaf adolescents attending a residential school. *Adolescent Psychiatry, 14,* 461–477.

Fields, B., Blum, E. J., & Scharfman, H. (1993). Mental health intervention with very young children and their parents: A model based on the infant deaf. In E. Fenichel & S. Provence (Eds.), *Development in jeopardy: Clinical responses to infants and families* (pp. 9–49). Madison, CT: International Universities Press.

Fields, T. E. (1994). Inclusion: Is it for all deaf children? *Volta Voices, 1* (5), 22–23.

Finn, G. (1995). Developing a concept of self. *Sign Language Studies, 86,* 1–18.

Fischler, I. (1985). Word recognition, use of context, and reading skill among deaf college students. *Reading Research Quarterly, 20,* 203–218.

Fisiloglu, A. G., & Fisiloglu, H. (1996). Turkish families with deaf and hard of hearing children: A systems approach in assessing family functioning. *American Annals of the Deaf, 141,* 231–235.

Fitzgerald, E. (1949). *Straight language for the deaf.* Washington, DC: The Volta Bureau.

Fitz-Gerald, M., & Fitz-Gerald, D. (1980). Sexuality and deafness. *British Journal of Sexual Medicine, 7,* 30–34.

Fitz-Gerald, M., & Fitz-Gerald, D. (1984). Adolescent sexuality: Trials, tribulations, and teaming. In G. B. Anderson & D. Watson (Eds.), *The habilitation and rehabilitation of deaf adolescents* (pp. 143–158). Washington, DC: Gallaudet College.

Fitz-Gerald, M., & Fitz-Gerald, D. (1985). Information on sexuality: Where does it come from? In D. Fitz-Gerald & M. Fitz-Gerald (Eds.), *Viewpoints: Sex education and deafness* (pp. 34–37). Washington, DC: Gallaudet College.

Fitz-Gerald, M., & Fitz-Gerald, D. R. (1987). Parents' involvement in the sex education of their children. *The Volta Review, 89,* 96–110.

Flaxbeard, R., & Toomey, W. (1987). No longer deaf to their needs. *British Journal of Special Education, 14,* 103–105.

Ford, N. M. (1984). Parent-education services for deaf adults. *Journal of Rehabilitation of the Deaf, 17*(4), 1–3.

Foster, S. (1987a). Employment experiences of deaf college graduates: An interview study. *Journal of Rehabilitation of the Deaf, 21*(1), 1–15.

Foster, S. (1987b, May). *The impact and outcome of mainstreamed and residential school programs.* New York: National Technical Institute for the Deaf, Rochester Institute of Technology. (ERIC Document Reproduction Service No. ED 296 524)

Foster, S. (1988). Life in the mainstream: Deaf college freshmen and their experiences in the mainstreamed high school. *Journal of the American Deafness and Rehabilitation Association, 22*(2), 27–35.

Foster, S. (1989a). Reflections of a group of deaf adults on their experiences in mainstream and residential school programs in the United States. *Disability, Handicap and Society, 4,* 37–56.

Foster, S. (1989b). Social alienation and peer identification: A study of the social construction of deafness. *Human Organization, 48,* 226–235.

Foster, S. (1991, April). *The role of education in the development of "nontechnical" job skills: What can or should we be doing?* Paper presented at the annual meeting of the American Educational Research Association, Chicago, Illinois.

Foster, S., & Elliot, L. (1986). *Alternatives in mainstreaming: A "range of options" model for the postsecondary hearing-impaired student.* (ERIC Document Reproduction Service No. ED 296 525)

Foster, S. B., & DeCaro, P. M. (1991). An ecological model of social interaction between deaf and hearing students within a postsecondary educational setting. *Disability, Handicap and Society, 6,* 181–201.

Frank, H. (1979). Psychodynamic conflicts in hearing children of deaf parents. *International Journal of Psychoanalytic Psychotherapy, 7,* 305–315.

Freeburg, J., Sendelbaugh, J., & Bullis, M. (1991). Barriers in school-to-community transition. *American Annals of the Deaf, 136,* 38–47.

Freeman, R., Malkin, S., & Hastings, J. (1975). Psychosocial problems of deaf children and their families: A comparative study. *American Annals of the Deaf, 120,* 391–405.

Freeman, S. T. (1989). Cultural and linguistic bias in mental health evaluations of deaf people. *Rehabilitation Psychology, 34,* 51–63.

Freeman, S. T., & Conoley, C. W. (1986). Training, experience, and similarity as factors of influence in preferences of deaf students for counselors. *Journal of Counseling Psychology, 33,* 164–169.

French, D. B. (1987). Validity, test bias, and the use of the Special Edition of the Stanford Achievement Test for the Hearing Impaired (SAT-HI) with Canadian students. *ACEHI, 13*(3), 104–116.

Fromkin, V., & Rodman, R. (1998). *An introduction to language* (6th ed.). Fort Worth, TX: Harcourt Brace.

Furstenberg, K., & Doyal, G. (1994). The relationship between emotional-behavioral functioning and personal characteristics on performance outcomes of hearing impaired students. *American Annals of the Deaf, 139,* 410–414.

Furth, H. G. (1966). *Thinking without language.* New York: Free Press.

Garrison, W., Long, G., & Dowaliby, F. (1997). Working memory capacity and comprehension processes in deaf readers. *Journal of Deaf Studies and Deaf Education, 2,* 78–94.

Garton, A., & Pratt, C. (1998). *Learning to be literate: The development of spoken and written language.* Oxford, England: Basil Blackwell.

Gaustad, M. G., & Kluwin, T. N. (1992). Patterns of communication among deaf and hearing adolescents. In T. N. Kluwin, D. F. Moores, & M. G. Gaustad (Eds.), *Toward effective public school programs for deaf students: Context, process, and outcomes* (pp. 107–128). New York: Teachers College.

Geers, A., & Moog, J. (1989). Factors predictive of the development of literacy in profoundly hearing-impaired adolescents. *The Volta Review, 91,* 69–86.

Geers, A. E., & Schick, B. (1988). Acquisition of spoken and signed English by hearing-impaired children of hearing-impaired or hearing parents. *Journal of Speech and Hearing Disorders, 53,* 136–143.

Geisser, M. J. (1990). Some people have names—false: Teaching children to think critically and logically. *Teaching English to Deaf and Second Language Students, 8*(2), 18–24.

Gentile, A., & DiFrancesca, S. (1969). *Academic achievement test performance of hearing-impaired students: United States, Spring, 1969.* (Series D, No. 1). Washington, DC: Gallaudet University, Center for Assessment and Demographic Studies.

Gerber, B. M. (1983). A communication minority: Deaf people and mental health care. *The American Journal of Social Psychiatry, 3*(2), 50–57.

Gerner de Garcia, B. (1995). Communication and language use in Spanish-speaking families with deaf children. In C. Lucas (Ed.), *Sociolinguistics in Deaf communities* (pp. 221–252). Washington, DC: Gallaudet University.

Gerstein, A. I. (1988). A psychiatric program for deaf patients. *Psychiatric Hospital, 19*, 125–128.

Gibbons, S. (1989). Use of the WISC-R Performance Scale and K-ABC Non-Verbal Scale with deaf children in the USA and Scotland. *School Psychology International, 10*, 193–197.

Gibson-Harmon, K., & Austin, G. F. (1985). A revised form of the Tennessee Self-Concept Scale for use with deaf and hard of hearing persons. *American Annals of the Deaf, 130*, 218–225.

Gilbertson, M., & Kamhi, A. G. (1995). Novel word learning in children with hearing impairment. *Journal of Speech and Hearing Research, 38*, 630–642.

Glass, L. E., & Elliott, H. (1993). Work place success for persons with adult-onset hearing impairment. *The Volta Review, 95*, 403–415.

Gleason, J. B. (1999). *The development of language* (4th ed.). Boston: Allyn and Bacon.

Glickman, N. S. (1996a). The development of culturally deaf identities. In N. S. Glickman & M. A. Harvey (Eds.), *Culturally affirmative psychotherapy with deaf persons* (pp. 115–153). Mahwah, NJ: Erlbaum.

Glickman, N. S. (1996b). What is culturally affirmative psychotherapy? In N. S. Glickman & M. A. Harvey (Eds.), *Culturally affirmative psychotherapy with deaf persons* (pp. 1–55). Mahwah, NJ: Erlbaum.

Glickman, N. S., & Zitter, S. M. (1989). On establishing a culturally affirmative psychiatric inpatient program for deaf people. *Journal of Rehabilitation of the Deaf, 23*(2), 46–59.

Goldin-Meadow, S., Butcher, C., Mylander, C., & Dodge, M. (1994). Nouns and verbs in a self-styled gesture system: What's in a name? *Cognitive Psychology, 27*, 259–319.

Goldin-Meadow, S., & Morford, M. (1985). Gesture in early child language: Studies of deaf and hearing children. *Merrill-Palmer Quarterly, 31*, 145–176.

Goldin-Meadow, S., Mylander, C., & Butcher, C. (1995). The resilience of combinatorial structure at the word level: Morphology in self-styled gesture systems. *Cognition, 56*, 195–262.

Goldstein, A. P., Sprafkin, R. P., Gershaw, N. J., & Klein, P. (1980). *Skillstreaming the adolescent*. Champaign, IL: Research Press.

Gordon, R. P., Stump, K., & Glaser, B. A. (1996). Assessment of individuals with hearing impairments: Equity in testing procedures and accommodations. *Measurement and Evaluation in Counseling and Development, 29*, 111–118.

Gough, D. (1987). Rational-emotive therapy: A discussion of its applicability for deaf clients. *Journal of Rational-Emotive Therapy, 5*, 162–182.

Graves, M. F. (1986). Vocabulary learning and instruction. In E. Z. Rothkopf (Ed.), *Review of research in education* (pp. 49–89). Washington, DC: American Educational Research Association.

Greenberg, J. (1972). *In this sign*. New York: Avon.

Greenberg, M. T., & Kusche, C. A. (1993). *Promoting social and emotional development in deaf children: The PATHS project*. Seattle: University of Washington.

Greenberg, M. T., Kusche, C. A., & Speltz, M. (1991). Emotional regulation, self-control, and psychopathology: The role of relationships in early childhood. In D.

Cicchetti & S. L. Toth (Eds.), *Internalizing and externalizing expressions of dysfunction* (Vol. 2) (pp. 21–55). Mahwah, NJ: Erlbaum.

Greenberg, M. T., & Marvin, R. S. (1979). Attachment patterns in profoundly deaf preschool children. *Merrill Palmer Quarterly, 25,* 265–279.

Gregory, S. (1991). Challenging motherhood: Mothers and their deaf children. In A. Phoenix, A. Woollett, & E. Lloyd (Eds.), *Motherhood: Meanings, practices, and ideologies* (pp. 123–142). London, England: Sage.

Gregory, S. (1992). The language and culture of deaf people: Implications for education. *Language and Education, 6,* 183–197.

Grieser, D. L., & Kuhl, P. K. (1988). Maternal speech to infants in a tonal language: Support for universal prosodic features in motherese. *Developmental Psychology, 24,* 14–20.

Grunblatt, H., & Daar, L. (1994). A support program: Audiological counseling. *Language, Speech, and Hearing Services in Schools, 25,* 112–114.

Gustason, G., Pfetzing, D., & Zawolkow, E. (1972). *Signing exact English.* Silver Spring, MD: National Association of the Deaf.

Guthmann, D., & Sandberg, K. (1998). Assessing substance abuse problems in deaf and hard of hearing individuals. *American Annals of the Deaf, 143,* 14–21.

Guthmann, D., & Sandberg, K. A. (1995). Clinical approaches in substance abuse treatment for use with deaf and hard of hearing adolescents. *Journal of Child and Adolescent Substance Abuse, 4*(3), 69–79.

Hadadian, A. (1995). Attitudes towards deafness and security of attachment relationships among young deaf children and their parents. *Early Education and Development, 6,* 181–191.

Hadadian, A., & Rose, S. (1991). An investigation of parents' attitudes and the communication skills of their deaf children. *American Annals of the Deaf, 136,* 273–277.

Hagborg, W. (1987). Hearing-impaired students and sociometric ratings. *The Volta Review, 89,* 221–228.

Hagborg, W. J. (1989a). A comparative study of parental stress among mothers and fathers of deaf school-age children. *Journal of Community Psychology, 17,* 220–224.

Hagborg, W. J. (1989b). A sociometric investigation of sex and race peer preferences among deaf adolescents. *American Annals of the Deaf, 134,* 265–267.

Haley, D. J., & Hood, S. B. (1986). Young adolescents' perceptions of their peers who wear hearing aids. *Journal of Communication Disorders, 19,* 449–460.

Haley, T. J., & Dowd, E. T. (1988). Responses of deaf adolescents to differences in counselor method of communication and disability status. *Journal of Counseling Psychology, 35,* 258–262.

Haller, B. (1992, August). *Paternalism and protest: The presentation of deaf persons in the New York Times and Washington Post.* Paper presented at the annual meeting of the Association for Education in Journalism and Mass Communication, Montreal, Quebec, Canada. (ERIC Document Reproduction Service No. ED 351 698)

Hanson, M. J., & Hanline, M. F. (1990). Parenting a child with a disability: A longitudinal study of parental stress and adaptation. *Journal of Early Intervention, 14,* 234–248.

Hanson, V. (1989). Phonology and reading: Evidence from profoundly deaf readers. In D. Shankweiler & I. Liberman (Eds.), *Phonology and reading disability: Solving the reading puzzle* (pp. 69–89). Ann Arbor: University of Michigan.

Hanson, V. L., & Wilkenfeld, D. (1985). Morphophonology and lexical organization in deaf readers. *Language and Speech, 28,* 269–280.

Harris, L. K., VanZandt, C. E., & Rees, T. H. (1997). Counseling needs of students who are deaf and hard of hearing. *The School Counselor, 44,* 271–279.

Harris, R. I. (1978). The relationship of impulse control to parent hearing status, manual communication, and academic achievement in deaf children. *American Annals of the Deaf, 123,* 52–67.

Harrison, M. F., Layton, T. L., & Taylor, T. D. (1987). Antecedent and consequent stimuli in teacher-child dyads. *American Annals of the Deaf, 132,* 227–231.

Harry, B. (1986). Interview, diagnostic, and legal aspects in the forensic psychiatric assessments of deaf persons. *Bulletin of the American Academy of Psychiatry and the Law, 14,* 147–162.

Harry, B., & Dietz, P. E. (1985). Offenders in a silent world: Hearing impairment and deafness in relation to criminality, incompetence, and insanity. *Bulletin of the American Academy of Psychiatry and the Law, 13,* 85–96.

Harvey, M. A. (1982). The influence and utilization of an interpreter for deaf persons in family therapy. *American Annals of the Deaf, 127,* 821–827.

Harvey, M. A. (1984). Family therapy with deaf persons: The systemic utilization of an interpreter. *Family Process, 23,* 205–213.

Harvey, M. A. (1985). Toward a dialogue between the paradigms of family therapy and deafness. *American Annals of the Deaf, 130,* 305–314.

Harvey, M. A., & Green, C. L. (1990). Looking into a deaf child's future: A brief treatment approach. *American Annals of the Deaf, 135,* 364–370.

Hayes, P. L. (1993). Clarifying the role of classroom interpreters. *Perspectives in Education and Deafness, 11*(5), 8–10, 24.

Hayes-Scott, F. C. (1987). Hearing-impaired college students' academic motivation, college degree plans, and locus of control—a relationship? *Journal of Rehabilitation of the Deaf, 21*(1), 39–32.

Haywood, H. C., Towery-Woolsey, J., Arbitman-Smith, R., & Aldridge, A. H. (1988). Cognitive education with deaf adolescents: Effects of instrumental enrichment. *Topics in Language Disorders, 8*(4), 23–40.

Heath, S. B. (1983). *Ways with words: Language, life, and work in communities and classrooms.* Cambridge, England: Cambridge University.

Heefner, D. L., & Shaw, P. C. (1996). Assessing the written narratives of deaf students using the Six-Trait Analytical Scale. *The Volta Review, 98,* 147–168.

Heinen, J. R., Cobb, L., & Pollard, J. W. (1976). Word imagery modalities and learning in the deaf and hearing. *Journal of Psychology, 93,* 191–195.

Heller, B. W., & Harris, R. I. (1987). Special considerations in the psychological assessment of hearing impaired persons. In B. W. Heller, L. M. Flohr, & L. S. Zegans (Eds.), *Psychosocial interventions with sensorially disabled persons* (pp. 53–77). Orlando, FL: Grune and Stratton.

Henggeler, S. W., Watson, S. M., Whelan, J. P., & Malone, C. M. (1990). The adaptation of hearing parents of hearing-impaired youths. *American Annals of the Deaf, 135,* 211–216.

Henwood, P. G., & Pope-Davis, D. B. (1994). Disability as cultural diversity: Counseling the hearing impaired. *Counseling Psychologist, 22,* 489–503.

Heward, W. L. (2000). *Exceptional children* (6th ed.). Columbus, OH: Merrill/Prentice Hall.

Hilburn, S., Marini, I., & Slate, J. R. (1997). Self-esteem among deaf versus hearing children with deaf versus hearing parents. *JADARA, 30*(2&3), 9–12.

Hills, C. G., Rappold, E. S., & Rendon, M. E. (1991). Binge eating and body image in a sample of the deaf college population. *Journal of the American Deafness and Rehabilitation Association, 25*(2), 20–28.

Hindley, P. (1997). Psychiatric aspects of hearing impairment. *Journal of Child Psychology, Psychiatry, and Allied Disciplines, 38,* 101–117.

Hirsch-Pasek, K. (1987). The metalinguistics of fingerspelling: An alternative way to increase reading vocabulary in congenitally deaf readers. *Reading Research Quarterly, 22,* 455–474.

Hirshoren, A., Hurley, O., & Kavale, K. (1979). Psychometric characteristics of the WISC-R Performance Scale with deaf children. *Journal of Speech and Hearing Disorders, 44,* 73–79.

Hittner, A., & Bornstein, H. (1990). Group counseling with older adults: Coping with late-onset hearing impairment. *Journal of Mental Health Counseling, 12,* 332–341.

Hodapp, R. M., & Krasner, D. V. (1994–1995). Families of children with disabilities: Findings from a national sample of eighth-grade students. *Exceptionality, 5*(2), 71–81.

Holland, C., & Rabbit, P. (1992). Effects of age-related reductions in processing resources on text recall. *Journal of Gerontology: Psychological Sciences, 47,* 129–137.

Holt, J. (1993). Stanford Achievement Test—8th edition: Reading comprehension subgroup results. *American Annals of the Deaf, 138,* 172–175.

Hood, L. J., & Berlin, C. I. (1996). Central auditory function and disorders. In J. L. Northern (Ed.), *Hearing disorders* (3rd ed.) (pp. 227–243). Boston: Allyn and Bacon.

Horovitz-Darby, E. G. (1991). Family art therapy within a deaf system. *The Arts in Psychotherapy, 18,* 251–261.

House, J. W. (1999). Hearing loss in adults. *The Volta Review Monograph, 99*(5), 161–166.

Huberty, T. J., & Koller, J. R. (1984). A test of the learning potential hypothesis with hearing and deaf students. *Journal of Educational Research, 78,* 22–28.

Hummel, J. W., & Schirmer, B. R. (1984). Review of research and description of programs for the social development of hearing-impaired students. *The Volta Review, 86,* 259–266.

Hurt, H. T., & Gonzalez, T. (1988). Communication apprehension and distorted self-disclosure: The hidden disabilities of hearing-impaired students. *Communication Education, 37,* 106–117.

Hyde, M., Power, D., & Cliffe, S. (1992). Teachers' communication with their deaf students: An Australian study. *Sign Language Studies, 75,* 159–166.

Isenberg, G. L., & Matthews, W. J. (1991). Working hypnotically with deaf people. *American Journal of Clinical Hypnosis, 34,* 91–99.

Isham, W. P., & Kamin, L. J. (1993). Blackness, deafness, IQ, and g. *Intelligence, 17,* 37–46.

Israelite, N. K. (1986). Hearing-impaired children and the psychological functioning of their normal-hearing siblings. *The Volta Review, 88,* 47–54.

Israelite, N. K., & Helfrich, M. A. (1988). Improving text coherence in basal readers: Effects of revision on the comprehension of hearing-impaired and normal-hearing readers. *The Volta Review, 90,* 261–273.

Jackson, D. W., Paul, P. V., & Smith, J. C. (1997). Prior knowledge and reading comprehension ability of deaf adolescents. *Journal of Deaf Studies and Deaf Education, 2,* 172–184.

Jacobs, R. (1987). Use of the Sixteen Personality Factor Questionnaire, form A, with deaf university students. *Journal of Rehabilitation of the Deaf, 21*(2), 19–26.

James, R. P. (1986). A comparison of social maturity between deaf and hearing children. *Indian Journal of Behaviour, 10*(10), 9–12.

Jamieson, J. R. (1994). Teaching as transaction: Vygotskian perspectives on deafness and mother-child interaction. *Exceptional Children, 60,* 434–449.

Jamieson, J. R. (1995). Interactions between mothers and children who are deaf. *Journal of Early Intervention, 19,* 108–117.

Janesick, V. J. (1990). Bilingual/multicultural education and the deaf: Issues and possibilities. *The Journal of Educational Issues of Language Minority Students, 7,* 99–109.

Jensema, C. J. (1994). Telecommunications for the deaf: Echoes of the past—a glimpse of the future. *American Annals of the Deaf, 139,* 22–27.

Jensen, A. R. (1985). The nature of the black-white difference on various psychometric tests: Spearman's hypothesis. *The Behavioral and Brain Sciences, 8,* 193–219.

Johansson, B., Zarit, S., & Berg, S. (1992). Changes in cognitive functioning of the oldest old. *Journal of Gerontology: Psychological Sciences, 47,* 75–80.

Johnson, G. S. (1989). Emotional indicators in the human figure drawings of hearing-impaired children: A small sample validation study. *American Annals of the Deaf, 134,* 205–208.

Johnson, H. A. (1995). Telecommunications: A strategy for teacher preparation and professional development. *Journal of Childhood Communication Disorders, 17,* 42–45.

Johnson, H. A., & Griffith, P. L. (1986). The instructional patterns of two fourth-grade spelling classes: A mainstreaming issue. *American Annals of the Deaf, 131,* 331–338.

Johnson, H. A., Padak, N. D., & Barton, L. E. (1994). Developmental spelling strategies of hearing-impaired children. *Reading and Writing Quarterly, 10,* 359–367.

Johnson, J. (1998). New program builds bridges for hearing impaired. *American Language Review, 2*(2), 21–22.

Johnson, K. (1991). Miscommunication in interpreted classroom interaction. *Sign Language Studies, 70,* 1–34.

Johnson, M. J. (1988, June). *Debugging the human computer: Instrumental enrichment.* Paper presented at the Annual Southeast Regional Summer Conference: New Directions in Resources for Special Needs Hearing Impaired Students, Cave Spring, Georgia. (ERIC Document Reproduction Service No. ED 312 845)

Johnson, R., Liddell, S., & Erting, C. (1989). *Unlocking the curriculum: Principles for achieving access in deaf education.* Gallaudet Research Institute Working Paper 89–3. Washington, DC: Gallaudet University.

Johnson, V. A. (1993). Factors impacting the job retention and advancement of workers who are deaf. *The Volta Review, 95,* 341–354.

Jones, E. G., & Dumas, R. E. (1996). Deaf and hearing parents' interactions with eldest hearing children. *American Annals of the Deaf, 141,* 278–283.

Jones, R. C., & Kretschmer, L. W. (1988). The attitudes of parents of Black hearing-impaired students. *Language, Speech, and Hearing Services in Schools, 19,* 41–50.

Jones, R. L. (1986). Can deaf students succeed in a public university? *ACEHI, 12*(1), 43–49.

Joseph, J. M., Sawyer, R., & Desmond, S. (1995). Sexual knowledge, behavior and sources of information among deaf and hard of hearing college students. *American Annals of the Deaf, 140,* 338–345.

Kalivoda, K. S., Higbee, J. L., & Brenner, D. C. (1997). Teaching students with hearing impairments. *Journal of Developmental Education, 20*(3), 10–16.

Kampfe, C. M. (1989). Parental reaction to a child's hearing impairment. *American Annals of the Deaf, 124,* 255–259.

Kasen, S., Ouellette, R., & Cohen, P. (1990). Mainstreaming and postsecondary educational and employment status of a rubella cohort. *American Annals of the Deaf, 135,* 22–26.

Katz, J., & White, M. A. (1992). Introduction to the handicap of hearing impairment. In R. H. Hull (Ed.), *Aural rehabilitation* (2nd ed.) (pp. 15–27). San Diego: Singular.

Keane, K. J., & Kretschmer, R. E. (1987). Effect of mediated learning intervention on cognitive task performance with a deaf population. *Journal of Educational Psychology, 79,* 49–53.

Keenan, S. K. (1993). Investigating deaf students' apologies: An exploratory study. *Applied Linguistics, 14,* 364–384.

Keith, R. W. (1996). The audiologic evaluation. In J. L. Northern (Ed.), *Hearing disorders* (3rd ed.) (pp. 45–56). Boston: Allyn and Bacon.

Kelly, D., Forney, J., Parker-Fisher, S., & Jones, M. (1993a). The challenge of attention deficit disorder in children who are deaf or hard of hearing. *American Annals of the Deaf, 138,* 343–348.

Kelly, D., Forney, J., Parker-Fisher, S., & Jones, M. (1993b). Evaluating and managing attention deficit disorder in children who are deaf or hard of hearing. *American Annals of the Deaf, 138,* 349–357.

Kelly, L. P. (1995). Processing of bottom-up and top-down information by skilled and average deaf readers and implications for whole language instruction. *Exceptional Children, 61,* 318–334.

Kelly, L. P. (1996). The interaction of syntactic competence and vocabulary during reading by deaf students. *Journal of Deaf Studies and Deaf Education, 1,* 75–90.

Kennedy, P., Northcott, W., McCauley, R., & Williams, S. N. (1976). Longitudinal sociometric and cross-sectional data on mainstreamed hearing impaired children: Implications for school planning. *The Volta Review, 78,* 71–81.

Kensicki, N. E. (1995). A dilemma for deaf teachers. *TELA Themes, 4* (4), 2–4.

Khan, F. J. (1991). Transitional services for hearing impaired young adults using the continuing education division of a community college. *Journal of the American Deafness and Rehabilitation Association, 25*(1), 16–27.

Klansek-Kyllo, V., & Rose, S. (1985). Using the scale of independent behavior with hearing-impaired students. *American Annals of the Deaf, 130,* 533–537.

Klima, E., & Bellugi, U. (1979). *The signs of language.* Cambridge, MA: Harvard University.

Kluwin, T. N. (1981). The grammaticality of manual representations of English in classroom settings. *American Annals of the Deaf, 126,* 417–421.

Kluwin, T. N. (1985). Profiling the deaf high school student who is a problem in the classroom. *Adolescence, 20,* 863–875.

Kluwin, T. N. (1989, March). *Effective teaching of hearing impaired students in different environments.* Paper presented at the annual meeting of the American Educational Research Association. (ERIC Document Reproduction Service No. ED 328 049)

Kluwin, T. N. (1993). Cumulative effects of mainstreaming on the achievement of deaf adolescents. *Exceptional Children, 60,* 73–81.

Kluwin, T. N. (1994a). The interaction of race, gender and social class effects in the education of deaf students. *American Annals of the Deaf, 139,* 465–471.

Kluwin, T. N. (1994b, April). *Interpreting services for deaf youngsters in local public school programs.* Paper presented at the annual meeting of the American Educational Research Association, New Orleans, Louisiana.

Kluwin, T. N., & Gaustad, M. G. (1992). How family factors influence school achievement. In T. N. Kluwin, D. F. Moores, & M. G. Gaustad (Eds.), *Toward effective public school programs for deaf students: Context, process, and outcomes* (pp. 66–82). New York: Teachers College.

Kluwin, T. N., & Gonsher, W. (1994). A single school study of social integration of children with and without hearing losses in a team taught kindergarten. *ACEHI, 20*(3), 74–87.

Kluwin, T. N., Gonsher, W., Silver, K., & Samuels, J. (1996). The E. T. class: Education together! Team teaching students with hearing impairments and students with normal hearing. *Teaching Exceptional Children, 29*(1), 11–15.

Kluwin, T. N., & Kelly, A. B. (1992a). Deaf adolescents who drop out of local public schools. *American Annals of the Deaf, 137,* 293–298.

Kluwin, T. N., & Kelly, A. B. (1992b). Implementing a successful writing program in public schools for students who are deaf. *Exceptional Children, 59,* 41–53.

Kluwin, T. N., & Moores, D. F. (1985). The effects of integration on the mathematics achievement of hearing impaired adolescents. *Exceptional Children, 52,* 153–160.

Kluwin, T. N., & Moores, D. F. (1989). Mathematics achievement of hearing impaired adolescents in different placements. *Exceptional Children, 55,* 327–335.

Kluwin, T. N., & Stinson, M. S. (1993). *Deaf students in local public high schools: Backgrounds, experiences, and outcomes.* Springfield, IL: Charles C Thomas.

Knutson, J. F., & Lansing, C. R. (1990). The relationship between communication problems and psychological difficulties in persons with profound acquired hearing loss. *Journal of Speech and Hearing Disorders, 55,* 656–664.

Koelle, W. H., & Convey, J. J. (1982). The prediction of the achievement of deaf adolescents from self-concept and locus of control measures. *American Annals of the Deaf, 127,* 769–779.

Koenigsfeld, A. S., Beukelman, D. R., & Stoefen-Fisher, J. M. (1993). Attitudes of severely hearing-impaired persons toward augmentative communication characteristics. *The Volta Review, 95,* 109–124.

Koester, L. S. (1995). Face-to-face interactions between hearing mothers and their deaf or hearing infants. *Infant Behavior and Development, 18,* 145–153.

Koester, L. S., Karkowski, A. M., & Traci, M. A. (1998). How do deaf and hearing mothers regain eye contact when their infants look away? *American Annals of the Deaf, 143,* 5–13.

Koester, L. S., & Meadow-Orlans, K. P. (1990). Parenting a deaf child: Stress, strength, and support. In D. F. Moores & K. P. Meadow-Orlans (Eds.), *Educational and developmental aspects of deafness* (pp. 299–320). Washington, DC: Gallaudet University.

Kolod, S. (1994). Lack of a common language: Deaf adolescents and hearing parents. *Contemporary Psychoanalysis, 30,* 634–650.

Konstantareas, M. M., & Lampropoulou, V. (1995). Stress in Greek mothers with deaf children: Effects of child characteristics, family resources and cognitive set. *American Annals of the Deaf, 140,* 264–270.

Kottke, J. L., Mellor, S., & Schmidt, A. C. (1987). Effects of information on attitudes toward and interpersonal acceptance of persons who are deaf. *Rehabilitation Psychology, 32,* 239–244.

Krakow, R., & Hanson, V. (1985). Deaf signers and serial recall in the visual modality: Memory for signs, fingerspelling and print. *Memory and Cognition, 13,* 265–272.

Kreimeyer, K., & Antia, S. (1988). The development and generalization of social interaction skills in preschool hearing-impaired children. *The Volta Review, 90,* 219–231.

Krinsky, S. G. (1990). The feeling of knowing in deaf adolescents. *American Annals of the Deaf, 135,* 389–395.

Kübler-Ross, E. (1969). *On death and dying.* New York: Simon and Schuster.

Kusche, C. A., Garfield, T. S., & Greenberg, M. T. (1983). The understanding of emotional and social attributions in deaf adolescents. *Journal of Clinical Child Psychology, 12,* 153–160.

Kusche, C. A., & Greenberg, M. T. (1983). Evaluative understanding and role-taking ability: A comparison of deaf and hearing children. *Child Development, 54,* 141–147.

Kusche, C. A., Greenberg, M. T., & Garfield, T. S. (1983). Nonverbal intelligence and verbal achievement in deaf adolescents: An examination of heredity and environment. *American Annals of the Deaf, 128,* 458–466.

Kyle, J. G., & Pullen, G. (1988). Cultures in contact: Deaf and hearing people. *Disability, Handicap and Society, 3,* 49–61.

Lachman, M., Weaver, S., Bandura, M., Elliot, E., & Lewkowics, C. (1992). Improving memory and control beliefs through cognitive restructuring and self-generated strategies. *Journal of Gerontology: Psychological Sciences, 47,* 293–299.

Lane, H. (1992). *The mask of benevolence: Disabling the deaf community.* New York: Knopf.

Lane, K. E. (1989). Substance abuse among the deaf population: An overview of current strategies, programs and barriers to recovery. *Journal of the American Deafness and Rehabilitation Association, 22*(4), 79–85.

Lang, H. G., & Conner, K. (1988). Faculty development: Meeting the needs of postsecondary educators of deaf students. *American Annals of the Deaf, 133,* 26–29.

Lang, H. G., Dowaliby, F. J., & Anderson, H. P. (1994). Critical teaching incidents: Recollections of deaf college students. *American Annals of the Deaf, 139,* 119–127.

Langholtz, D. J., & Rendon, M. E. (1991–1992). The deaf gay/lesbian client: Some perspectives. *Journal of the American Deafness and Rehabilitation Association, 25*(3), 31–34.

LaSasso, C., & Davey, B. (1987). The relationship between lexical knowledge and reading comprehension for prelingually, profoundly hearing impaired students. *The Volta Review, 89,* 211–220.

LaSasso, C. J., & Mobley, R. T. (1997). National survey of reading instruction for deaf or hard-of-hearing students in the U.S. *The Volta Review, 99,* 31–58.

Laughton, J. (1988). Strategies for developing creative abilities of hearing-impaired children. *American Annals of the Deaf, 133,* 258–263.

Laughton, J. (1989). The learning disabled, hearing impaired student: Reality, myth, or overextension? *Topics in Language Disorders, 9*(4), 70–79.

Lederberg, A. R. (1991). Social interaction among deaf preschoolers: The effects of language ability and age. *American Annals of the Deaf, 136,* 53–59.

Lederberg, A. R., Chapin, S. L., Rosenblatt, V., & Vandell, D. L. (1986). Ethnic, gender, and age preferences among deaf and hearing preschool peers. *Child Development, 57,* 375–386.

Lederberg, A. R., & Mobley, C. E. (1990). The effects of hearing impairment on the quality of attachment and mother-toddler interaction. *Child Development, 61,* 1590–1604.

Lederberg, A. R., Rosenblatt, V., & Vandell, D. L. (1985, April). *Stable and unstable frienships: An observational study of hearing and deaf preschoolers.* Paper presented at the biennial meeting of the Society for Research in Child Development, Toronto, Ontario, Canada. (ERIC Document Reproduction Service No. ED 262 870)

Lederberg, A. R., Rosenblatt, V., Vandell, D. L., & Chapin, S. L. (1987). Temporary and long-term friendships in hearing and deaf preschoolers. *Merrill-Palmer Quarterly, 33,* 515–533.

Lederberg, A. R., Ryan, H. B., & Robbins, B. L. (1986). Peer interaction in young deaf children: The effect of partner hearing status and familiarity. *Developmental Psychology, 22,* 691–700.

Leigh, I. W., Corbett, C. A., Gutman, V., & Morere, D. A. (1996). Providing psychological services to deaf individuals: A response to new perceptions of diversity. *Professional Psychology: Research and Practice, 27,* 364–371.

Leigh, I. W., Robins, C. J., & Welkowitz, J. (1990). Impact of communication on depressive vulnerability in deaf individuals. *Journal of Rehabilitation of the Deaf, 23*(3), 68–73.

Leigh, I. W., Robins, C. J., Welkowitz, J., & Bond, R. N. (1989). Toward greater understanding of depression in deaf individuals. *American Annals of the Deaf, 134,* 249–254.

Lemanek, K. L., & Gresham, F. M. (1984). Social skills training with a deaf adolescent: Implications for placement and programming. *School Psychology Review, 13,* 385–390.

Lemanek, K. L., Williamson, D. A., Gresham, F. M., & Jensen, B. J. (1986). Social skills training with hearing-impaired children and adolescents. *Behavior Modification, 10,* 55–71.

Levy, B., & Langer, E. (1994). Aging free from negative stereotypes: Successful memory in China and among the American Deaf. *Journal of Personality and Social Psychology, 66,* 989–997.

Leybaert, J. (1993). Reading in the deaf: The roles of phonological codes. In M. Marschark & M. D. Clark (Eds.), *Psychological perspectives on deafness* (pp. 269–309). Mahwah, NJ: Erlbaum.

Liddell, S. K., & Johnson, R. E. (1989). American Sign Language: The phonological base. *Sign Language Studies, 64,* 195–277.

Lieberth, A. K. (1991). Use of scaffolded dialogue journals to teach writing to deaf students. *Teaching English to Deaf and Second-Language Students, 9*(1), 10–13.

Lieberth, A. K. (1992). Literacy training for deaf adults. *Teaching English to Deaf and Second-Language Students, 10*(1), 4–10.

Light, L., & Burke, D. (1988). Patterns of language and memory in old age. In L. Light & D. Burke (Eds.), *Language, memory and aging* (pp. 244–271). New York: Cambridge University.

Lillo-Martin, D. C., Hanson, V. L., & Smith, S. T. (1992). Deaf readers' comprehension of relative clause structures. *Applied Psycholinguistics, 13,* 13–30.

Limbrick, E. A. (1991). The reading development of deaf children: Critical factors associated with success. *Teaching English to Deaf and Second-Language Students, 9*(1), 4–9.

Ling, D. (1976). *Speech and the hearing-impaired child.* Washington, DC: Alexander Graham Bell Association for the Deaf.

Ling, D. (1989). *Foundations of spoken language for hearing-impaired children.* Washington, DC: Alexander Graham Bell Association for the Deaf.

Liu, A. (1995). Full inclusion and deaf education—redefining equality. *Journal of Law and Education, 24,* 241–266.

Livingston, S. (1997). *Rethinking the education of deaf students.* Portsmouth, NH: Heinemann.

Livneh, H., & Antonak, R. F. (1997). *Psychosocial adaptation to chronic illness and disability.* Gaithersburg, MD: Aspen.

Loeb, R., & Sarigiani, P. (1986). The impact of hearing impairment on self-perceptions of children. *The Volta Review, 88,* 89–100.

Lombardino, L. J., & Sproul, C. J. (1984). Patterns of correspondence and non-correspondence between play and language in developmentally delayed preschoolers. *Education and Training of the Mentally Retarded, 19,* 5–14.

Long, G., Stinson, M. S., & Braeges, J. (1991). Students' perceptions of communication ease and engagement: How they relate to academic success. *American Annals of the Deaf, 136,* 414–421.

Long, N. M. (1992). Overview of services to traditionally underserved persons who are deaf: An historical perspective. In N. M. Long, N. Carr, & K. J. Carlstrom (Eds.), *Provision of services to traditionally underserved persons who are deaf* (pp. 8–11). DeKalb, IL: Northern Illinois University. (ERIC Document Reproduction Service No. ED 355 736)

Love, E. (1983). Parental and staff attitudes toward instruction in human sexuality for sensorially impaired students at the Alabama Institute for Deaf and Blind. *American Annals of the Deaf, 128,* 45–47.

Luckner, J. (1988). Expanding personal limits—Outward Bound and the hearing impaired. *The Volta Review, 90,* 233–235.

Luckner, J. L. (1987). Strategies for building your students' self-esteem. *Perspectives for Teachers of the Hearing Impaired, 6*(2), 9–11.

Luckner, J. L. (1989). Effects of participation in an outdoor adventure education course on the self-concept of hearing-impaired individuals. *American Annals of the Deaf, 134,* 45–49.

Luckner, J. L. (1991a). The competencies needed for teaching hearing-impaired students: A comparison of elementary and secondary school teacher perceptions. *American Annals of the Deaf, 136,* 17–20.

Luckner, J. L. (1991b). Mainstreaming hearing-impaired students: Perceptions of regular educators. *Language, Speech, and Hearing Services in Schools, 22,* 302–307.

Luckner, J. L. (1992). Problem solving: A comparison of hearing-impaired and hearing individuals. *Journal of the American Deafness and Rehabilitation Association, 25*(4), 21–27.

Luckner, J. L., & Gonzales, B. R. (1993). What deaf and hard-of-hearing adolescents know and think about AIDS. *American Annals of the Deaf, 138,* 338–342.

Luckner, J. L., & Isaacson, T. L. (1990). Teaching expressive writing to hearing-impaired students. *Journal of Childhood Communication Disorders, 13,* 135–152.

Luckner, J. L., & McNeill, J. H. (1994). Performance of a group of deaf and hard-of-hearing students and a comparison group of hearing students on a series of problem-solving tasks. *American Annals of the Deaf, 139,* 371–377.

Luckner, J. L., & Miller, K. J. (1994). Itinerant teachers: Responsibilities, perceptions, preparation, and students served. *American Annals of the Deaf, 139,* 111–118.

Luckner, J. L., Schauermann, D., & Allen, R. (1994). Learning to be a friend. *Perspectives in Education and Deafness, 12*(5), 2–7.

Ludders, B. B. (1987). Communication between health care professionals and deaf patients. *Health and Social Work, 12,* 303–310.

Luetke-Stahlman, B. (1988). Documenting syntactically and semantically incomplete bimodal input to hearing-impaired subjects. *American Annals of the Deaf, 133,* 230–234.

Luetke-Stahlman, B., Griffith, C., & Montgomery, N. (1998). Development of text structure knowledge as assessed by spoken and signed retellings of deaf second-grade students. *American Annals of the Deaf, 143,* 337–346.

Luetke-Stahlman, B., & Luckner, J. (1991). *Effectively educating students with hearing impairments.* New York: Longman.

Luey, H. S. (1980). Between worlds: The problems of deafened adults. *Social Work in Health Care, 5,* 253–265.

Lundeen, C., & Lundeen, D. J. (1993, November). *Effectiveness of mainstreaming with collaborative teaching.* Paper presented at the annual convention of the American Speech-Language-Hearing Association. (ERIC Document Reproduction Service No. ED 368 127)

Luterman, D. (1987). *Deafness in the family.* Boston: College-Hill.

Lutes, J. W. (1987). The struggles of being hard of hearing. *ACEHI, 13* (2), 71–78.

Lytle, R. R. (1987). A social skills training program for deaf adolescents. *Perspectives for Teachers of the Hearing Impaired, 6*(2), 19–22.

Lytle, R. R., Feinstein, C., & Jonas, B. (1987). Social and emotional adjustment in deaf adolescents after transfer to a residential school for the deaf. *Journal of the American Academy of Child and Adolescent Psychiatry, 26,* 237–241.

MacDonald, M., & McLaughlin, J. (1987). The peer support team at the Alberta School for the Deaf. *ACEHI, 13*(3), 117–127.

Macklin, G. F., & Matson, J. L. (1985). A comparison of social behaviors among non-handicapped and hearing impaired children. *Behavioral Disorder, 11* , 60–65.

MacLeod-Gallinger, J. (1992). The career status of deaf women: A comparative look. *American Annals of the Deaf, 137,* 315–325.

MacLeod-Gallinger, J. (1993, April). *Deaf ethnic minorities: Have they a double liability?* Paper presented at the annual meeting of the American Educational Research Association.

MacNeil, B. (1990). Educational needs for multicultural hearing-impaired students in the public school system. *American Annals of the Deaf, 135,* 75–82.

MacTurk, R. H., Meadow-Orlans, K. P., Koester, L. S., & Spencer, P. E. (1993). Social support, motivation, language, and interaction: A longitudinal study of mothers and deaf infants. *American Annals of the Deaf, 138,* 19–25.

Madell, J. R. (1998). *Behavioral evaluation of hearing in infants and young children.* New York: Thieme.

Magen, Z. (1990). Positive experiences and life aspirations among adolescents with and without hearing impairments. *International Journal of Disability, Development and Education, 37,* 57–69.

Malcolm, R. (1990). My sister is deaf, and what about me? Meeting the needs of siblings. *Perspectives in Education and Deafness, 9*(1), 12–14.

Maller, S. J. (1997). Deafness and WISC-III item difficulty: Invariance and fit. *Journal of School Psychology, 35,* 299–314.

Maller, S. J., & Ferron, J. (1997). WISC-III factor invariance across deaf and standardization samples. *Educational and Psychological Measurement, 57,* 987–994.

Mallory, B. L., Schein, J. D., & Zingle, H. W. (1992). Hearing offspring as visual language mediators in deaf-parented families. *Sign Language Studies, 76,* 193–213.

Mallory, B. L., Zingle, H. W., & Schein, J. D. (1993). Intergenerational communication modes in deaf-parented families. *Sign Language Studies, 78,* 73–92.

Markoulis, D., & Christoforou, M. (1991). Sociomoral reasoning in congenitally deaf children as a function of cognitive maturity. *Journal of Moral Education, 20,* 79–93.

Markoulis, D., & Christoforou, M. (1993). Sociomoral reasoning of deaf children: A rejoinder to Paul Arnold. *Journal of Moral Education, 22,* 167–169.

Marmor, G., & Pettito, L. (1979). Simultaneous communication in the classroom: How well is English grammar represented? *Sign Language Studies, 23,* 99–136.

Marschark, M. (1994). Gesture and sign. *Applied Psycholinguistics, 15,* 209–236.

Martin, D. S. (1983, April). *Cognitive education for the hearing-impaired adolescent.* Paper presented at the annual conference of the American Educational Research Association, Montreal, Canada. (ERIC Document Reproduction Service No. ED 233 511)

Martin, D. S. (1984). Cognitive modification for the hearing impaired adolescent: The promise. *Exceptional Children, 51,* 235–242.

Martin, D. S. (1987). Reducing ethnocentrism. *Teaching Exceptional Children, 20,* 5–8.

Martin, D. S. (1992). Maximizing intellectual potential in today's learner: Can we really improve student thinking? *Focus on Learning Problems in Mathematics, 14* (3), 3–13.

Martin, D. S. (1993). Reasoning skills: A key to literacy for deaf learners. *American Annals of the Deaf, 138,* 82–86.

Martin, D. S., & Jonas, B. S. (1989). Improving thinking skills in deaf college students. *Research and Training in Developmental Education, 6,* 33–47.

Martin, D. S., Rohr, C., & Innes, J. (1982, February). *Teaching thinking skills to hearing-impaired adolescents.* Paper presented at the Washington Regional Conference of Educators of the Hearing-Impaired, Kendall Demonstration Elementary School, Washington, DC. (ERIC Document Reproduction Service No. ED 221 969)

Martin, J. E., & Prickett, H. T. (1992). Black deaf children: Culture and education. *Perspectives in Education and Deafness, 10*(4), 6–8, 24.

Marzano, R. J., Brandt, R. S., Hughes, C. S., Jones, B. F., Presseisen, B. Z., Rankin, S. C., & Suhor, C. (1988). *Dimensions of thinking: A framework for curriculum and instruction.* Alexandria, VA: Association for Supervision and Curriculum Development.

Masataka, N. (1992). Motherese in a signed language. *Infant Behavior and Development, 15,* 453–460.

Masataka, N. (1996). Perception of motherese in a signed language by 6-month-old deaf infants. *Developmental Psychology, 32,* 874–879.

Masino, L. L., & Hodapp, R. M. (1996). Parental educational expectations for adolescents with disabilities. *Exceptional Children, 62,* 515–523.

Masters, B. A. (1994, May 13). Hearing cultures clash at Gallaudet. *The Washington Post, A10,* 1, 8–9.

Matthews, W. J., & Isenberg, G. L. (1992). Hypnotic inductions with deaf and hearing subjects—an initial comparison. *International Journal of Clinical and Experimental Hypnosis, 40,* 7–11.

Mattock, L., & Crist, P. (1989). Hearing impairment: Implications for mother-daughter interaction. *The Volta Review, 91,* 333–340.

Mauk, G. W., & Mauk, P. P. (1992). Somewhere out there: Preschool children with hearing impairment and learning disabilities. *Topics in Early Childhood Special Education, 12,* 174–195.

Maxon, A. B., Brackett, D., & van den Berg, S. A. (1991). Self perception of socialization: The effects of hearing status, age, and gender. *The Volta Review, 93,* 7–17.

Mayer, C., & Wells, G. (1996). Can the linguistic interdependence theory support a bilingual-bicultural model of literacy education for deaf students? *Journal of Deaf Studies and Deaf Education, 1,* 93–107.

Mayer, P., & Lowenbraun, S. (1990). Total communication use among elementary teachers of hearing-impaired children. *American Annals of the Deaf, 135,* 257–263.

McAnally, P. L., Rose, S., & Quigley, S. P. (1998). *Language learning practices with deaf children* (2nd ed.). Austin, TX: Pro-Ed.

McCallem, F. C. (1994). Robarts School parents support total communication. *American Annals of the Deaf, 139,* 317–318.

McCartney, B. (1987). Factors contributing to the lives of the hearing impaired: Perspective of oral deaf adults. *The Volta Review, 89,* 325–338.

McCauley, R. W., & Bruninks, R. H. (1976). Behavior interactions of hearing impaired children in regular classrooms. *Journal of Special Education, 10,* 277–284.

McCrone, W. P. (1983). Reality therapy with deaf rehabilitation clients. *Journal of Rehabilitation for the Deaf, 17*(2), 13–15.

McCrone, W. P. (1984). Alice in rehabland: Teachers can make a difference. *Perspectives for Teachers of the Hearing Impaired, 2*(4), 9–11.

McEntee, M. K. (1993). Accessibility of mental health services and crisis intervention to the deaf. *American Annals of the Deaf, 138,* 26–30.

McKellin, W. H. (1995). Hearing impaired families: The social ecology of hearing loss. *Social Science and Medicine, 40,* 1469–1480.

McKnight, T. K. (1989). The use of cumulative cloze to investigate contextual build-up in deaf and hearing readers. *American Annals of the Deaf, 134,* 268–272.

McLaughlin, B., White, D., McDevitt, T., & Raskin, R. (1983). Mothers' and fathers' speech to their young children: Similar or different? *Journal of Child Language, 10,* 245–252.

Meadow, K. P. (1983). An instrument for assessment of social-emotional adjustment in hearing-impaired preschoolers. *American Annals of the Deaf, 128,* 826–834.

Meadow, K. P., & Dyssegaard, B. (1983). Social-emotional adjustment of deaf students. *International Journal of Rehabilitation Research, 6,* 345–348.

Meadow, K. P., Greenberg, M. T., & Erting, C. (1983). Attachment behavior of deaf children with deaf parents. *Journal of the American Academy of Child Psychiatry, 22,* 23–28.

Meadow, K. P., Karchmer, M. A., Petersen, L. M., & Rudner, L. (1980). *Meadow/Kendall Social-Emotional Assessment Inventory for Deaf Students: Manual.* Washington, DC: Gallaudet College.

Meadow-Orlans, K. (1985). Social and psychological effects of hearing loss in adulthood. In H. Orlans (Ed.), *Adjustment to hearing loss* (pp. 35–57). San Diego: College Hill.

Meadow-Orlans, K. P. (1987). An analysis of the effectiveness of early intervention programs for hearing-impaired children. In M. J. Guralnick & F. C. Bennett (Eds.), *The effectiveness of early intervention for at-risk and handicapped children* (pp. 325–362). Orlando, FL: Academic.

Meadow-Orlans, K. P. (1990). The impact of a child's hearing loss on the family. In D. F. Moores & K. P. Meadow-Orlans (Eds.), *Educational and developmental aspects of deafness* (pp. 321–338). Washington, DC: Gallaudet University.

Meadow-Orlans, K. P. (1994). Stress, support, and deafness: Perceptions of infants' mothers and fathers. *Journal of Early Intervention, 18,* 91–102.

Meadow-Orlans, K. P. (1995). Sources of stress for mothers and fathers of deaf and hard of hearing infants. *American Annals of the Deaf, 140,* 352–357.

Meadow-Orlans, K. P., Mertens, D. M., Sass-Lehrer, M. A., & Scott-Olson, K. (1997). Support services for parents and their children who are deaf or hard of hearing: A national survey. *American Annals of the Deaf, 142,* 278–288.

Meadow-Orlans, K. P., & Sass-Lehrer, M. (1995). Support services for families with children who are deaf: Challenges for professionals. *Topics in Early Childhood Special Education, 15,* 314–334.

Meadow-Orlans, K. P., & Steinberg, A. G. (1993). Effects of infant hearing loss and maternal support on mother-infant interactions at 18 months. *Journal of Applied Developmental Psychology, 14,* 407–426.

Melton, W. C. (1987). Trends and directions in vocational rehabilitation and their influence upon the education of deaf people. *American Annals of the Deaf, 132,* 315–316, 354.

Mertens, D. M. (1989). Social experiences of hearing-impaired high school youth. *American Annals of the Deaf, 134,* 15–19.

Mertens, D. M. (1990). A conceptual model for academic achievement: Deaf student outcomes. In D. F. Moores & K. P. Meadow-Orlans (Eds.), *Educational and developmental aspects of deafness* (pp. 11–72). Washington, DC: Gallaudet University.

Messenheimer-Young, T., & Kretschmer, R. R. (1994). "Can I play?" A hearing-impaired preschooler's requests to access maintained social interaction. *The Volta Review, 96,* 5–18.

Meyer, D. J., Vadasy, P. F., & Fewell, R. R. (1985a). *Living with a brother or sister with special needs: A book for sibs.* Seattle: University of Washington.

Meyer, D. J., Vadasy, P. F., & Fewell, R. R. (1985b). *Sibshops: A handbook for implementing workshops for siblings of children with special needs.* Seattle: University of Washington.

Meyers, J. E., & Bartee, J. W. (1992). Improvements in the signing skills of hearing parents of deaf children. *American Annals of the Deaf, 137,* 257–260.

Minnett, A., Clark, K., & Wilson, G. (1994). Play behavior and communication between deaf and hard of hearing children and their hearing peers in an integrated preschool. *American Annals of the Deaf, 139,* 420–429.

Misiaszek, J., Dooling, J., Gieseke, M., Melman, H., Misiaszek, J. G., & Jorgensen, K. (1985). Diagnostic considerations in deaf patients. *Comprehensive Psychiatry, 26,* 513–521.

Moaven, I. D., Gilbert, G. L., Cunningham, A. L., & Rawlinson, W. D. (1995). Amniocentesis to diagnose congenital cytomegalovirus infection. *Medical Journal of Australia, 162,* 334–335.

Moores, D. F. (1993). Total inclusion/zero reject models in general education: Implications for deaf children. *American Annals of the Deaf, 138,* 251.

Moores, D. F. (1996). *Educating the deaf: Psychology, principles, and practices* (4th ed.). Boston: Houghton Mifflin.

Morford, J. P. (1996). Insights to language from the study of gesture: A review of research on the gestural communication of non-signing deaf people. *Language and Communication, 16,* 165–178.

Morford, J. P., & Goldin-Meadow, S. (1997). From here and now to there and then: The development of displaced reference in homesign and English. *Child Development, 68,* 420–435.

Morgan, A., & Vernon, M. (1994). A guide to the diagnosis of learning disabilities in deaf and hard-of-hearing children and adults. *American Annals of the Deaf, 139,* 358–370.

Mottez, B. (1990). Deaf identity. *Sign Language Studies, 68,* 195–216.

Mowry, R. L., & Anderson, G. B. (1993). Deaf adults tell their stories: Perspectives on barriers to job advancement and on-the-job accommodations. *The Volta Review, 95,* 367–377.

Murphy, J., & Slorach, N. (1983). The language development of pre-preschool hearing children of deaf parents. *British Journal of Disorders of Communication, 18,* 118–126.

Murphy, J. S., & Newlon, B. J. (1987). Loneliness and the mainstreamed hearing impaired college student. *American Annals of the Deaf, 132,* 21–25.

Murphy-Berman, V., Stoefen-Fisher, J., & Mathias, K. (1987). Factors affecting teachers' evaluations of hearing-impaired students' behavior. *The Volta Review, 89,* 145–156.

Murphy-Berman, V., & Whobrey, L. (1982). Educational materials designed to promote hearing-impaired children's social and affective skills. *Journal of Special Education Technology, 5*(2), 60–68.

Murphy-Berman, V., Witters, L., & Harding, R. (1985). Effect of giftedness, sex, and bottle shape on hearing impaired adolescents' performance on the water line task. *Journal for the Education of the Gifted, 8,* 273–283.

Murphy-Berman, V., Witters, L., & Harding, R. (1986). The effect of bottle shape, bottle position, and subject gender on intermediate-aged hearing-impaired students' performance on the water line task. *The Volta Review, 88,* 37–46.

Musatti, T. (1986). Representational and communicative abilities in early social play: A case study. *Human Development, 29,* 49–60.

Musselman, C., & Churchill, A. (1991). Conversational control in mother-child dyads. *American Annals of the Deaf, 136,* 5–16.

Musselman, C., & Churchill, A. (1992). The effects of maternal conversational control on the language and social development of deaf children. *Journal of Childhood Communication Disorders, 14,* 99–117.

Musselman, C., MacKay, S., Trehub, S. E., & Eagle, R. S. (1996). Communicative competence and psychosocial development in deaf children and adolescents. In J. H. Beitchman, N. J. Cohen, M. M. Konstantareas, & R. Tannock (Eds.), *Language, learning, and behavior disorders* (pp. 555–570). Cambridge, England: Cambridge University.

Musselman, C., Mootilal, A., & MacKay, S. (1996). The social adjustment of deaf adolescents in segregated, partially integrated, and mainstreamed settings. *Journal of Deaf Studies and Deaf Education, 1,* 52–63.

Myers, P. C., & Danek, M. M. (1989). Deafness mental health needs assessment: A model. *Journal of the American Deafness and Rehabilitation Association, 22*(4), 72–78.

Myers, P. C., & Danek, M. M. (1990). Deaf employment assistance network: A model for employment service delivery. *Journal of the American Deafness and Rehabilitation Association, 24*(2), 59–67.

Myers, R. R. (1993). Model mental health state plan (MMHSP) of services for persons who are deaf or hard-of-hearing. *Journal of the American Deafness and Rehabilitation Association, 26*(4), 19–28.

Myklebust, H. (1964). *The psychology of deafness.* New York: Grune and Stratton.

Naglieri, J. A., & Das, J. P. (1988). Planning-attention-simultaneous-successive (PASS): A model for assessment. *Journal of School Psychology, 26,* 35–48.

Naglieri, J. A., & Das, J. P. (1990). Planning, attention, simultaneous, successive cognitive processes as a model for intelligence. *Journal of Psychoeducational Assessment, 8,* 303–337.

Naglieri, J. A., Welch, J. A., & Braden, J. (1994). Performance of hearing-impaired students on planning, attention, simultaneous, and successive (PASS) cognitive processing tasks. *Journal of School Psychology, 32,* 371–383.

National Association of State Directors of Special Education. (1994). *Deaf and hard of hearing students: Educational service guidelines.* Alexandria, VA: Author.

National Center for Education Statistics. (1999). [www.nces.ed.gov]

National Center for Health Statistics. (1999). [www.edc.gov/nchswww/fastats/disable/htm]

Neuroth-Gimbrone, C., & Logiodice, C. M. (1992). A cooperative bilingual language program for deaf adolescents. *Sign Language Studies, 74*, 74–91.

Niver, J. M., & Schery, T. K. (1994). Deaf children's spoken language output with a hearing peer and with a hearing mother. *American Annals of the Deaf, 139*, 103.

Nohara, M., MacKay, S., & Trehub, S. E. (1995). Analyzing conversations between mothers and their hearing and deaf adolescents. *The Volta Review, 97*, 123–134.

Nolen, S. B., & Wilbur, R. B. (1985). The effects of context on deaf students' comprehension of difficult sentences. *American Annals of the Deaf, 130*, 231–235.

Nordeng, H., Martinsen, H., & von Tetzchner, S. (1985). Forced language change as a result of acquired deafness. *International Journal of Rehablitation Research, 8*(1), 71–74.

Northern, J. L. (1996). *Hearing disorders* (3rd ed.). Boston: Allyn and Bacon.

Northern, J. L., & Downs, M. P. (1991). *Hearing in children* (4th ed.). Baltimore: Williams and Wilkins.

Nower, B. (1985). Scratching the itch: High school students and their topic choices for writing. *The Volta Review, 87*, 171–185.

Oblowitz, N., Green, L., & de V. Heyns, I. (1991). A self-concept scale for the hearing-impaired. *The Volta Review, 93*, 19–29.

O'Brien, D. H. (1987). Reflection-impulsivity in total communication and oral deaf and hearing children: A developmental study. *American Annals of the Deaf, 132*, 213–217.

O'Connor, N., & Hermelin, B. (1976). Backward and forward recall by deaf and hearing children. *Journal of Experimental Psychology, 28*, 83–92.

Orlans, H. (1988). Confronting deafness in an unstilled world. *Society, 25*(4), 32–39.

Orlans, H. (1989). The revolution at Gallaudet. *Change, 21*(1), 8–18.

Orlansky, M. D., & Bonvillian, J. D. (1985). Sign language acquisition: Language development in children of deaf parents and implications for other populations. *Merrill-Palmer Quarterly, 31*, 127–143.

Otis-Wilborn, A. (1992). Developing oral communication in students with hearing impairments: Whose responsibility? *Language, Speech, and Hearing Services in Schools, 23*, 71–77.

Ouellette, S. E. (1988). The use of projective drawing techniques in the personality assessment of prelingually deafened young adults: A pilot study. *American Annals of the Deaf, 133*, 212–218.

Oyler, R. F., Oyler, A. L., & Matkin, N. D. (1988). Unilateral hearing loss: Demographics and educational impact. *Language, Speech, and Hearing Services in Schools, 19*, 201–210.

Paal, N., Skinner, S., & Reddig, C. (1988). The relationship of non-verbal intelligence measures to academic achievement among deaf adolescents. *Journal of Rehabilitation of the Deaf, 21*(3), 8–11.

Padden, C., & Humphries, T. (1988). *Deaf in America: Voices from a culture*. Cambridge, MA: Harvard University.

Padmapriya, V., & Mythili, S. P. (1988). A comparative study of deaf and normal children: Cognitive factors and academic achievement. *Journal of Indian Psychology, 7*(1), 27–36.

Page, J. M. (1993). Ethnic identity in deaf Hispanics of New Mexico. *Sign Language Studies, 80*, 185–222.

Page, L. (1996). What do deaf students see for their future? A national vision project. *Perspectives on Education and Deafness, 15*(2), 8–10, 21.

Paquin, M. M., & Braden, J. P. (1990). The effect of residential school placement on deaf children's performance IQ. *School Psychology Review, 19,* 350–355.

Parasnis, I. (1983). Effects of parental deafness and early exposure to manual communication on the cognitive skills, English language skill, and field independence of young deaf adults. *Journal of Speech and Hearing Research, 26,* 588–594.

Parasnis, I., Samar, V. J., Bettger, J. G., & Sathe, K. (1996). Does deafness lead to enhancement of visual spatial cognition in children? Negative evidence from deaf nonsigners. *Journal of Deaf Studies and Deaf Education, 1,* 145–152.

Passmore, D. L. (1982). Vocational and economic implications of deafness. *The Journal of Epsilon Pi Tau, 8*(2), 34–38.

Patterson, K., & Berry, V. (1987). The older hearing-impaired student: Managing obstacles to learning. *Educational Gerontology, 13,* 505–509.

Paul, P. V. (1996). Reading vocabulary knowledge and deafness. *Journal of Deaf Studies and Deaf Education, 1,* 3–15.

Paul, P. V. (1998). *Literacy and deafness: The development of reading, writing, and literate thought.* Boston: Allyn and Bacon.

Pearson, P. D., & Johnson, D. D. (1978). *Teaching reading comprehension.* New York: Holt, Rinehart and Winston.

Perske, R. (1988). *Circle of friends.* Nashville, TN: Abingdon.

Pervin, L. A. (1996). *Personality: Theory and research* (7th ed.). New York: John Wiley.

Peterson, C. C., & Peterson, J. L. (1989). Positive justice reasoning in deaf and hearing children before and after exposure to cognitive conflict. *American Annals of the Deaf, 134,* 277–282.

Peterson, C. C., & Peterson, J. L. (1990). Sociocognitive conflict and spatial perspective-taking in deaf children. *Journal of Applied Developmental Psychology, 11,* 267–281.

Peterson, C. C., & Siegal, M. (1997). Domain specificity and everyday biological, physical, and psychological thinking in normal, autistic, and deaf children. *New Directions for Child Development, 75,* 55–70.

Peterson, D. B., & Gough, D. L. (1995). Applications of Gestalt therapy in deafness rehabilitation counseling. *Journal of the American Deafness and Rehabilitation Association, 29*(1), 17–31.

Petitto, L. A. (1987). On the autonomy of language and gesture: Evidence from the acquisition of personal pronouns in American Sign Language. *Cognition, 27,* 1–52.

Phaneuf, J. (1987). Considerations on deafness and homosexuality. *American Annals of the Deaf, 132,* 52–55.

Phelps, L., & Branyan, B. J. (1988). Correlations among the Kiskey, K-ABC Nonverbal Scale, Leiter, and WISC-R Performance Scale with public-school deaf children. *Journal of Psychoeducational Assessment, 6,* 354–358.

Phelps, L., & Branyan, B. J. (1990). Academic achievement and nonverbal intelligence in public school hearing-impaired children. *Psychology in the Schools, 27,* 210–217.

Phelps, L., & Ensor, A. (1987). The comparison of performance by sex of deaf children on the WISC-R. *Psychology in the Schools, 24,* 209–214.

Phillippe, T., & Auvenshine, D. (1985). Career development among deaf persons. *Journal of Rehabilitation of the Deaf, 19*(1–2), 9–17.

Piaget, J. (1962). *Play, dreams, and imitation.* New York: Norton.

Plapinger, D., & Kretschmer, R. (1991). The effect of context on the interactions between a normally-hearing mother and her hearing-impaired child. *The Volta Review, 93,* 75–87.

Plapinger, D., & Sikora, D. (1990). Diagnosing a learning disability in a hearing-impaired child. *American Annals of the Deaf, 135,* 285–292.

Pogoda-Ciccone, N. (1994). The writing process in 55 minutes. *Perspectives in Education and Deafness, 13*(1), 6–9.

Poon, B. (1996). Attitudes toward deaf or hard of hearing individuals: Factors and strategies. *ACEHI, 22*(2/3), 130–139.

Power, D. J., Wood, D. J., Wood, H. A., & Macdougall, J. (1990). Maternal control over conversations with hearing and deaf infants and young children. *First Language, 10,* 19–35.

Powers, A. R., Elliott, R. N., Patterson, D., Shaw, S., & Taylor, C. (1995). Family environment and deaf and hard-of-hearing students with mild additional disabilities. *Journal of Childhood Communication Disorders, 17,* 15–19.

Powers, G. W., & Saskiewicz, J. A. (1998). A comparison study of educational involvement of hearing parents of deaf and hearing children of elementary school age. *American Annals of the Deaf, 143,* 35–39.

Prendergast, S. G., & McCollum, J. A. (1996). Let's talk: The effect of maternal hearing status on interactions with toddlers who are deaf. *American Annals of the Deaf, 141,* 11–18.

Preston, P. (1994). *Mother father deaf: Living between sound and silence.* Cambridge, MA: Harvard University.

Prinz, P., & Prinz, E. (1979). Simultaneous acquisition of ASL and spoken English (in a hearing child of a deaf mother and hearing father): Phase I, early lexical development. *Sign Language Studies, 25,* 283–296.

Prinz, P., & Prinz, E. (1981). Acquisition of ASL and spoken English by a hearing child of a deaf mother and a hearing father: Phase II, early combinatorial patterns. *Sign Language Studies, 30,* 78–88.

Prinz, P. M., & Prinz, E. A. (1985). If only you could hear what I see: Discourse development in sign language. *Discourse Processes, 8,* 1–19.

Pugh, B. L. (1955). *Steps in language development for the deaf.* Washington, DC: The Volta Bureau.

Pyke, J. M., & Littmann, S. K. (1982). A psychiatric clinic for the deaf. *Canadian Journal of Psychiatry, 27,* 384–389.

Quedenfeld, C., & Farrelly, F. (1983). Provocative therapy with the hearing impaired client. *Journal of Rehabilitation of the Deaf, 17*(2), 1–12.

Quigley, S. P., King, C. M., McAnally, P. L., & Rose, S. (1993). *Reading milestones* (2nd ed.). Austin, TX: Pro-Ed.

Quittner, A. L., Glueckauf, R. L., & Jackson, D. N. (1990). Chronic parenting stress: Moderating versus mediating effects of social support. *Journal of Personality and Social Psychology, 59,* 1266–1278.

Rachford, D., & Furth, H. G. (1986). Understanding of friendship and social rules in deaf and hearing adolescents. *Journal of Applied Developmental Psychology, 7,* 391–402.

Rasing, E. J. (1993). Effects of a multifaceted training procedure on the social behaviors of hearing-impaired children with severe language disabilities: A replication. *Journal of Applied Behavior Analysis, 26,* 405–406.

Rasing, E. J., & Duker, P. C. (1992). Effects of multifaceted training procedures on the acquisition and generalization of social behaviors in language-disabled deaf children. *Journal of Applied Behavior Analysis, 25,* 723–734.

Rasing, E. J., & Duker, P. C. (1993). Acquisition and generalization of social behaviors in language-disabled deaf children. *American Annals of the Deaf, 138,* 362–369.

Raths, L. E., Wassermann, S., Jonas, A., & Rothstein, A. (1986). *Teaching for thinking: Theory, strategies, and activities for the classroom* (2nd ed.). New York: Teachers College.

Rea, C. A., Bonvillian, J. D., & Richards, H. C. (1988). Mother-infant interactive behaviors: Impact of maternal deafness. *American Annals of the Deaf, 133,* 317–324.

Reagan, T. (1985). The deaf as a linguistic minority: Educational considerations. *Harvard Educational Review, 55,* 265–277.

Reagan, T. (1995). Neither easy to understand nor pleasing to see: The development of manual sign codes as language planning activity. *Language Problems and Language Planning, 19,* 133–150.

Reed, S. K. (1995). *Cognition: Theory and applications* (4th ed.). Pacific Grove, CA: Brooks/Cole.

Reilly, J. S., & Bellugi, U. (1996). Competition on the face: Affect and language in ASL motherese. *Journal of Child Language, 23,* 219–239.

Reiman, J., Bullis, M., Davis, C., & Cole, A. B. (1991). "Lower-achieving" deaf people: Overview and case study. *The Volta Review, 93,* 99–120.

Rendon, M. E. (1992). Deaf culture and alcohol and substance abuse. *Journal of Substance Abuse Treatment, 9,* 103–110.

Rice, D. N. (1984). Relationships: Marriage and family life of hearing-impaired people living in the mainstream. *The Volta Review, 86*(5), 17–27.

Rice, M. L., & Kemper, S. (1984). *Child language and cognition.* Baltimore: University Park.

Rienzi, B. M. (1990). Influence and adaptability in families with deaf parents and hearing children. *American Annals of the Deaf, 135,* 402–408.

Rienzi, B. M., Levinson, K. S., & Scrams, D. J. (1992). University students' perceptions of deaf parents. *Psychological Reports, 71,* 764–766.

Rittenhouse, R. (1981). The effect of instructional manipulation on the cognitive performance of normal-hearing and deaf children. *Journal of Childhood Communication Disorders, 5*(1), 14–22.

Rittenhouse, R., Kenyon, P., Leitner, J., & Baechle, C. (1989). Conservation and metaphor in deaf children: Cued speech, manually-coded English and oral-aural comparisons. *Journal of Childhood Communication Disorders, 11*(2), 1–8.

Rittenhouse, R., & Spiro, R. (1979). Conservation interrogation of deaf and normal-hearing children. *Journal of Childhood Communication Disorders, 3*(2), 120–127.

Rittenhouse, R. K. (1987a). The attitudes of deaf and normal hearing high schoolers toward school, each other, and themselves: Mainstreamed and self-contained comparisons. *Journal of Rehabilitation of the Deaf, 21*(1), 24–28.

Rittenhouse, R. K. (1987b). Piagetian conservation in deaf children. *Journal of Childhood Communication Disorders, 10*(2), 95–106.

Rittenhouse, R. K., & Blough, L. K. (1995). Gifted students with hearing impairments: Suggestions for teachers. *Teaching Exceptional Children, 17*(4), 51–53.

Rittenhouse, R. K., & Kenyon, P. L. (1991). Conservation and metaphor acquisition in hearing-impaired children: Some relationships with communication mode, hearing acuity, schooling, and age. *American Annals of the Deaf, 136,* 313–320.

Roark, R., & Berman, S. (1996). Otitis media. In J. L. Northern (Ed.), *Hearing disorders* (3rd ed.) (pp. 127–137). Boston: Allyn and Bacon.

Roberts, S. D., & Wharton, L. K. (1991). Audiologic counseling and work-readiness program for deaf and hard of hearing young adults. *Journal of the Academy of Rehabilitative Audiology, 24,* 143–155.

Robinshaw, H. M. (1996). The pattern of development from non-communicative behavior to language by hearing-impaired and hearing infants. *Early Child Development and Care, 120,* 67–93.

Robinshaw, H. M., & Evans, R. (1995). Caregivers' sensitivity to the communicative and linguistic needs of their deaf infants. *Early Child Development and Care, 109,* 23–41.

Robinson, L. D., Olethia, M. D., & Weathers, O. D. (1974). Family therapy of deaf parents and hearing children: A new dimension in psychotherapeutic intervention. *American Annals of the Deaf, 119,* 325–330.

Romaine, S. (1989). *Bilingualism.* Oxford, England: Basil Blackwell.

Rosenfeld, M., Mounty, J., Ehringhaus, M., & Klem, L. (1993, April). *Pursuing equity in licensing and certification examinations: What we have learned in the process of developing a test for teaching deaf and hard of hearing students.* Paper presented at the annual meeting of the American Educational Research Association, Atlanta, Georgia.

Ross, M. (1994). The price of the ticket. *American Annals of the Deaf, 139,* 463–464.

Roth, V. (1991). Students with learning disabilities and hearing impairment: Issues for the secondary and postsecondary teacher. *Journal of Learning Disabilities, 24,* 391–397.

Rottenberg, C. J. (1992). Integration of the handicapped: A comparative review. *B. C. Journal of Special Education, 16,* 59–68.

Rottenberg, C. J., & Searfoss, L. W. (1992). Becoming literate in a preschool class: Literacy development of hearing-impaired children. *Journal of Reading Behavior, 24,* 463–479.

Roush, J., Harrison, M., & Palsha, S. (1991). Family-centered early intervention: The perceptions of professionals. *American Annals of the Deaf, 136,* 360–366.

Rutherford, S. D. (1988). The culture of American Deaf people. *Sign Language Studies, 59,* 12–147.

Rutman, D. (1989). The impact and experience of adventitious deafness. *American Annals of the Deaf, 134,* 305–311.

Sabin, M. C. (1988). Responses of deaf high school students to an "Attitude toward Alcohol" scale: A national survey. *American Annals of the Deaf, 133,* 199–203.

Sachs, J., Bard, B., & Johnson, M. (1981). Language learning with restricted input: Case studies of two hearing children of deaf parents. *Applied Psycholinguistics, 2,* 33–54.

Salend, S. J., & Longo, M. (1994). The roles of the educational interpreter in mainstreaming. *Teaching Exceptional Children, 26*(4), 22–28.

Salladay, S., & San Agustin, T. (1984). Special needs of the deaf dying patient. *Death Education, 8,* 257–269.

Salvia, J., & Ysseldyke, J. E. (1998). *Assessment* (7th ed.). Boston: Houghton Mifflin.

Sam, A., & Wright, I. (1988). The structure of moral reasoning in hearing-impaired students. *American Annals of the Deaf, 133,* 264–269.

Sanders, G. (1985). The perception and decoding of expressive emotional information by hearing and hearing-impaired children. *Early Child Development and Care, 21,* 11–26.

Sands, D. J. (1992). Validity of the National Independent Living Skills Screening Instrument. *Exceptionality, 3,* 133–145.

Sarti, D. M. (1993). Reaching the deaf child: A model for diversified intervention. *Smith College Studies in Social Work, 63,* 187–198.

Sass-Lehrer, M. (1983). Competencies critical to teachers of hearing-impaired students in two settings. *American Annals of the Deaf, 128,* 867–872.

Sass-Lehrer, M. (1986a). Competencies critical to teachers of hearing-impaired students in two settings: Supervisors' views. *American Annals of the Deaf, 131,* 9–12.

Sass-Lehrer, M. (1986b). Competencies for effective teaching of hearing impaired students. *Exceptional Children, 53,* 230–234.

Sass-Lehrer, M., Cohen-Silver, L. G., & Bodner-Johnson, B. (1990). Training for equity and excellence for college teachers of hearing-impaired students. *American Annals of the Deaf, 135,* 54–58.

Saunders, J. (1997). Educating deaf and hearing children in a bilingual/bicultural environment. *CAEDHH, 23*(1), 61–68.

Saur, R. E., & Stinson, M. S. (1986). Characteristics of successful mainstreamed hearing-impaired students: A review of selected research. *Journal of Rehabilitation of the Deaf, 20*(1), 15–21.

Saville-Troike, M. (1979). Culture, language, and education. In H. T. Trueba & C. Barnett-Mizrahi (Eds.), *Bilingual and multicultural education and the professional: From theory to practice* (pp. 139–156). Rowley, MA: Newbury House.

Schaper, M. W., & Reitsma, P. (1993). The use of speech-based recoding in reading by prelingually deaf children. *American Annals of the Deaf, 138,* 46–54.

Schein, J. D. (1989). *At home among strangers.* Washington, DC: Gallaudet University.

Schessel, D. A. (1999). Ménière's disease. *The Volta Review Monograph, 99*(5), 177–193.

Schiff-Myers, N. (1982). Sign and oral language development of preschool hearing children of deaf parents in comparison with their mothers' communication system. *American Annals of the Deaf, 127,* 322–330.

Schiff-Myers, N., & Ventry, I. (1976). Communication problems in hearing children of deaf parents. *Journal of Speech and Hearing Disorders, 41,* 348–358.

Schildroth, A., Rawlings, B., & Allen, T. (1991). Deaf students in transition: Education and employment issues for deaf adolescents. *The Volta Review, 93,* 41–53.

Schildroth, A. N., & Hotto, S. A. (1994). Inclusion or exclusion? Deaf students and the inclusion movement. *American Annals of the Deaf, 139,* 239–243.

Schildroth, A. N., Rawlings, B. W., & Allen, T. E. (1989). Hearing-impaired children under age 6: A demographic analysis. *American Annals of the Deaf, 134,* 63–69.

Schirmer, B. R. (1985). An analysis of the language of young hearing-impaired children in terms of syntax, semantics, and use. *American Annals of the Deaf, 130,* 15–19.

Schirmer, B. R. (1989). Relationship between imaginative play and language development in hearing-impaired children. *American Annals of the Deaf, 134,* 219–222.

Schirmer, B. R. (1993). Constructing meaning from narrative text: Cognitive processes of deaf children. *American Annals of the Deaf, 138,* 397–403.

Schirmer, B. R. (2000). *Language and literacy development in children who are deaf* (2nd ed.). Boston: Allyn and Bacon.

Schirmer, B. R., Bailey, J., & Fitzgerald, S. M. (1999). Using a writing assessment rubric for writing development of children who are deaf. *Exceptional Children, 65,* 383–397.

Schirmer, B. R., & Bond, W. L. (1990). Enhancing the hearing impaired child's knowledge of story structure to improve comprehension of narrative text. *Reading Improvement, 27,* 242–254.

Schirmer, B. R., Busch, W. L., & Classen, M. M. (1988, March). *Development of empathy in brothers and sisters of exceptional children: Insights from the children.* Paper presented at the annual convention of the Council for Exceptional Children.

Schirmer, B. R., & Winter, C. R. (1993). Use of cognitive schema by children who are deaf for comprehending narrative text. *Reading Improvement, 30,* 26–34.

Schirmer, B. R., & Woolsey, M. L. (1997). Effect of teacher questions on the reading comprehension of deaf children. *Journal of Deaf Studies and Deaf Education, 2,* 47–56.

Schleper, D. R. (1996). Write that one down! Using anecdotal records to inform our teaching. *The Volta Review, 98,* 201–208.

Schlesinger, H. S., & Meadow, K. P. (1972). *Sound and sign: Childhood deafness and mental health.* Berkeley, CA: University of California.

Schloss, P. J., Selinger, J., Goldsmith, L., & Morrow, L. (1983). Classroom-based approaches to developing social competence among hearing-impaired youth. *American Annals of the Deaf, 128,* 842–850.

Schloss, P. J., & Smith, M. A. (1990). *Teaching social skills to hearing-impaired students.* Washington, DC: Alexander Graham Bell Association for the Deaf.

Schloss, P. J., Smith, M. A., & Schloss, C. N. (1984). Empirical analysis of a card game designed to promote consumer-related social competence among hearing-impaired youth. *American Annals of the Deaf, 129,* 417–423.

Schmidt, M. J., & Haydu, M. L. (1992). The older hearing-impaired adult in the classroom: Real-time closed captioning as a technological alternative to the oral lecture. *Educational Gerontology, 18,* 273–276.

Schroedel, J. G. (1991). Improving the career decisions of deaf seniors in residential and day high schools. *American Annals of the Deaf, 136,* 330–338.

Schroedel, J. G., & Carnahan, S. (1991). Parental involvement in career development. *Journal of the American Deafness and Rehabilitation Association, 25*(2), 1–12.

Schultz, C. B., & Pomerantz, M. (1976). Achievement motivation, locus of control, and academic behavior. *Journal of Personality, 33,* 428–442.

Schwartz, N. S., Mebane, D. L., & Malony, H. N. (1990). Effects of alternate modes of administration on Rorschach performance of deaf adults. *Journal of Personality Assessment, 54,* 671–683.

Scott, S. (1984). Deafness in the family: Will the therapist listen? *Family Process, 23,* 214–216.

Seal, B. C., & Hammett, L. A. (1995). Language intervention with a child with hearing whose parents are deaf. *American Journal of Speech-Language Pathology, 4,* 15–21.

Searls, J. M. (1993). Self-concept among deaf and hearing children of deaf parents. *Journal of the American Deafness and Rehabilitation Association, 27*(1), 25–37.

Serwatka, T. S., Anthony, R. A., & Simon, S. C. (1986). A comparison of deaf and hearing teacher effectiveness. *American Annals of the Deaf, 131,* 339–343.

Sharpe, S. L. (1985). The primary mode of human communication and complex cognition. *American Annals of the Deaf, 130,* 39–46.

Shaw, J., & Jamieson, J. (1995). Interactions of an integrated deaf child with his hearing partners: A Vygotskian perspective. *ACEHI, 21*(1), 4–29.

Shroyer, E. H., & Compton, M. V. (1994). Educational interpreting and teacher preparation: An interdisciplinary model. *American Annals of the Deaf, 139,* 472–479.

Siedlecki, T., Votaw, M. C., Bonvillian, J. D., & Jordan, I. K. (1990). The effects of manual interference and reading level on deaf subjects' recall of word lists. *Applied Psycholinguistics, 11,* 185–199.

Silverman, F. H., & Largin, K. (1993). Do children's reactions to peers who wear visible hearing aids always tend to be negative? *Journal of Communication Disorders, 26,* 205–207.

Sinkkonen, J. (1998). Mental health problems and communication of children with hearing loss in Finnish special schools. In A. Weisel (Ed.), *Issues unresolved: New perspectives on language and deaf education* (pp. 197–205). Washington, DC: Gallaudet University.

Siple, P., Fischer, S. D., & Bellugi, U. (1977). Memory for nonsemantic attributes of American Sign Language signs and English words. *Journal of Verbal Learning and Verbal Behavior, 16,* 561–574.

Sisco, F. H., & Anderson, R. J. (1980). Deaf children's performance on the WISC-R relative to hearing status of parents and child-rearing experiences. *American Annals of the Deaf, 125,* 923–930.

Sloman, L., & Springer, S. (1987). Strategic family therapy interventions with deaf member families. *Canadian Journal of Psychiatry, 32,* 558–562.

Smith, M. C. A., & Hasnip, J. H. (1991). The lessons of deafness: Deafness awareness and communication skills training with medical students. *Medical Education, 25,* 319–321.

Smith-Gray, S., & Koester, L. S. (1995). Defining and observing social signals in deaf and hearing infants. *American Annals of the Deaf, 140,* 422–427.

Snow, C. E. (1986). Conversations with children. In P. Fletcher & M. Garman (Eds.), *Language acquisition: Studies in first language development* (pp. 69–89). Cambridge, England: Cambridge University.

Spandel, V., & Stiggins, R. J. (1997). *Creating writers: Linking writing assessment and instruction* (2nd ed.). New York: Addison-Wesley-Longman.

Spencer, P., Koester, L. S., & Meadow-Orlans, K. (1994). Communicative interactions of deaf and hearing children in a day care center. *American Annals of the Deaf, 139,* 512–518.

Spencer, P. E., Bodner-Johnson, B. A., & Gutfreund, M. K. (1992). Interacting with infants with a hearing loss: What can we learn from mothers who are deaf? *Journal of Early Intervention, 16,* 64–78.

Spencer, P. E., & Gutfreund, M. (1990). Characteristics of "dialogues" between mothers and prelinguistic hearing-impaired and normally-hearing infants. *The Volta Review, 92,* 351–360.

Stach, B. A. (1998). *Clinical audiology: An introduction.* San Diego: Singular.

Staton, J. (1985). Using dialogue journals for developing thinking, reading, and writing with hearing-impaired students. *The Volta Review, 87,* 127–154.

Steinberg, A. (1991). Issues in providing mental health services to hearing-impaired persons. *Hospital and Community Psychiatry, 42,* 380–389.

Steinberg, A. G., Davila, J. R., Collazo, J., Loew, R. C., & Fischgrund, J. E. (1997). "A little sign and a lot of love...": Attitudes, perceptions, and beliefs of Hispanic families with deaf children. *Qualitative Health Research, 7,* 202–222.

Stevens, J. M. (1982). Some psychological problems of acquired deafness. *British Journal of Psychiatry, 140,* 453–456.

Stevens, R. P. (1987). Deaf teenagers and family alcohol problems. *American Annals of the Deaf, 132,* 289–290.

Stewart, D. A. (1984). Mainstreaming deaf children: A different perspective. *ACEHI, 10*(2), 91–104.

Stewart, D. A. (1986). Deaf sport in the community. *Journal of Community Psychology, 14,* 196–205.

Stewart, D. A. (1992). Initiating reform in total communication programs. *The Journal of Special Education, 26,* 68–84.

Stewart, D. A. (1993a). Bi-Bi to MCE? *American Annals of the Deaf, 138,* 331–337.

Stewart, D. A. (1993b). Participating in deaf sport: Characteristics of deaf spectators. *Adapted Physical Activity Quarterly, 10,* 146–156.

Stewart, D. A., & Akamatsu, C. T. (1988). The coming of age of American Sign Language. *Anthropology and Education Quarterly, 19,* 235–252.

Stewart, D. A., Akamatsu, C. T., Bennett, D., Corwin, S., Frank, J., Hull, B., & Gustafson, L. (1989). Monitoring communication behavior in English and ASL. *Teaching English to Deaf and Second Language Students, 7*(2), 4–8.

Stewart, D. A., Akamatsu, C. T., & Bonkowski, N. (1988). Factors influencing simultaneous communication behaviors in teachers. *ACEHI, 14*(2), 43–58.

Stewart, D. A., & Benson, G. (1988). Dual cultural negligence: The education of Black deaf children. *Journal of Multicultural Counseling and Development, 16,* 98–109.

Stewart, D. A., McCarthy, D., & Robinson, J. (1988). Participation in deaf sport: Characteristics of deaf sport directors. *Adapted Physical Activity Quarterly, 5,* 233–244.

Stewart, D. A., Robinson, J., & McCarthy, D. (1991). Participation in deaf sport: Characteristics of elite deaf athletes. *Adapted Physical Activity Quarterly, 8,* 136–145.

Stewart, D. A., & Stinson, M. S. (1992). The role of sport and extracurricular activities in shaping socialization patterns. In T. N. Kluwin, D. F. Moores, & M. G. Gaustad (Eds.), *Toward effective public school programs for deaf students: Context, process, and outcomes* (pp. 129–148). New York: Teachers College.

Stinson, M. S., & Kluwin, T. N. (1996). Social orientations toward deaf and hearing peers among deaf adolescents in local public high schools. In P. C. Higgins & J. E. Nash (Eds.), *Understanding deafness socially: Continuities in research and theory* (2nd ed.) (pp. 113–134). Springfield, IL: Charles C Thomas.

Stinson, M. S., Liu, Y., Saur, R., & Long, G. (1995, April). *Deaf college students' perceptions of communication in mainstream classes.* Paper presented at the annual meeting of the American Educational Research Association, San Francisco, California.

Stinson, M. S., & Walter, G. G. (1992). Persistence in college. In S. B. Foster & G. G. Walter (Eds.), *Deaf students in postsecondary education* (pp. 43–64). London: Routledge.

Stinson, M. S., & Whitmire, K. (1992). Students' views of their social relationships. In T. N. Kluwin, D. F. Moores, & M. G. Gaustad (Eds.), *Toward effective public school programs for deaf students: Context, process, and outcomes* (pp. 149–174). New York: Teachers College.

Stoefen-Fisher, J. M. (1987–1988). Hearing impaired adolescents' comprehension of anaphoric relationships within conjoined sentences. *Journal of Special Education, 21,* 85–98.

Stoefen-Fisher, J. M., & Balk, J. (1992). Educational programs for children with hearing loss: Least restrictive environment. *The Volta Review, 94,* 19–28.

Stokoe, W. (1971). *The study of sign language.* Silver Spring, MD: National Association of the Deaf.

Strassman, B. K. (1997). Metacognition and reading in children who are deaf: A review of the research. *Journal of Deaf Studies and Deaf Education, 2,* 140–149.

Strauss, M. (1999). Hearing loss and cytomegalovirus. *The Volta Review Monograph, 99* (5), 71–74.

Strickland, D. S. (1982). Comprehending what's new in comprehension. *Reading Instruction Journal, 25,* 9–12.

Strong, C. J., Clark, T. C., Johnson, D., Watkins, S., Barringer, D. G., & Walden, B. E. (1994). SKI*HI home-based programming for children who are deaf or hard of hearing: Recent research findings. *Infant-Toddler Intervention, 4,* 25–36.

Strong, M. (1995). A review of bilingual/bicultural programs for deaf children in North America. *American Annals of the Deaf, 140,* 84–94.

Stuckless, E., & Birch, J. (1966). The influence of early manual communication on the linguistic development of deaf children. *American Annals of the Deaf, 111,* 425–460, 499–504.

Sue, D. W., Arredondo, P., & McDavis, R. (1992). Multicultural counseling competencies and standards: A call to the profession. *Journal of Counseling and Development, 70,* 477–486.

Sullivan, P. M., & Montoya, L. A. (1997). Factor analysis of the WISC-III with deaf and hard-of-hearing children. *Psychological Assessment, 9,* 317–321.

Sullivan, P. M., & Scanlan, J. M. (1990). Psychotherapy with handicapped sexually abused children. *Developmental Disabilities Bulletin, 18*(2), 21–34.

Sullivan, P. M., Scanlan, J. M., Brookhouser, P. E., Schulte, L. E., & Knutson, J. F. (1992). The effects of psychotherapy on behavior problems of sexually abused deaf children. *Child Abuse and Neglect, 16,* 297–307.

Sullivan, P. M., & Schulte, L. E. (1992). Factor analysis of WISC-R with deaf and hard-of-hearing children. *Psychological Assessment, 4,* 537–540.

Sullivan, P. M., Vernon, M., & Scanlan, J. M. (1987). Sexual abuse of deaf youth. *American Annals of the Deaf, 132,* 256–262.

Sulzby, E. (1992). Research directions: Transitions from emergent to conventional writing. *Language Arts, 69,* 290–297.

Summers, M., Bridge, J., & Summers, C. R. (1991). Sibling support groups. *Teaching Exceptional Children, 23*(4), 20–25.

Swink, D. F. (1983). The use of psychodrama with deaf people. *Journal of Group Psychotherapy, Psychodrama, and Sociometry, 36,* 23–29.

Swink, D. F. (1985). Psychodramatic treatment for deaf people. *American Annals of the Deaf, 130,* 272–277.

Sylvester, R. A. (1987). Treatment of the deaf alcoholic: A review. *Alcoholism Treatment Quarterly, 3*(4), 1–23.

Tanksley, C. K. (1993). Interactions between mothers and normal-hearing or hearing-impaired children. *The Volta Review, 95,* 33–47.

Taska, R., & Rhoads, J. (1981). Psychodynamic issues in a hearing woman raised by deaf parents. *The Psychiatric Forum, 10,* 11–16.

Taylor, R. L. (1997). *Assessment of exceptional students* (4th ed.). Boston: Allyn and Bacon.

Tebo, G. (1984). Using a dramatization/discussion model in educating deaf adults. *Journal of Rehabilitation of the Deaf, 18*(2), 25–26.

Terrell, B. Y., Schwartz, R. G., Prelock, P. A., & Messick, C. K. (1984). Symbolic play in normal and language-impaired children. *Journal of Speech and Hearing Research, 27,* 424–429.

Thomas, A. J. (1984). *Acquired hearing loss: Psychological and psychosocial implications.* London: Academic.

Tidball, K. (1990). Application of coping strategies developed by older deaf adults to the aging process. *American Annals of the Deaf, 135,* 33–40.

Tomlinson-Keasey, C., & Smith-Winberry, C. (1990). Cognitive consequences of congenital deafness. *The Journal of Genetic Psychology, 151,* 103–115.

Tripp, A. W. (1993). Turning students into grownups: Values and decision-making. *Perspectives in Education and Deafness, 11*(4), 2–6.

Tripp, A. W., & Kahn, J. V. (1986). Comparison of the sexual knowledge of hearing impaired and hearing adults. *Journal of Rehabilitation of the Deaf, 19*(3–4), 15–18.

Truax, R. (1985). Linking research to teaching to facilitate reading-writing-communication connections. *TheVolta Review, 87,* 155–169.

Truax, R. (1992). Becoming literate: A sketch of a neverending cycle. *The Volta Review, 94,* 395–410.

Truax, R. R. (1987). Literacy learning in a secondary writing studio. *Teaching English to Deaf and Second-Language Students, 5*(3), 17–23.

Trueba, H. T. (1979). Bilingual-education models: Types and designs. In H. T. Trueba & C. Barnett-Mizrahi (Eds.), *Bilingual multicultural education and the professional: From theory to practice* (pp. 54–73). Rowley, MA: Newbury House.

Trybus, R., & Karchmer, M. (1977). School achievement scores of hearing impaired children: National data on achievement status and growth patterns. *American Annals of the Deaf, 122,* 62–69.

Tsui, H. F., & Rodda, M. (1990). Memory and metamemory in deaf students. *ACEHI, 16*(1), 20–42.

Tzuriel, D., & Caspi, N. (1992). Cognitive modifiability and cognitive performance of deaf and hearing preschool children. *The Journal of Special Education, 26,* 235–252.

Updegraff, D. R. (1992). Deafness and psychological development. In S. B. Friedman, M. Fisher, & S. K. Schonberg (Eds.), *Comprehensive adolescent health care* (pp. 818–823). St. Louis: Quality Medical.

U.S. Department of Education. (1996). *Eighteenth annual report to Congress on the implementation of the Individuals with Disabilities Act* (p. 69). Washington, DC: Author.

Valli, C., & Lucas, C. (1995). *Linguistics of American Sign Language.* Washington, DC: Gallaudet University.

Vandell, D. L., Anderson, L. D., Ehrhardt, G., & Wilson, K. S. (1982). Integrating hearing and deaf preschoolers: An attempt to enhance hearing children's interactions with deaf peers. *Child Development, 53,* 1354–1363.

Vandenberg, B. (1981). Play: Dormant issues and new perspectives. *Human Development, 24,* 357–365.

van Eldik, T. T. (1994). Behavior problems with deaf Dutch boys. *American Annals of the Deaf, 139,* 394–399.

van Gurp, S. (1996). Self-concept measurement with deaf students: A revised SDQ-1 with sign language support. *B. C. Journal of Special Education, 20,* 41–59.

van Uden, A. (1968). *A world of language for deaf children, part 1.* St. Michielsgestel, The Netherlands: The Institute for the Deaf.

Vernon, M. (1967a). Characteristics associated with post-rubella deaf children. *The Volta Review, 69,* 176–185.

Vernon, M. (1967b). The relationship of language to the thinking process. *Archives of General Psychiatry, 16,* 325–333.

Vernon, M. (1968). Fifty years of research on the intelligence of deaf and hard of hearing children: A review of literature and discussion of implications. *Journal of Rehabilitation of the Deaf, 1*(4), 1–12.

Vernon, M., & Daigle-King, B. (1999). Historical overview of inpatient care of mental patients who are deaf. *American Annals of the Deaf, 144,* 51–61.

Vernon, M., & Hicks, W. (1983). A group counseling and educational program for students with Usher's Syndrome. *Journal of Visual Impairment and Blindness, 77*(2), 64–66.

Vernon, M., & Koh, S. (1970). Effects of manual communication on deaf children's educational achievement, linguistic competence, oral skills, and psychological development. *American Annals of the Deaf, 115*, 527–536.

Vernon, M., & LaFalce-Landers, E. (1993). A longitudinal study of intellectually gifted deaf and hard of hearing people: Educational, psychological, and career outcomes. *American Annals of the Deaf, 138*, 427–434.

Vernon, M., & Wallrabenstein, J. M. (1984). The diagnosis of deafness in a child. *Journal of Communication Disorders, 17*(1), 1–8.

Volterra, V., & Erting, C. J. (Eds.). (1990). *From gesture to language in hearing and deaf children.* Berlin, Germany: Springer-Verlag.

Wall, S. G. (1991). Treatment of a deaf multiple personality disorder. *American Journal of Clinical Hypnosis, 34*, 68–69.

Wallace, G., & Corballis, M. (1973). Short-term memory and coding strategies in the deaf. *Journal of Experimental Psychology, 99*, 334–343.

Walsh, C., & Eldredge, N. (1989). When deaf people become elderly: Counteracting a lifetime of difficulties. *Journal of Gerontological Nursing, 15*(12), 27–31.

Walter, G. G. (1987, May). *Outcomes of increased access to postsecondary education by deaf persons.* Paper presented at the annual meeting of the American Deafness and Rehabilitation Association, Minneapolis, Minnesota. (ERIC Document Reproduction Service No. ED 296 522)

Walter, G. G. (1993). Some strategies for enhancing career advancement prospects: A reactant paper. *The Volta Review, 95*, 417–420.

Walter, G. G., & Welsh, W. A. (1986, October). *Providing for the needs of handicapped students in a postsecondary environment.* Paper presented at the annual conference of the Northeast Association for Institutional Research, Philadelphia, Pennsylvania. (ERIC Document Reproduction Service No. ED 286 517)

Warner, H. C. (1987). Community service centers for deaf people: Where are we now? *American Annals of the Deaf, 132*, 237–238.

Warren, C., & Hasenstab, S. (1986). Self-concept of severely and profoundly hearing-impaired children. *The Volta Review, 88*, 289–295.

Watson, B., Goldgar, D., Kroese, J., & Lotz, W. (1986). Nonverbal intelligence and academic achievement in the hearing impaired. *The Volta Review, 88*, 151–158.

Watt, J. D., & Davis, F. E. (1991). The prevalence of boredom proneness and depression among profoundly deaf residential school adolescents. *American Annals of the Deaf, 136*, 409–413.

Wax, T. M. (1990). Deaf community leaders as liaisons between mental health and deaf cultures. *Journal of the American Deafness and Rehabilitation Association, 24*(2), 33–40.

Wax, T. M. (1993). Matchmaking among cultures: Disability culture and the larger marketplace. In R. L. Guralnick, L. B. Sechrest, G. R. Bond, & E. C. McDonel (Eds.), *Improving assessment in rehabilitation and health* (pp. 156–175). Newbury Park, CA: Sage.

Waxman, R. P., Spencer, P. E., & Poisson, S. S. (1996). Reciprocity, responsiveness, and timing in interactions between mothers and deaf and hearing children. *Journal of Early Intervention, 20*, 341–355.

Weaver, C. B., & Bradley-Johnson, S. (1993). A national survey of school psychological services for deaf and hard of hearing students. *American Annals of the Deaf, 138*, 267–274.

Weber, J. (1997). Teacher support in mainstreaming deaf and hard of hearing students in rural Saskatchewan, Canada: A pilot project. *CAEDHH, 23*(1), 40–48.

Weinberg, N., & Sterritt, M. (1986). Disability and identity: A study of identity patterns in adolescents with hearing impairments. *Rehabilitation Psychology, 31,* 95–102.

Weisel, A. (1985). Deafness and perception of nonverbal expression of emotion. *Perceptual and Motor Skills, 61,* 515–522.

Weisel, A. (1988a). Contact with mainstreamed disabled children and attitudes towards disability: A multi-dimensional analysis. *Educational Psychology, 8,* 161–168.

Weisel, A. (1988b). Parental hearing status, reading comprehension skills and social-emotional adjustment. *American Annals of the Deaf, 133,* 356–359.

Weisel, A., & Bar-Lev, H. (1992). Role taking ability, nonverbal sensitivity, language and social adjustment of deaf adolescents. *Educational Psychology, 12,* 3–13.

Weisel, A., Dromi, E., & Dor, S. (1990). Exploration of factors affecting attitudes towards sign language. *Sign Language Studies, 68,* 257–276.

Wells, G. (1986). *The meaning makers: Children learning language and using language to learn.* Portsmouth, NH: Heinemann.

Welsh, W. A., & Walter, G. G. (1988). The effect of postsecondary education on the occupational attainments of deaf adults. *Journal of the American Deafness and Rehabilitation Association, 22*(1), 14–22.

White, A. (1990). Differences in teacher expectations. *The Volta Review, 92,* 131–143.

White, K. R. (1982). Defining and prioritizing the personal and social competencies needed by hearing-impaired students. *The Volta Review, 84,* 266–274.

Wilbur, R. B. (1987). *American Sign Language: Linguistic and applied dimensions* (2nd ed.). Austin, TX: Pro-Ed.

Wilbur, R. B., & Goodhart, W. C. (1985). Comprehension of indefinite pronouns and quantifiers by hearing-impaired students. *Applied Psycholinguistics, 6,* 417–434.

Wilbur, R. B., Goodhart, W. C., & Montandon, E. (1983). Comprehension of nine syntactic structures by hearing-impaired students. *The Volta Review, 85,* 328–345.

Wilcox, P., Schroeder, F., & Martinez, T. (1990). A commitment to professionalism: Educational interpreting standards within a large public school system. *Sign Language Studies, 68,* 277–286.

Williams, C. C. (1970). Some psychiatric observations on a group of maladjusted deaf children. *Journal of Child Psychology and Psychiatry, 11,* 1–18.

Williams, C. L. (1993). Learning to write: Social interaction among preschool auditory/oral and total communication children. *Sign Language Studies, 80,* 267–284.

Williams, C. L. (1994). The language and literacy worlds of three profoundly deaf children. *Reading Research Quarterly, 29,* 125–155.

Williams, C. L., & McLean, M. M. (1997). Young deaf children's response to picture book reading in a preschool setting. *Research in the Teaching of English, 31,* 337–366.

Williams, R. L., & Bonvillian, J. D. (1989). Early childhood memories in deaf and hearing college students. *Merrill-Palmer Quarterly, 35,* 483–497.

Wilson, C. (1997). Mainstream or "deaf school?" Both! Say deaf students. *Perspectives in Education and Deafness, 16*(2), 10–13.

Winter, S. M., & Van Reusen, A. K. (1997). Inclusion and kindergartners who are deaf or hard of hearing: Comparing teaching strategies with recommended guidelines. *Journal of Research in Childhood Education, 11,* 114–134.

Witters-Churchill, L. J., Kelly, R. P., & Witters, L. A. (1983). Hearing-impaired students' perception of liquid horizontality: An examination of the effects of gender, development, and training. *The Volta Review, 85,* 211–225.

Wittrock, M. C. (1982). Three studies of generative reading comprehension. In J. A. Niles & L. A. Harris (Eds.), *New inquiries in reading research and instruction* (pp. 85–88). Rochester, NY: National Reading Conference.

Wolk, S. (1985). The attributional beliefs of hearing-impaired students concerning academic success and failure. *American Annals of the Deaf, 130,* 32–38.

Wolk, S., & Allen, T. E. (1984). A 5-year follow-up of reading comprehension achievement of hearing-impaired students in special education programs. *The Journal of Special Education, 18,* 161–176.

Wolk, S., & Beach, R. (1986). Perception of cause and solution for personal problems by a hearing-impaired student population: The significance of situation-defined attributions for control. *Journal of Rehabilitation of the Deaf, 20*(2), 17–23.

Wolk, S., & Ziezula, F. R. (1985). Reliability of the 1973 edition of the SAT-HI over time: Implications for assessing minority students. *American Annals of the Deaf, 130,* 285–290.

Wood, D. (1991). Communication and cognition. *American Annals of the Deaf, 136,* 247–251.

Wood, T. E. (1987). Communicating with hearing-impaired patients. *Journal of the American Optometric Association, 58,* 62–65.

Woodward, J. (1972). Implications for sociolinguistic research among the Deaf. *Sign Language Studies, 1,* 1–7.

Woodward, J., & Allen, T. (1988). Classroom use of artificial sign systems by teachers. *Sign Language Studies, 61,* 405–418.

Woodward, J., & Allen, T. (1993). Sociolinguistic differences: U.S. teachers in residential schools and non-residential schools. *Sign Language Studies, 81,* 361–374.

Wright, D. (1993). *Deafness: An autobiography.* London, England: Mandarin.

Wyatt, T. L., & White, L. J. (1993). Counseling services for the deaf adult: Much demand, little supply. *Journal of the American Deafness and Rehabilitation Association, 27*(2), 8–12.

Yachnik, M. (1986). Self-esteem in deaf adolescents. *American Annals of the Deaf, 131,* 305–310.

Yacobacci-Tam, P. (1987). Interacting with the culturally different family. *The Volta Review, 89,* 46–58.

Yewchuk, C. R., & Bibby, M. A. (1988). A comparison of parent and teacher nomination of gifted hearing-impaired students. *American Annals of the Deaf, 133,* 344–348.

Yewchuk, C. R., & Bibby, M. A. (1989). Identification of giftedness in severely and profoundly hearing impaired students. *Roeper Review, 12,* 42–48.

Yewchuk, C. R., Bibby, M. A., & Fraser, B. (1989). Identifying giftedness in the hearing impaired: The effectiveness of four nomination forms. *Gifted Education International, 6*(2), 87–97.

Yoshinago-Itano, C., & Downey, D. M. (1986). A hearing-impaired child's acquisition of schemata: Something's missing. *Topics in Language Disorders, 7,* 45–57.

Yoshinago-Itano, C., & Stredler-Brown, A. (1992). Learning to communicate: Babies with hearing impairments make their needs known. *The Volta Review, 94,* 107–129.

Zahn, S. B., & Kelly, L. J. (1995). Changing attitudes about the employability of the deaf and hard of hearing. *American Annals of the Deaf, 140,* 381–385.

Zalewska, M. (1989). Non-verbal psychotherapy of deaf children with disorders in personality development. *Journal of the American Deafness and Rehabilitation Association, 22* (4), 65–71.

Zieziula, F. R., & Harris, G. (1998). National survey of school counselors working with deaf and hard of hearing children: Two decades later. *American Annals of the Deaf, 143,* 40–45.

Zinser, E. A. (1988). Reflections on revolution and leadership by surprise. *Educational Record, 69*(2), 22–25.

Zwiebel, A. (1987). More on the effects of early manual communication on the cognitive development of deaf children. *American Annals of the Deaf, 132,* 16–20.

Zwiebel, A., & Mertens, D. M. (1985). A comparison of intellectual structure in deaf and hearing children. *American Annals of the Deaf, 130,* 27–31.

Zwiebel, A., & Wolff, A. B. (1988). "Draw-A-Person" as a reliable test for deaf children: Cross-cultural and deaf-hearing comparisons. *ACEHI, 14*(3), 91–104.

INDEX